Ward C8.

Lecture Notes on Urology

Lecture Notes on Urology Third edition

JOHN BLANDY MA, DM, MCh, FRCS, FACS

Professor of Urology in The University of London
at The London Hospital Medical College,
Consultant Urologist, St Peter's Hospital, London

BLACKWELL SCIENTIFIC PUBLICATIONS

OXFORD LONDON EDINBURGH

BOSTON PALO ALTO MELBOURNE

First published 1976
Second edition 1977
Reprinted 1979
Third edition 1982
Reprinted 1984, 1986, 1988

Printed and bound in Great Britain
at the Alden Press, Oxford

DISTRIBUTORS

USA
  Year Book Medical Publishers
  200 North LaSalle Street,
  Chicago, Illinois 60601

Canada
  The C.V. Mosby Company
  5240 Finch Avenue East,
  Scarborough, Ontario

Australia
  Blackwell Scientific Publications
    (Australia) Pty Ltd.
  107 Barry Street,
  Carlton, Victoria 3053

British Library
Cataloguing in Publication Data

Blandy, John P.
  Lecture notes on urology.–3rd ed.
  1. Urology
  I. Title
  616.6   RC871

ISBN 0-632-00688-9

Contents

Preface to the Third Edition

One of the excitements of Urology is that it grows so quickly: indeed, there have been so many and such important advances even in the last five years that it has been necessary to make this into a new book rather than a new edition. All the text has been rewritten, and most of my pictures have been drawn again—I hope, more clearly. Much new material has been put in, and a lot taken out to make room. I hope students will find the new chapter on the management of common urological problems helpful when they start off as house-surgeons. It must again be pointed out that the section on operations is not intended for the FRCS student—it is there only to make clinical experience more interesting for the medical student, who ought at least to understand what patients have to undergo. These lecture notes started off as duplicated sheets of notes, embellished with cartoons, for my students on the urology 'firm', hoping that they would learn something without becoming too bored. It has grown rather—but it still aims to offer the maximum of information with the minimum of boredom.

J.P.B.

Preface

This book has been written for the undergraduate medical student. About a quarter of all the operations of surgery concern the genitourinary system: about 15% of all doctors suffer at some time or other from a stone in the urinary tract: one in ten of all males have to have an operation on their prostate before they reach the end of their days. The management of haematuria, of impotence, of infertility, and of urinary tract infections: the investigation of hypertension, and the evaluation of albuminuria—no doctor, however recondite his speciality—is not at some time touched by one or other of these common problems. Of all diseases in the world, in prevalence second only to malaria, schistosomiasis affects more human beings, and those more miserably, than any other. The author makes no apology therefore for the claim that the speciality of urology encompasses some of the most important, and arguably the most fascinating of all the topics of medicine and surgery. My object has been to communicate my own interest and enthusiasm to my students, for unlike some topics which they have to learn, there ought to be nothing boring or dull in this, the oldest and most vigorous of all the specialities. It is for this reason that the solemn minded reader may not approve of some of my pictures, or my omission of the customary protracted dissertation about body fluids and electrolytes for which he will have to consult those other of his textbooks which deal with them in a way which I could not imitate even if I understood. Sexually transmitted diseases are not covered in this book, not because I find them tedious, but because they are too important to be dealt with by other than an expert. On the other hand I found it impossible not to trespass from time to time on the ground normally and correctly assigned to my colleagues in nephrology from whom I crave forgiveness if, in an attempt to make an understandable and unified presentation of the subject, my ignorance has led me into too many and too barbarous errors concerning the esoteric mysteries of nephritis and hypertension. The last chapter about the operations of urology is there simply to make the students' visits to the operating theatre more interesting: they should not attempt to learn surgical technique—though I hope they may find watching operations helps in the understanding of living pathology. For the same reason the little glossary, of jargon, eponyms and gobbledygook is added for fun, not because students need learn any of it.

Preface to Second Edition

The need for a second edition so soon after the first gives me an opportunity to revise it thoroughly, to correct some mistakes, to bring the text and references up to date, and to try to improve some of my sketches in order to make them more clear.

J.P.B.

Begin at the beginning: how old is your patient, and what is his or her occupation? If he is retired, what did he do before? Could he ever have been in contact with rubber, chemicals, plastics, tar, pitch, or any other occupational hazard known to concern the urinary tract. Do not accept vague terms like 'company director' or 'process worker'—the company he directed may have been manufacturing naphthylamine, or the process the mixing of raw rubber with noxious antioxidants. If your patient is female, ask when she was married, how many and how old are her children, and whether there was any complication during pregnancy or delivery that may have necessitated the passing of a catheter e.g. the use of forceps in delivery, or the stitching of a torn perineum.

Turn to the trouble which brings the patient to your clinic. Try to determine when the symptoms began, and what they were like to start with, before any treatment was given. As you listen—and listening is the key to taking a useful history—try to make clear in your own mind how the pattern of the illness has changed over the years. At the end, be sure you understand what it is that bothers the patient right now, and never end your enquiry without asking whether the patient has noticed blood in the urine: haematuria is the most important symptom in the whole of urology.

Note-taking (Fig. 1.1)

Although you must set down all the relevant facts in the history, it is no good writing down a host of irrelevant twaddle in the hope that somebody, sometime, will be able to make sense out of it. It is better to try to keep your notes as brief and as clear as possible. Remember that you are not merely writing them down for your own benefit, but in order that another doctor can understand the problem, and take up the care of the patient where you have left off. So do write legibly and if you don't write clearly, teach yourself to use a typewriter. A drawing may save you lines of prose. If the patient has pain, note on your sketch where the patient says the pain starts and where it radiates to, and add a word or two to specify the character of the pain, e.g. was it sharp, dull, colicky and so forth.

Avoid phoney Greek or Latin terms unless they are clear, short, and unambiguous. Never use them, like an undertaker's top hat, to adorn your work with pretentious respectability. Shun the word *dysuria*—it can mean pain or difficulty or both, and it is more clear to say which it is that you had in mind. *Micturition* is a tiresome euphemism for passing urine, and in most languages in most parts of the world, this physiological function is briefly and explicitly set down by the letter *p*—or if you insist—*pee. Frequency* is more clearly expressed by finding out how often your patient pees by day and by night: and it can be easily written D = 6, N = 3 if your patient has to void six times by day and thrice at night. Avoid *polyuria, nocturia, pollakiuria* and *enuresis*—they are all open to misinterpretation. If you mean the patient *wets the bed*, say so.

Blood noticed by the patient in the urine is allowably and more briefly noted

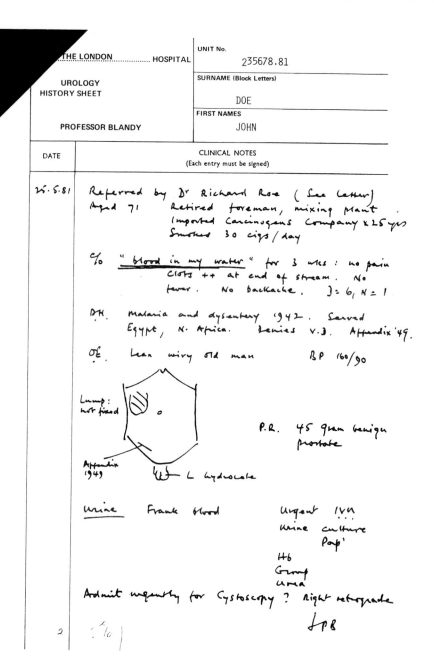

| | THE LONDON HOSPITAL | UNIT No. | 235678.81 |

THE LONDON HOSPITAL

UNIT No. 235678.81

UROLOGY HISTORY SHEET

SURNAME (Block Letters) DOE

FIRST NAMES JOHN

PROFESSOR BLANDY

DATE	CLINICAL NOTES (Each entry must be signed)

25·5·81 — Referred by Dr Richard Roe (See Letter) Aged 71 Retired foreman, mixing plant Imported Carcinogens Company × 25 yrs Smoked 30 cigs/day

C/o "blood in my water" for 3 wks: no pain Clots ++ at end of stream. No fever. No backache. }= 6, N = 1

P.H. Malaria and dysentery 1942. Served Egypt, N. Africa. Denies V.D. Appendix '49.

O.E. Lean wiry old man BP 160/90

Lump: not fixed

Appendix 1949 — L hydrocele

P.R. 45 gram benign prostate

Urine Frank blood

Urgent IVU Urine culture Pap' Hb Group urea

Admit urgently for Cystoscopy ? right retrograde J P B

Fig. 1.1. Keep your notes as brief as possible.

as *haematuria*, but even this can be confusing, for blood detected in the urine on microscopy is no less important an indication for further investigation. Whether the blood was well mixed with the urine, had formed clots, and appeared at the beginning or the end of urination is (in my opinion) of little importance, though it is often made much of in taking a history. Blood trickling away in between the acts of urination is usually coming from the urethra itself.

Do not be put off by a history of taking anticoagulants: haematuria on anticoagulation therapy must be investigated with equal diligence.

Previous history

Ask if your patient has lived in a hot climate, especially in Africa and those parts of the world where schistosomiasis is common. Ask if he or she has been under treatment for rheumatism or sciatica in the course of which analgesics may have been given—analgesic nephropathy is surprisingly common, and will not be disclosed unless you ask indirectly about the possibility of over-consumption of pain-killing tablets. Direct questions on this score will usually not be answered truthfully.

In women, enquire about the menstrual history, not only because of the obvious possible confusion between menstrual loss and haematuria, but also because you must not have unnecessary X-rays taken if there is the slightest possibility of your patient being pregnant. Note the date of the last menstrual period on the X-ray request form.

Students often feel awkward when asking about venereal disease. In fact most men are secretly flattered at the suggestion that they may have been gay dogs in their youth, and a tactful question referring to when they were youngsters will seldom be taken amiss.

DO NOT WASTE TIME

Even before you have finished listening to the patient's story, it will have become obvious that certain investigations are going to be needed. Unobtrusive filling in of the relevant forms should not stop you listening attentively, but will save time, and more important—will prevent you from writing down too many irrelevant details. *Listening is far more important than writing.*

PHYSICAL EXAMINATION

Your physical examination begins as the patient comes into your room. Does he look ill, has he obviously lost weight, does he walk in a way that suggests he may be in pain, or suffer from Parkinsonism? Does he bring with him that faint scent of urine that may suggest uraemia, or perhaps wet trousers? As you shake your patient's hand, remember this is not mere politeness, but may give you useful information. Never forget that you are a doctor first, and a urologist second, and that your first task is to look at the patient as a whole. In an ideal world, where no doctor was ever pushed for time, and no patient was ever in a hurry to get back to his work or her children, you could spend all day over one case, getting to know the patient in depth, and making a thorough and complete physical examination of every system. Such a thorough clerking will of course apply to patients admitted to the ward, but in the clinic this method of working, however ideal, would be cruelly slow. At the same time if you do notice some feature that draws attention to disorder in another system, by all means examine that system as well.

In most patients who attend the urological clinic you will be looking for evidence of enlargement of a kidney or bladder, for disorders in the inguinal region and genitalia, for hypertension, and evidence of pelvic disease detectable

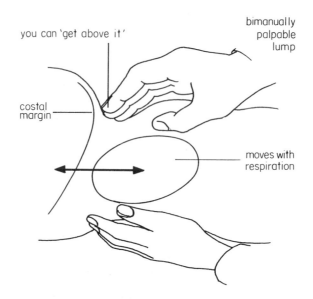

Fig. 1.2. Physical signs of an enlarged kidney.

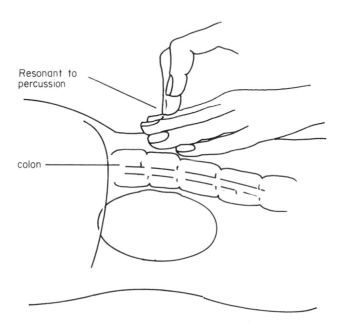

Fig. 1.3. A band of resonance may be found in front of the kidney.

Chapter 1/*History and Examination*

by internal examination per rectum or per vaginam. It is to these features then that your attention will primarily be directed.

Abdominal examination

The physical signs of an *enlarged kidney* (Fig. 1.2) are classically a rounded lump in the loin, bimanually palpable, that moves on respiration, above which one can get the hand between the lump and the edge of the costal margin, and in front of which there is resonance from gas in the bowel (Fig. 1.3). In fact these supposedly classical signs (however often they may be asked for in qualifying examinations) are notoriously misleading and should never be trusted. On the right side the supposed 'kidney' may well turn out to be the gall-bladder or the liver; on the left, it often proves to be the spleen despite being able to slide your hand under the costal margin. A large mass may display the colon and so there is no resonance in front of the kidney, or it may in fact be arising from the colon. The notorious 'kidney punch'—hitting the patient in the loin over the 12th rib—is never needed. Kind doctors do not need to strike their patients: gentle palpation is much more useful (Fig. 1.4).

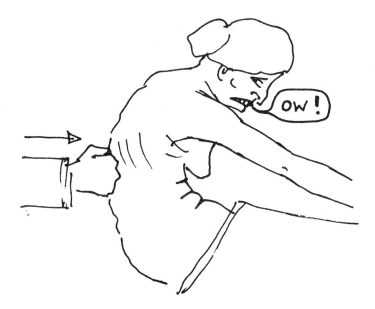

Fig. 1.4. The notorious kidney punch—gentle palpation is just as informative.

The physical signs of an *enlarged bladder* (Figs 1.5 and 1.6) are equally misleading at times, though classically a rounded swelling arising from the pelvis that is dull to percussion ought to be the bladder. In practice a floppy, over-distended bladder may feel rather soft, and it does not always rise up in the midline but may be more on one side than the other (Fig. 1.7). The most useful

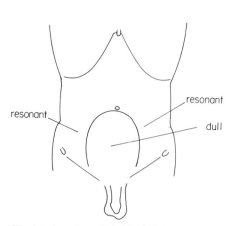

Fig. 1.5. An enlarged bladder is dull to percussion while the flanks are resonant.

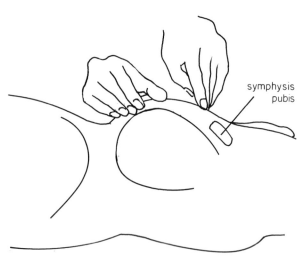

Fig. 1.6. Bimanual examination may show the fluid-filled bladder even when it is atonic and floppy.

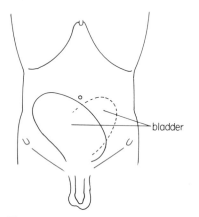

Fig. 1.7. The bladder may not enlarge in the midline, but lean over to one side or the other.

physical sign here is that the swelling goes away when the urine is let out with a catheter.

Examination of the *inguinal regions* is concerned with three hernial orifices on each side (Figs 1.8 and 1.9). Each one needs to be felt both in the supine and erect positions, with and without the patient coughing. An *inguinal hernia* may be direct or indirect; the difference between them is that the hernial orifices are

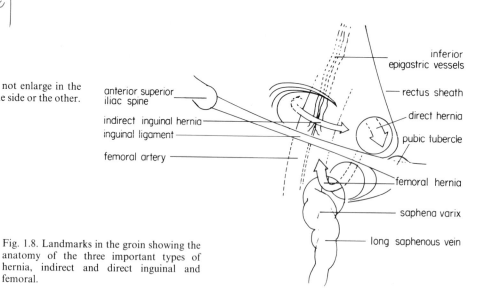

Fig. 1.8. Landmarks in the groin showing the anatomy of the three important types of hernia, indirect and direct inguinal and femoral.

Chapter 1/*History and Examination*

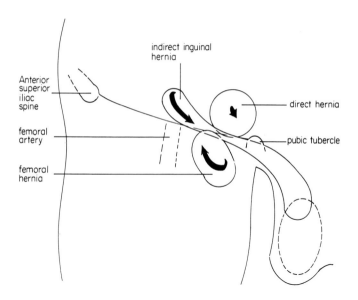

Fig. 1.9. The indirect inguinal hernia slides obliquely down the course of the spermatic cord towards the scrotum; the direct hernia pushes straight out in front; the femoral hernia rises upwards and laterally, and is covered by several layers of fat.

separated by the line of the inferior epigastric vessels. In practice also the *indirect hernia* in a male slides indirectly and obliquely along the line of the spermatic cord towards the scrotum, whereas the *direct hernia* pushes out anteriorly and seldom enters the scrotum. In practice you should never be surprised to find your pre-operative diagnosis proved wrong when the hernia is exposed at operation. It is not at all uncommon to find a direct sac accompanied by an indirect one—the so called saddlebag or pantaloon hernia.

Do not forget to search for *femoral herniae*. The neck of the sac is always rather narrow, and its fundus is surrounded by layer upon layer of fat, like an onion. The hernia pushes out below the inguinal ligament and medial to the femoral vein, but then it bulges out through the fossa ovalis—the gap in the deep fascia where the saphenous vein turns backwards to enter the femoral vein. In practice, unless a femoral hernia is strangulated, it feels like a lipoma and the cough impulse is often very hard to elicit. In the standing-up position a *saphena varix* can mimic a femoral hernia, but it vanishes when the patient lies down, and usually feels 'thin' rather than the fatty lump so typical of a femoral hernia. It has a very obvious cough impulse that coincides with the impulse and thrill running down the rest of the saphenous vein.

The scrotum and its contents

By tradition the term 'testicle' is taken to include both testis and epididymis. When examining the scrotum, the first thing to make sure is that the swelling is not a hernia, i.e. coming down along the cord from above. If you can 'get above' the swelling, then you know it is arising from the testicle (Fig. 1.10).

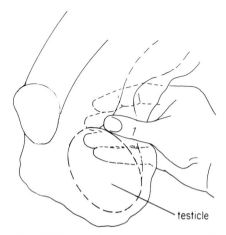

Fig. 1.10. First step in examination of a scrotal swelling: can you get above it?

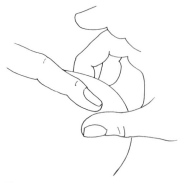

Fig. 1.11. Second step in examination of a scrotal swelling: is it fluctuant or solid? Fluctuation is determined in two planes as shown.

The second step is to ascertain whether the swelling is solid or fluctuant (Fig. 1.11). If the swelling is fluctuant, it must either be made up of fluid in the sac of the tunica vaginalis around the testis (i.e. a hydrocele), or fluid in one or more cysts of the epididymis. Since the epididymis usually lies behind the testis (Fig. 1.12), fluid-filled cysts usually lie behind the body of the testis, and a *hydrocele* envelopes the testis, making it difficult to feel clearly, but when the testis can be distinguished, it lies posteriorly (Fig. 1.13). In practice, *cysts of the epididymis* often coexist with hydroceles and again, it is not at all uncommon for a confident pre-operative diagnosis to be disproved at operation. Traditionally it is usual to shine a light through a hydrocele or an epididymal cyst. If the wall of the cyst or the hydrocele has become thickened, or if the contents has been rendered opaque by haemorrhage or the accumulation of debris, then it will no longer be translucent.

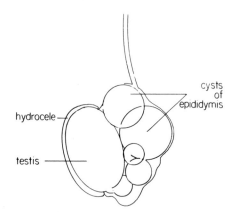

Fig. 1.12. Cysts of the epididymis are multi-locular, flutuant swellings behind the testis. There may be an associated hydrocele.

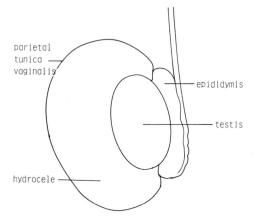

Fig. 1.13 Hydroceles tend to surround and hide the testicle: when it can be found, it lies behind the hydrocele.

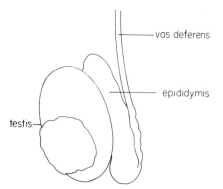

Fig. 1.14. Non-fluctuant (solid) swellings in the testis are usually due to malignant tumour, and always demand to be explored.

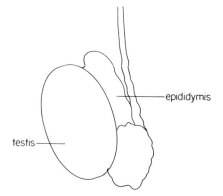

Fig. 1.15. Solid lumps in the epididymis are usually due to chronic inflammation.

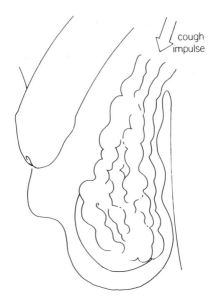

Fig. 1.16. A varicocele is formed by enlarged and tortuous spermatic veins. It feels like a 'bag of worms'. There is usually a cough impulse.

If the lump is not fluctuant, but solid, then the next step is to decide whether it is in the testis or the epididymis. If it is in the testis (Fig. 1.14), then it is a malignant tumour until proved otherwise. If there is a solid lump in the epididymis (Fig. 1.15), then it is a sperm granuloma, tuberculosis, or else a rare tumour.

SWELLINGS IN THE SPERMATIC CORD

The veins draining the testicle may become varicose and distended. It is still widely believed that this condition—*varicocele*—is an important cause of infertility though the matter is in doubt. By tradition a varicocele feels like a 'bag of worms' (Fig. 1.16). Like the reader, the author has never actually felt a bag of worms, but that does not stop him from knowing what one would feel like, and it is certainly a very apt description. A varicocele goes away when the patient lies down.

The vas deferens lies posterior to the cord. If the vas is inflamed, or has been injured (e.g. by previous vasectomy) one may feel knots along its course. Multiple, knotty swellings along the vas are characteristic of tuberculosis (Fig. 1.17). Inflammatory swellings in the cord are seen in the tropical conditions of schistosomiasis and filariasis.

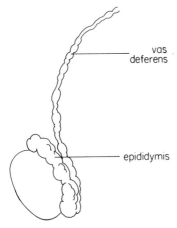

Fig. 1.17. Multiple, knotty swellings along the course of the vas deferens are typical of tuberculosis.

Pelvic examination

Rectal examination in either sex may be carried out either in the supine position, the knee elbow position, or the left lateral position. It is important to introduce the finger slowly and gently. Few readers have never experienced the discomfort

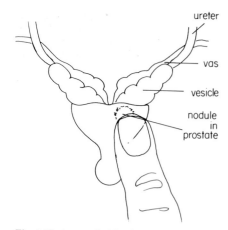

ureter

vas

vesicle

nodule
in
prostate

Fig. 1.18. Anatomical landmarks that may be felt per rectum.

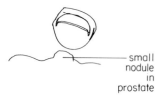

small
nodule
in
prostate

Fig. 1.19. Small nodules protruding from the surface of the prostate may be caused by cancer, and call for biopsy.

of passing a constipated stool, and all should understand the need to introduce the finger slowly. Once inside the rectum, feel the prostate and the rest of the wall of the rectum carefully (Fig. 1.18). Occasionally you will detect a cancer of the rectum. More often, the prostate can be felt, bulging backwards. It may bulge down because the bladder is distended with urine, or because the gland is swollen from the formation of benign nodular hyperplasia. It is not possible to distinguish one from the other on rectal examination.

More important is it to find a discrete hard irregular mass in the prostate, for this may signify carcinoma (Fig. 1.19). A clinical suspicion of prostatic carcinoma must always be confirmed by histology if active treatment is contemplated.

The most experienced surgeons are misled by rectal examination. It is notoriously fallible, and the beginner should, wherever possible, take the opportunity of learning what the normal and abnormal prostate feels like in the anaesthetized patient.

FURTHER READING

Hamilton Bailey W. (1973) In A. Clain (ed.), *Demonstrations of Physical Signs in Clinical Surgery*, 15th edn. Wright, Bristol.

Chapter 1/*History and Examination*

TESTING THE URINE

For centuries physicians have learned much useful information by careful examination of the patient's urine. In times past he would look at it, measure it, smell it, and taste it. Today he should still look at it and smell it, and there are many occasions when the diagnosis rests, not upon sophisticated tests, but upon the simple recording of the time and the volume of urine passed on each occasion—*the fluid chart*.

pH

The pH indicator dye impregnated on a paper test strip is sufficiently accurate for most purposes: a very acid urine should make you consider uric acid stone formation, and a very alkaline urine usually signifies infection with an urea-splitting organism such as *Proteus mirabilis*.

Protein

Paper impregnated with another indicator dye—Bromphenol blue—usually turns blue in the pH range normally found in human urine, but the presence of protein alters this reaction, turning it increasingly yellow the greater the concentration of protein present. Because the dye is essentially an indicator, extremes of acidity or alkalinity render it unreliable. An alternative test for protein is to add 25% salicylsulphonic acid to the urine: protein is precipitated as a cloud unless it is exceptionally dilute. One can still test for protein without special apparatus by boiling it, checking with a drop of a dilute acid that the first cloud thrown down by boiling is not phosphatic. When protein has been discovered in the urine, and there is good clinical reason to want to know whether the quantity present is significant or not, the urine should be collected over a 24 hour period and the protein measured in the laboratory accurately: more than 150 mgm of protein per 24 hours is abnormal and calls for further investigation.

Reducing substances

Today it is customary and convenient to use cheap paper strips impregnated with indicator that changes colour from specific enzymatic hydrolysis of glucose. If these are not available one may use Fehling's or Benedict's solution—glucose and other reducing substances will precipitate orange copper oxide.

Red cells in the urine

Several commercial 'stix' texts for urine rely on the oxidation of orthotoluidine by cumene peroxidase which is catalysed by haemoglobin to give a blue colour.

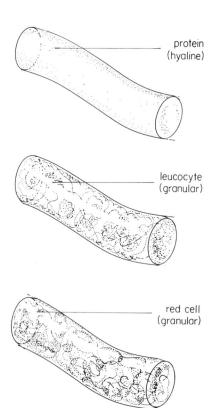

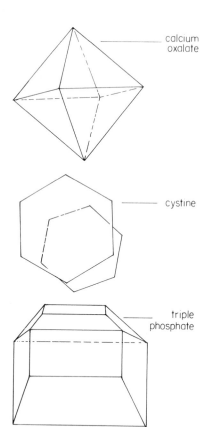

Fig. 2.1. Casts in the urine are extrusions from collecting tubules and may contain protein, pus, or blood.

It detects free haemoglobin and numbers of red cells as low as 5–10 per high power field. This is very close to the number present in centrifuged urine in healthy males so that the test is apt to give rise to false positives. It is always necessary to confirm the positive 'stix' test with a count of the centrifuged urine using standard conditions. False positive results may be found if the urine is slightly contaminated with povidone iodine or hypochlorite.

Examination of the deposit

In busy clinical practice one often requires to know if there is blood or pus in the urine. Do not forget how useful it can be to examine a drop of urine on a microscope slide covered with a cover-slip: significant amounts of pus and blood can easily be seen without the need for a centrifuge or for special staining.

However, more information is obtained after gently centrifuging the urine and placing a drop of the sediment on a slide under a cover-slip. Now you might be able to see *casts*, *crystals* and *bacteria*.

Casts are squeezed-out contents of the collecting tubules from the kidney:

Fig. 2.2. Crystals have characteristic shapes in the urine of which oxalate, cystine and triple phosphate are some of the more common types.

Chapter 2/*Investigations*

they are clear or granular. Clear ones (*hyaline casts*) are formed from protein. *Granular* casts are made up either of red cells or white cells or both, and you may need to stain the deposit to determine which is which (Fig. 2.1).

Crystals are common, and can often give useful leads in diagnosis: the octahedral diamonds of calcium oxalate are characteristic as are the hexagonal plates of cystine or the dodecahedrons of triple phosphate (Fig. 2.2).

The ova of *Schistosoma haematobium* may be found in urine of people who have visited Africa (Fig. 2.3).

In most cases of urinary infection numerous bacteria will be seen in the centrifuged deposit, which may be stained with the Gram stain to help detect the organism responsible for urinary infection (this can be a most useful clue in a very severe illness). If searching for *Mycobacterium tuberculosis* the urine is stained with the *Ziehl–Neelsen method*, and it is customary to send the laboratory at least three specimens of the first urine passed in the morning.

If searching for cancer in the urinary tract any urine specimen *except* the early morning one will do, but must immediately be fixed (e.g. with an equal volume of 10% formalin solution) and then centrifuged, fixed and stained with one of the variations on the *Papanicolaou* stain.

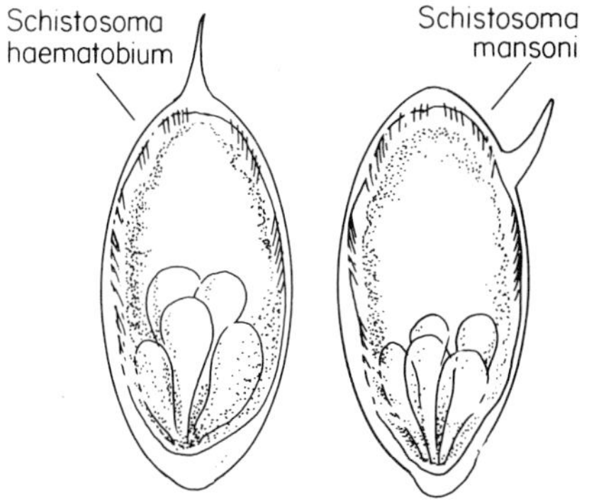

Fig. 2.3. Ova of *Schistoma* contain live *Miracidia* which will hatch out in freshwater. A terminal spine is typical of *S. haematobium*, a lateral spine of *S. mansoni*.

Culture of the urine

Urine is readily contaminated from the wall of the urethra, prepuce or vulva or from air-borne dust entering the specimen bottle. At room temperature these contaminants will grow rapidly, so that it is important that specimens of urine should be cultured at once, or, if there is to be delay, kept in the refrigerator. It is

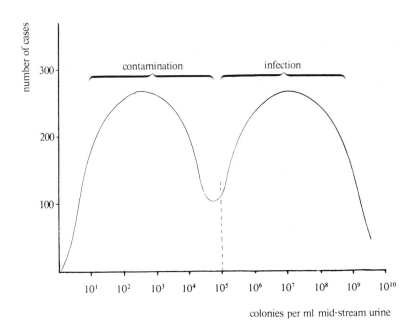

Fig. 2.4. Quantitative differences between urinary contamination and infection.

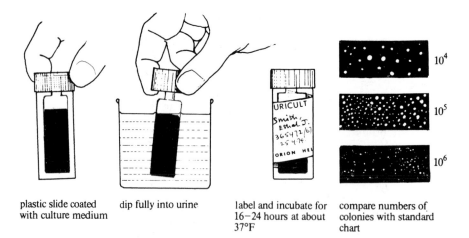

Fig. 2.5. Use of the dip inoculum slide.

plastic slide coated with culture medium

dip fully into urine

label and incubate for 16–24 hours at about 37°F

compare numbers of colonies with standard chart

a mistake to allow a specimen of urine to stand around at room temperature for several hours before it reaches the laboratory bench, and even more futile to send it through the mail. Even when urine is examined at once, some of the organisms that appear in the culture medium will be contaminants. It has been shown that if the urine is mixed up with the medium, each organism present will produce a colony, and by counting the colonies one can quantify the numbers of organisms originally present. By making colony counts in this way one can distinguish contaminants from significant infections (Fig. 2.4).

For use in the busy general practitioner's surgery a simple way to make a fairly accurate 'colony count' on freshly voided urine is to use the 'dip-slide' (Fig. 2.5). The slide coated with culture medium is dipped into the urine, the surplus drained off, replaced in the sterile bottle, and put in a warm place (e.g. an incubator, or near a radiator) for 24 hours. A glance at a chart supplied with the dip-slide will show with tolerable accuracy, whether there are more than 10^5 colonies per ml present or not.

When it is really vital to know whether there is an infection or not, then it is useful to obtain it from the bladder by direct suprapubic puncture (Fig. 2.6). This is almost painless and usually safe, though as with any invasive investigation there are always some complications including osteomyelitis of the symphysis, and so it should only be employed when really necessary.

RADIOLOGICAL EXAMINATIONS

The plain abdominal radiograph ('scout film', 'KUB')

All radiological examinations begin with a plain radiograph before any contrast medium is injected, and it is often very informative by itself in urinary surgery (Fig. 2.7). A good drill to use when studying the preliminary plain radiograph is that of the '4 Ss': *S*ide?, *S*keleton, *S*oft tissues, *S*tones?

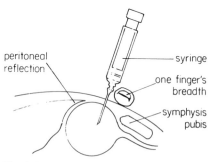

peritoneal reflection

syringe

one finger's breadth

symphysis pubis

Fig. 2.6. Method of obtaining urine from the bladder by direct suprapubic puncture. This avoids errors due to contamination. *Any* colonies, however few, obtained from this specimen are significant.

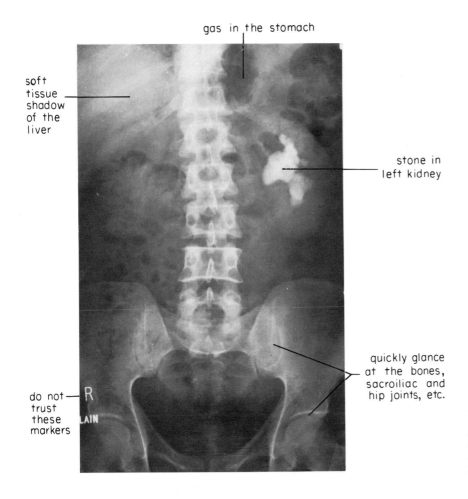

gas in the stomach

soft tissue shadow of the liver

stone in left kidney

quickly glance at the bones, sacroiliac and hip joints, etc.

do not trust these markers

R

LAIN

Fig. 2.7. The plain film: check the 4 Ss. Is the *side* correctly marked (look for the liver and gastric air-bubble as well as the radiographer's sign)? Is the *skeleton* normal? Is there any obvious abnormality in the *soft tissue* shadows? Are there any radio-opaque shadows that might be *stones*?

SIDE?

Radiographers are only human, and it is very easy to put the wrong letter on the film. Always check that the soft tissue shadow of the liver is on the right side and the gastric air bubble on the left. (One day you will be deceived by a patient with *situs inversus*—but then, the Deity is allowed to make mistakes!)

SKELETON

Carefully examine the appearances of the spine, ribs, hips and sacroiliac joints. Look for osteoblastic and osteoclastic metastatic deposits, for evidence of arthritis, ankylosing spondylitis, disease in the hip joints, etc.

SOFT TISSUES

Especially in a fat person, when the kidneys are surrounded by radiolucent adipose tissue, one can make out their outline, though this should always be checked carefully later on with the appearance in the nephrogram phase of the urogram. Look in the pelvis for the soft tissue shadow of a distended bladder, for that of an enlarged uterus, and do not neglect to observe an enlarged Riedel's lobe of the liver or the typical shadow of an enlarged spleen.

STONES?

To the urologist any radiodense shadow in the line of the urinary tract must raise the suspicion of a calculus. If there is some doubt, when the shadow lies in front of the soft tissue shadow of the kidney, films may be taken in inspiration and expiration to move the kidneys up and down: adjacent tissues containing calcified material will change their position with respect to the kidney. Note gall stones, calcified fibroids, and the presence of phleboliths in the pelvis—often a cause of confusion with calculi in the line of the ureter. Calcified nodes are common in the mesentery, and calcification in the costal cartilages a common finding in the vicinity of the renal shadows.

The intravenous urogram (IVU, IVP)

This is the most common and most useful of urological investigations but to get the best out of it, one needs to understand some of its underlying principles.

A family of compounds based on benzoic acid attached to three iodine atoms (Fig. 2.8) may be safely given intravenously: some are given as the sodium salt, others as the methylglucamine salt. It is thought that the latter are less toxic, but they are more viscous. In these modern contrast media there is virtually no free iodine. If given rapidly intravenously they often give rise to discomfort in the arm along the line of the vein, to nausea and sometimes vomiting.

More serious toxic reactions are less common: of these an urticarial rash comes on within a few minutes of beginning the injection, and is readily amenable to an antihistamine. Far more serious, and alas, sometimes deadly, are the angioneurotic oedema of glottis and trachea, or the widespread vasodilatation that leads to hypotension and cardiac arrest. These two severe reactions are manifestations of allergy to the whole iodinated molecule, not to free iodine, and so it is of no value to perform skin testing with iodine previous to the injection. Many physicians give the first few ml of the injection very slowly on this account, but even this may not prevent a fatal reaction. Of far more consequence is it to make sure, whenever you are asked to give an injection for a urogram, that the essentials for resuscitation and for countering the reaction are instantly available. If oedema develops, or peripheral vasodilatation and shock occur, 200 mgm of hydrocortisone are injected intravenously at once; oxygen is given by positive pressure using a face mask and if necessary an endotracheal tube, and it may be necessary to proceed to cardiac massage and defibrillation. Although these fatal reactions only occur in 1 in 100 000

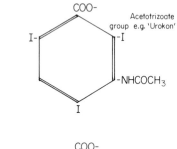

Fig. 2.8. All the commonly used contrast media employed for urography are based on benzoic acid.

Chapter 2/*Investigations*

urograms, to fail to provide the appropriate means of resuscitation and to acquaint yourself with their position in the room, is negligent.

HANDLING OF CONTRAST MEDIA BY THE KIDNEY

Today the standard dose of contrast medium contains about 300 mgm iodine/kg body weight (as provided in about 1 ml/kg body weight of most currently used commercial preparations). In renal failure larger doses are required. In such a dose the majority of the contrast medium is filtered in the glomerulus, and thereafter concentrated by reabsorption of water.

It will take 15–20 seconds for the intravenously injected contrast medium to reach the kidney (the usual circulation time) so that films taken in the first 1–3 minutes will catch the contrast lying in the glomeruli and proximal tubule. Most of the tubular reabsorption of water takes place, it will be remembered, in the proximal tubule, and so the early pictures of the urographic series will give a clear image of the renal parenchyma. This is called the 'nephrogram' phase (Fig. 2.9). When it is particularly important to get a good image of the outline of the kidney, e.g. when you suspect scarring, or a lump due to a tumour, it is common to supplement the early nephrogram pictures by one or two tomographic cuts judged to slice through the kidney and eliminate unwanted shadows due to gas in the bowel.

In conditions which slow the rate of circulation through the renal parenchyma, or which hold up the rate at which the filtrate flows down the tubule, the nephrogram is more pronounced, more dense, and more long-lasting. In obstruction, for example from a stone in the ureter, one may obtain a dense nephrogram many hours after the original injection of contrast medium.

In the normal patient the flow of contrast in the filtrate soon begins to opacify the calices and pelvis, and the accumulation of contrast medium in the renal parenchyma is succeeded by the 'pyelogram' phase, during which most of the contrast medium outlines the calices, pelvis, and ureter. It is customary therefore to take pictures at 15 and 20 minutes to show the full length of the urinary tract, including the bladder, which by now is usually fairly well filled with contrast medium (Fig. 2.10).

The pyelogram films may also be supplemented, when necessary, by films taken in the oblique or lateral position, especially when there is some doubt about the nature of a small calcified shadow in the line of the ureter.

The patient is then asked to empty his or her bladder. If one needs to show the urethra (e.g. when one suspects a urethral stricture) it is often useful to obtain pictures of the urethra during the act of micturition (*a voiding urethrogram*). In patients with suspected obstruction to the outflow from the bladder a *postmicturition* film is taken as soon as possible after the patient has emptied the bladder. This gives an image of the contrast retained in the bladder, the *residual urine*, which has repeatedly been shown to correlate very accurately with the volume of urine left behind in the bladder.

Knowing how the kidney handles the contrast medium allows us to modify

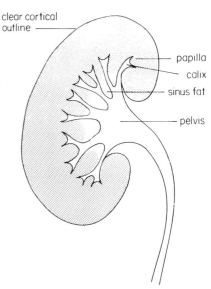

clear cortical outline

papilla
calix
sinus fat
pelvis

Fig. 2.9. The 'nephrogram phase' of the IVU. The contrast medium has just reached the glomeruli and proximal tubule.

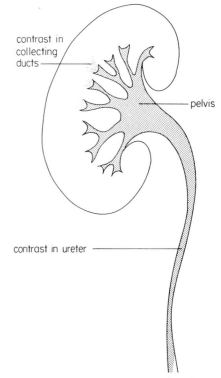

contrast in collecting ducts

pelvis

contrast in ureter

Fig. 2.10. The 'pyelogram phase' of the IVU. Most of the contrast has now reached the calices and pelvis.

the urogram when we need special answers to special questions. For example, in renal failure, one can still obtain a useful answer to the anatomical questions, 'Is the kidney small, is it scarred, or is it obstructed?', but one needs to use a very large dose of contrast medium, and one needs to be patient and take the pictures after 6–12 hours so as to obtain a *delayed nephrogram* and a *delayed pyelogram*. The density of the picture will not be so great, and one may need careful tomography to eliminate bone and gas shadows from the background.

Similarly, one must not fall into the trap of imagining that a good radiographic image implies good renal function. For example, if one kidney is small and diseased, but the other one is normal, the good kidney will eliminate the solute load, and the bad kidney will give quite a good picture since the small amount of contrast filtering into its proximal tubules can be concentrated there, for what little that is worth. The tiny diseased kidney 'which seems to have good function' is all too often diagnosed in the urogram, and one must beware not to copy this mistake.

Because the density of the image depends on concentration of the filtered contrast medium in the proximal and the collecting tubules of the cortex, one may (slightly) improve the picture by having the patient deprived of fluid for 6–8 hours before the examination. This is of course quite futile when the patient is in renal failure, and cannot concentrate urine anyway.

The large dose of contrast medium that enters the glomerular filtrate must act as an osmotic diuretic; however if there is doubtful obstruction to be investigated, one can distend the urinary tract upstream of the obstruction by adding a water or frusemide diuresis to that of the contrast medium—the 'water-load IVU'.

Antegrade urography

From time to time, even with all the tricks of using high dose urography and tomography, one still cannot see exactly what is the anatomy of the kidney and ureter. If a fine needle is inserted through the skin over the kidney into the lumen of the renal pelvis (Fig. 2.11) (first locating the distended pelvis with an intravenous urogram or perhaps with ultrasound) contrast medium can be injected so as to outline the pelvis and ureter. If the needle is replaced with a polyethylene cannula, and connected to a pressure-measuring recorder, contrast can be run in at a certain rate, the pressure in the upper tract can be recorded, and one can not only get good pictures of the anatomy of the system, but can also diagnose whether it is truly obstructed or merely baggy and distended (Whitaker's test). If there is any question of tumour inside the renal pelvis or ureter, fluid can be aspirated and sent for Papanicolaou stain for malignant cells. If the patient is in renal failure and the system is obstructed, the polyethylene tube may be left in position and used to drain away the urine until the patient has dialysed himself into a better condition (*medical nephrostomy*).

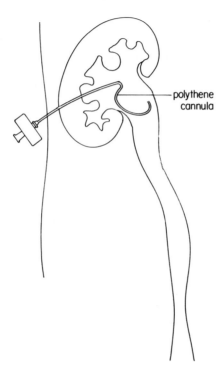

Fig. 2.11. Antegrade urography and the 'medical nephrostromy'; the cannula may be left in the kidney to keep it decompressed.

Retrograde urography

It is usually very easy to see the ureteric orifices through a cystoscope and pass a fine tube into them. The ureteric catheter is marked in centimetres, and in most adults the kidney lies about 25 cm up from the ureteric orifice (Fig. 2.12). The catheter is easily passed up into the renal pelvis, if one needs to get urine from the pelvis for Papanicolaou staining, or for culture for tuberculosis, and contrast can be injected—usually 2–5 ml at a time. This is the standard 'retrograde pyelogram' and gives good pictures of the renal pelvis and calices. It has largely been supplanted by using the image intensifier screen and television, and by pushing a bulb-ended catheter into the ureteric orifice before injecting the contrast medium (Fig. 2.13). This 'ascending ureterography' allows the surgeon to watch the active movement of the kidney, calices and ureter, and observe the way the contrast medium trickles over and around tumours or stones in the ureter and upper tract.

Cystogram

Radiographs taken when the bladder is filled with contrast medium are

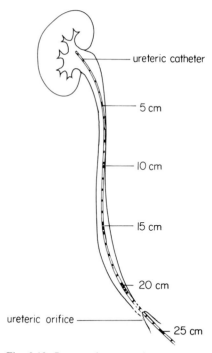

Fig. 2.12. Retrograde urography: a ureteric catheter is passed by means of the operating cystoscope up the ureter to the kidney. Urine may be aspirated from the kidney and examined for TB or malignant cells, and contrast injected to give a clear radiograph.

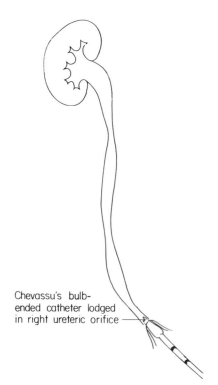

Chevassu's bulb-
ended catheter lodged
in right ureteric orifice

Fig. 2.13. Retrograde ureterography using a bulb-ended catheter which is lodged in the ureteric orifice: the contrast runs up and down the ureter and is usually observed with an image intensifier.

routinely used when one suspects that there are defective ureterovesical valves and that reflux of urine from bladder to kidney is carrying infection up to them. Usually these cystograms are performed with image intensification so that fleeting reflux from bladder to kidney which might be missed in a static film can be observed.

Cystograms of a different kind are used in the investigation of people with incontinence. Lateral and oblique films are obtained in women with descent of the neck of the bladder associated with stress incontinence. Others are taken in conjunction with simultaneous recording of pressure inside the bladder when investigating disorders of bladder function related to neuropathy. Static films of the bladder are used to show diverticula and may be supplemented by double contrast films using gas as well as contrast medium when one suspects carcinoma in the bladder or in diverticula.

From all this it is clear that the clinician must discuss the problem with his radiodiagnostic colleague and not merely fill in a form for a 'cystogram'. Since all these investigations require the passage of a catheter and a certain amount of indignity and discomfort, they should never be ordered without good reason, and without carefully considering whether some other more simple investigation would not answer the diagnostic question just as well.

Urethrography

To display the urethra in the male, a Knutsson's syringe is inserted into the external meatus, and contrast mixed with a fairly viscous gel ('Umbradil viscous') is gently injected into the urethra. As an alternative one may lodge a thin Foley catheter just inside the external meatus and inject water-soluble contrast. Lateral and oblique films are then taken to show the urethra.

In females, a similar technique using a balloon catheter wedged against the external meatus may be employed to delineate urethral diverticula.

Angiography

To show diseases of the renal artery, and to distinguish benign swellings of the renal parenchyma from malignant ones, a Seldinger catheter is placed in the orifice of the renal artery, and contrast is injected into it. Films are then taken in rapid sequence to show the early 'arterial' phase, which shows the parenchyma, followed by less frequent succeeding pictures of the arterial, and later on, the venous circulation of the kidney and the suspicious area. Similar methods are used to display narrowings of the renal artery thought to cause hypertension.

Cavography

Contrast may be injected into the vena cava to display indentations of its contour caused by tumour spreading from the kidney into the renal vein and on into the vena cava. At this investigation one may also pass a catheter into the renal vein in patients with hypertension to aspirate blood and have its renin measured.

Lymphangiography

A drop of patent blue violet (an innoccuous dye) is injected into the first two web spaces of the foot. After one hour, the dye has found its way into lymphatics. Under local anaesthetic, a small incision is made over a lymphatic which is cannulated and then slowly filled with an oily contrast medium that runs up the lymphatics of the leg, fills the lymph nodes first in the groin and then the iliac and para-aortic groups. Metastases are detected if a normal lymphatic pathway is unexpectedly blocked off, or if a filling defect is seen in an otherwise well-filled lymph node (Fig. 2.14). Lymphangiography is commonly used in the evaluation of testicular tumours to help to tell how far the tumour has spread, and also to guide the radiotherapist in directing his field of fire. It has been found to be disappointing in determining the spread of cancer of the bladder and prostate. It is very unpleasant for the patient, very time-consuming, and by no means accurate. Since the oily contrast medium ends up in the thoracic duct and lung fields, and since the oil impairs lung function, a general anaesthetic must be avoided for a week after a lymphangiogram has been done.

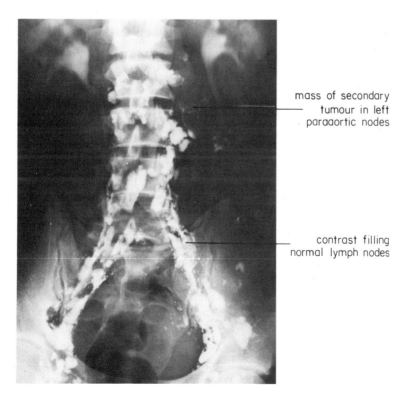

mass of secondary tumour in left paraaortic nodes

contrast filling normal lymph nodes

Fig. 2.14. Lymphangiogram used to reveal abdominal metastases from testicular tumour. Here the large mass of growth has displaced the lymphatics.

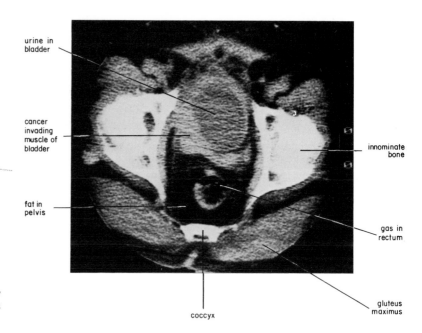

urine in
bladder

cancer
invading
muscle of
bladder

fat in
pelvis

innominate
bone

gas in
rectum

gluteus
maximus

coccyx

Fig. 2.15. Computer Assisted Tomography (CAT or EMI scan). A 'slice' of a pelvis in a patient with an invasive bladder cancer.

Computer Assisted Tomography (CAT scan, EMI scan) (Fig. 2.15)

Just as the conventional tomogram provides a clear image of a slice through one part of the body, and eliminates unwanted information from slices above and below the one to be examined, so in principle, does the CAT scan. However, by means of a battery of detectors and a rotating source, it is able to obtain information about thousands of tiny slices and present this information in the form of a cross-section, the mass of information being hoarded and processed by computer. Of course, ultimately, each item of information is a measure of the absorption of X-rays at a certain point. An arbitrary scale of these absorption values, the Hounsfield number (appropriately celebrating the Nobel prize-winning inventor of the machine), is used to measure the nature of the tissue at any one point: thus air has a Hounsfield number -1000, dense bone $+1000$, fat -100 and water 0. In the urinary tract one often makes use of the ordinary excretion urogram contrast medium to show up dilated renal pelves and ureters and so on. It is too soon to be sure how useful this wonderful invention will be in diagnosis and treatment of disorders of the urinary tract. It is in competition with other, less expensive diagnostic techniques, and even the exactness and refinement of the Hounsfield number cannot distinguish fibrosis from cancer, if they each absorb X-rays to the same extent. It looks likely to prove the most accurate and least unpleasant of all techniques for detecting hidden lymph node metastases. It is certainly the most sensitive method of finding small metastases in the lungs that would otherwise escape diagnosis. It can probably show with accuracy and precision when cancer has invaded outside the renal capsule and into the arterial wall or vein, but it remains to be seen whether this will influence the surgeon's decision to explore or not to explore.

ultrasound

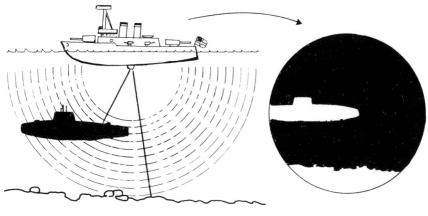

echoes detect submarine on ship's Asdic

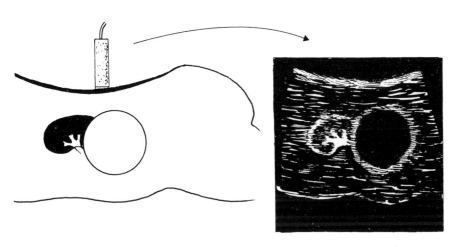

renal cyst is seen in sonar scan as a trans-sonic mass without echoes

Fig. 2.16. Ultrasound.

Ultrasound (Fig. 2.16)

Sonar, used to detect submarines in the Second World War, or today, to find shoals of fish for factory ships, has been adapted to medicine with wonderful results. Thanks to the use of a technological advance—the grey scale ultrasound—it is now possible to detect internal structure in some organs, particularly the liver. In the kidney, to date, these differences are not very useful. In the bladder it seems very likely that one will shortly be able to tell how far a bladder cancer has invaded its muscular wall (the T stage), and it shows great promise in the diagnosis of lymph node enlargement in the pelvis. Its great advantage is that it is entirely safe and does not hurt. No needles are involved and there are no unpleasant injections. There is no radiation hazard. It is routine practice to use ultrasound to distinguish a benign cyst from a cancer of the kidney, and to use ultrasound as a guide whenever it is necessary to pass a needle into a dilated renal pelvis, or aspirate a renal cyst. At operation, ultrasound helps to detect tiny particles of stone lodged in the kidney parenchyma. It is exceedingly accurate in detecting metastases in the liver. For finding and following other collections of fluid, e.g. pus near the kidney, or collections of lymph near a transplant kidney, ultrasound is useful, can be repeated frequently, and above all, does not hurt at all.

ISOTOPE STUDIES

Overall renal function

Instead of the standard measure of renal function—creatinine clearance—which measures the clearance from blood to urine (but depends on the accurate collection of the entire 24 hour specimen of urine) we rely increasingly on a different measure, namely, the clearance from blood to kidney of a substance given intravenously. More conveniently one may use ^{51}Cr ethylenediamine tetra-acetic acid (EDTA). After giving a dose of the isotope intravenously serial measurements of the radioactivity in the blood are measured. One may select

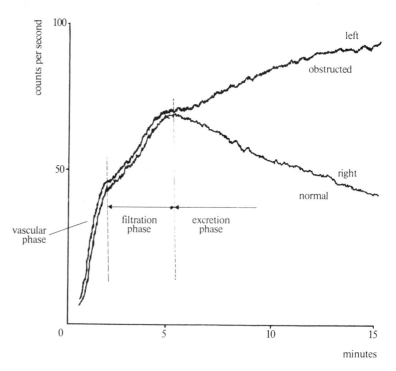

Fig. 2.17. Diagram of a I^{131} hippuran renogram showing the effect of obstruction on the left side.

Chapter 2/*Investigations*

the ^{51}Cr EDTA activity at 75 minutes as an arbitrary time against which serial measurements may be compared on later occasions. This is a particularly useful technique for measurement of renal function in patients from whom it may be very difficult to obtain a complete 24 hour urine collection. A modification of this principle employs a sensitive counter over the forearm rather than serial sampling of the blood.

Individual renal function

If a radiation counter is pointed over the kidneys, or a battery of counters (gamma camera) aimed over both of them, and an isotope is given intravenously, one can compare the way it is handled by each kidney with its fellow (Fig. 2.17).

RENOGRAM

The uptake of radioactivity over the kidney falls into three phases. Phase 1 records the arrival of the isotope in the bloodstream to the kidney and shows as a rapidly rising curve over about 30 seconds; Phase 2 rises more slowly, since some of the isotope starts to leave the parenchyma as some is still arriving. In Phase 3 the bolus of isotope is beginning to leave the calices and pelvis and pass down the ureter. These three phases reflect four distinct functions of the kidney. First, there is the *uptake function* of the kidney from the blood: obviously if there is less blood getting to the kidney, this function will be diminished.

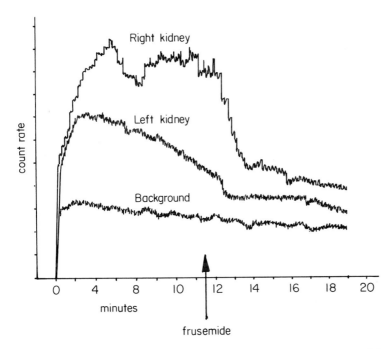

Fig. 2.18. Example of the use of renography. This patient had a small (previously scarred) left kidney, hence the lower peak at the end of the filtration phase. But on the right side there was a big baggy pelvis which seemed to be obstructed. As the isotope collected in the big pelvis the count rate continued to stay high, but when frusemide was given, the diuresis rapidly carried the contrast away down the ureter, thereby proving that there was no obstruction.

Secondly, it reflects the *transit* of isotope through the nephron to the pelvis. This will be slowed when the perfusion pressure falls for any reason. Thirdly, there is the *removal function*, i.e. the ability of the kidney to pass the isotope into the renal pelvis. Fourthly, its ability to transfer the isotope from the pelvis down the ureter—the *pelvic transit function*. After giving the isotope intravenously some of it will be carried in the bloodsteam to the soft tissues behind and in front of the kidney, and to allow for these non-renal tissues, a counter may be placed over an adjacent part of the loin and its count subtracted from that recorded over the kidney (Fig. 2.18).

GAMMA CAMERA

Using a gamma camera rather than a single counter over the kidney it is possible to measure the count over the renal pelvis distinct from the parenchyma and so measure the rate of transit of the isotope through the kidney. If there is significant obstruction to the upper urinary tract this transit rate is impaired. By giving a diuretic such as frusemide one can get a big, floppy, renal pelvis to empty out, and so make the distinction between the big, extrarenal pelvis and the one that is obstructed at the pelvi-ureteric junction.

IMAGING

Different isotopes may be used for different purposes. For measuring the different renal functions listed above, it is customary to use 99^{m}Tc-labelled diethylene triamine pentacetic acid (DTPA). If one is particularly interested in obtaining a clear image of the renal parenchyma rather than in measuring its various functions, one can photograph the image on the gamma camera early in the 'nephrogram' phase of the renogram using 99^{m}Tc-DTPA or a different substance that is taken up and held in the renal tubules—the mercurial substance 99^{m}Tc dimercaptosuccinic acid (DMSA). The latter is photographed after one hour, and gives clear pictures of scarring, cysts, infarcts and so on.

Again the clinician must bring his colleague in nuclear medicine into the clinical picture: it is no good just filling in a form and asking for a 'renal scan'.

BONE SCAN

One of the most useful and practical indications for isotope scanning is found in the evaluation of carcinoma of the prostate. Using 99^{m}TC MDP the isotope is taken up by the more vascular parts of the bone, and since most metastases are hypervascular, they are detectable in the scan even before they can be seen in conventional radiographs. In following men with prostatic cancer this isotope scan has the additional advance that it gives a very useful image of the kidneys, ureters and bladder (Fig. 2.19).

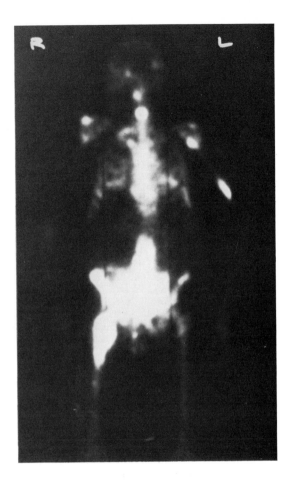

Fig. 2.19. Bone scan after giving 99^mTc MDP in a patient riddled with bony metastases from prostatic cancer.

CLINICAL TESTS OF KIDNEY FUNCTION

Glomerular filtration rate

Inulin clearance is the standard method, but seldom used in clinical practice. Creatinine clearance is more commonly asked for, but in practice, depends for its accuracy upon the complete collection of all the urine passed by the patient over a 24 hour period—an ideal often difficult to achieve in a busy surgical ward. The plasma creatinine is measured at a convenient time during the period of urine collection and clearance is given by the formula UV/P where U = urine creatinine/100 ml, V = urine volume ml/minute and P = plasma creatinine mgm/100 ml, and the answer is expressed in ml/minute. For most purposes the level of plasma creatinine provides a good enough working guide to the normality of renal glomerular function. Urea and urea clearance used to be asked for, but the plasma urea is readily elevated (e.g. by vomiting or a hearty protein meal) and is less accurately measured than creatinine.

Tests of tubular function

None of the conventional clinical tests of tubular function are easy to apply, and it seems likely that they will be supplanted by isotope measurements before very long. One may measure the *response to acid load*, which is a rough index of the function of the distal tubule. After collecting two specimens of urine over a period of two hours the patient is given an acid load in the form of NH_4Cl (as gelatin coated capsules 0.1 g/kg body weight) with a litre of water over a period of one hour. Three hours later an hour collection of urine is made. If the tubules are healthy they should respond to this acid load by secreting urine with a pH les than 5.3, a titratable acidity more than 25 mEq/minute and more than 35 mEq/minute of ammonium.

The urine concentration test measures the ability of the kidney to respond to antidiuretic hormone. One may deprive the patient of water, or give him pitressin tannate (5 units subcutaneously) and then follow the specific gravity in each specimen of urine passed thereafter. This test should never be used in patients in renal failure.

ENDOSCOPY

It is no exaggeration to say that the speciality of urology really began with the invention of the *cystoscope*, and has been revolutionized in the last decade thanks to the invention by Professor Harold Hopkins of the flexible fibre light and the rod-lens telescope. Thanks to these two inventions it is now possible to examine the interior of the bladder (by *cystoscopy*), urethra (*urethroscopy*) and, at operation, the inside of the kidney (*nephroscopy*). Another of his inventions, the flexible fibre-optic endoscope, has been adapted to the human ureter, so that one may pass the ureteroscope via a cystoscope right up to the renal pelvis. Added to these optical wonders are complete sets of transurethral instruments which permit the surgeon to remove bladder and prostatic tumours, perform biopsies, crush stones and catheterize the ureters. What is being done can be demonstrated to colleagues on endoscopic television and recorded, measured, and studied at leisure. Again, it is no good merely requesting 'a cystoscopy'— nowadays each endoscopic investigation sets out to answer a specific question, and merely to look around the inside of the bladder is in most cases only the first step, which will be followed by a biopsy or some other transurethral manoeuvre.

FURTHER READING

Abrams H.L. (1978) Computed tomography of the kidney. In J.H. Harrison *et al.* (eds), *Campbell's Urology*, Vol. 1, 4th edn, p. 292. W.B. Saunders Co., Philadelphia.
Barratt T.M. (1976) Fundamentals of renal physiology. In D.I. Williams & G.D. Chisholm (eds), *Scientific Foundations of Urology*, p. 19. Heinemann, London.

Britton K. (1978) Radionuclides in renal imaging. *British Journal of Hospital Medicine*, **20,** 140.

Gow J.G. (1976) The cystoscope. *British Journal of Hospital Medicine*, **16,** 16.

Macleod M.A., Sampson W.F. & Houston A.S. (1977) Urinary clearance of [113m]In-DTPA and [99m]Tc-(Sn)DTM measured by external arm counting. *Urological Research*, **5,** 71.

O'Reilly P.H., Lawson R.S., Shields R.A., Testa H.J., Charlton-Edwards E. & Carroll R.N.P. (1977) Dynamic scintigraphy in clinical urology. *British Journal of Urology*, **49,** 575.

Siegle R.L. & Lieberman P. (1978) A review of untoward reactions to iodinated contrast material. *Journal of Urology* **119,** 581.

Whitfield H.N., Britton K.E., Hendry W.F., Nimmon C.C. & Wickham J.E.A. (1978) The distinction between obstructive uropathy and nephropathy by radioisotope transit times. *British Journal of Urology*, **50,** 433.

Chapter 3
The Kidney—
Structure and
Function

SURGICAL RELATIONS OF THE KIDNEYS

The posterior relations of each kidney are to the twelfth rib, diaphragm, pleura and lung, and below the rib, to the quadratus lumborum muscle and psoas muscle. The ilioinguinal and iliohypogastric nerves cross obliquely on the front of the quadratus lumborum muscle. The hilum of the kidney is closely related to the tips of the transverse processes of the upper lumbar vertebrae (Fig. 3.1).

On the left side the kidney is covered in front by the spleen and tail of the pancreas, the duodenojejunal flexure and the descending colon, and any of these structures may be densely adherent to the kidney when it is malignant or inflamed, and are therefore easily injured during nephrectomy (Figs 3.2, 3.3).

On the right side lying in front of the kidney are the ascending colon and the second part of the duodenum (Figs 3.4, 3.5).

Medial to the left kidney lies the aorta; medial to the right one lies the vena cava. Above and medial to each kidney lies its suprarenal.

The importance of these surgical relations is that they govern the choice of

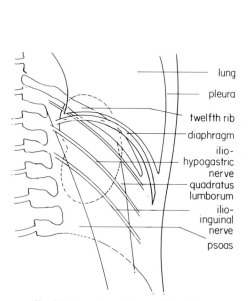

Fig. 3.1. Posterior relations of the kidney.

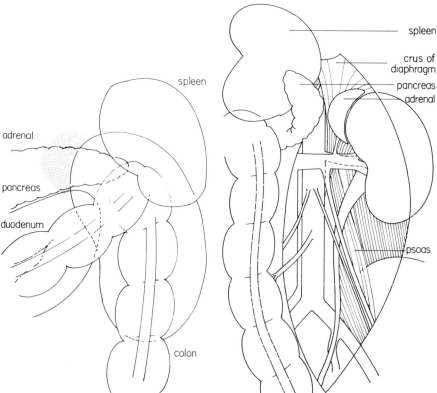

Fig. 3.2. The left kidney lies behind the colon, duodenum, pancreas and spleen.

Fig. 3.3. By mobilizing the colon medially, and detaching the spleen from the diaphragm, the kidney can be exposed completely.

30   Chapter 3/*The Kidney—Structure and Function*

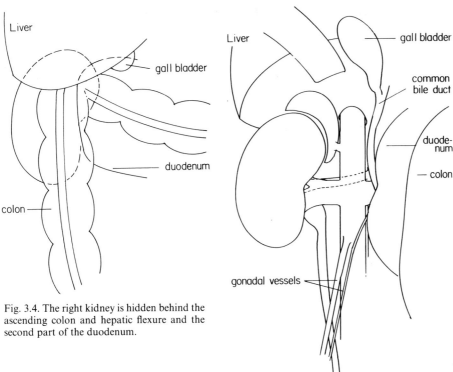

Fig. 3.4. The right kidney is hidden behind the ascending colon and hepatic flexure and the second part of the duodenum.

Fig. 3.5. When the right colon and hepatic flexure are mobilized medially the right kidney is exposed.

the surgical route to the kidney, and to some extent, what complications are likely to occur after an operation on it.

SURGICAL APPROACH TO THE KIDNEY

1. Posterior incisions

A. TWELFTH RIB APPROACH

The majority of operations on the kidney are performed through an incision which passes through the bed of the twelfth rib (which may or may not be resected). The incision thus skirts the pleura (which may be opened) and is carried forward in the gap between the eleventh and twelfth subcostal neuro-vascular bundles, cutting the latissimus dorsi and the external and internal oblique muscles, and splitting the transversus in the line of its fibres (Fig. 3.6).

B. VERTICAL LUMBOTOMY

One may reach the kidney through a more or less vertical incision along the

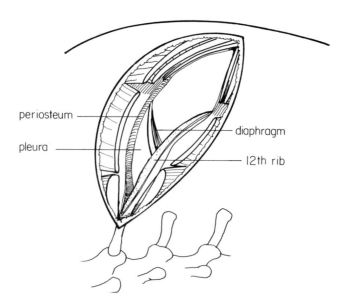

periosteum

pleura

diaphragm

12th rib

Fig. 3.6. Twelfth rib-bed exposure of the right kidney through the periosteum of the rib. Note the close relationship to the pleura.

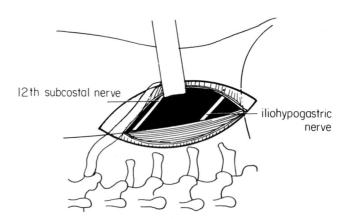

12th subcostal nerve

iliohypogastric nerve

Fig. 3.7. Vertical lumbotomy approach to the right kidney.

lateral border of sacrospinalis, detaching the fascial attachments of the abdominal muscles from the lumbar fascia (Fig. 3.7). This incision is mainly used for small kidneys.

2. Anterior incisions

One may use a transverse incision to approach the kidney in a short, broad person (Fig. 3.8) or in a long, thin one, a long paramedian (Fig. 3.9). The colon and duodenum have to be reflected medially to give access to the renal vessels (Figs 3.10, 3.11). Anterior incisions are mainly used for carcinoma of the kidney.

Chapter 3/*The Kidney—Structure and Function*

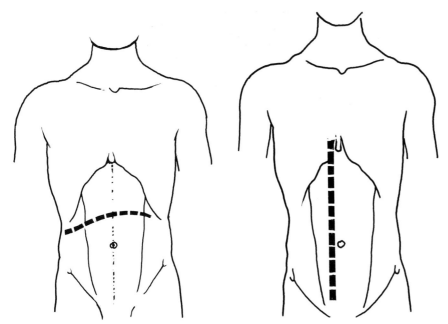

Fig. 3.8. Transverse approach to the right kidney for transabdominal nephrectomy.

Fig. 3.9. Long paramedian approach to right kidney in a long, thin patient.

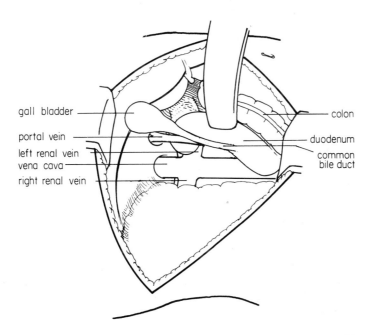

gall bladder

portal vein

left renal vein

vena cava

right renal vein

colon

duodenum

common bile duct

Fig. 3.10. Right kidney displayed through transverse incision after mobilizing the colon and duodenum.

Chapter 3/*The Kidney—Structure and Function*

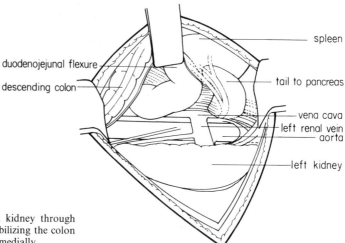

duodenojejunal flexure

descending colon

spleen

tail to pancreas

vena cava

left renal vein

aorta

left kidney

Fig. 3.11. Exposure of left kidney through transverse incision after mobilizing the colon and the tail of the pancreas medially.

Complications

The surgical relations of the kidney explain most of the common postoperative complications; they fall into two main groups: (a) those involving the chest, and (b) those involving the bowel. Because all the posterior incisions give rise afterwards to pain on breathing and coughing, *collapse of the basal segments* of the lung is common. This is made more likely if the pleura has been opened, when there is often a *pneumothorax* that may need to be aspirated or drained with an underwater system. Because most operations involve mobilizing the colon or duodenum to give access to the kidney, and frequently there is some postoperative leakage of urine or blood into the retroperitoneal space, a disturbance of intestinal transport (*paralytic ileus*) is almost inevitable, though usually of brief duration. In days gone by, when operations on the kidney were left to the last moment and when anaesthesia was less expert, accidental injury to the duodenum or colon was a common and much-feared complication of renal surgery.

STRUCTURE OF THE KIDNEY

The renal pyramid

Each kidney is formed of about a dozen *pyramids* (Fig. 3.12) and each pyramid is formed of a bundle of collecting ducts of Bellini arranged like a bunch of flowers (Fig. 3.13): the flowers are the glomeruli and their stems the collecting ducts (Fig. 3.14). The vase is the calix. The collecting ducts open onto the papilla obliquely so that when pressure increases inside the collecting system, they close off as if by a valve action. When papillae are fused to form

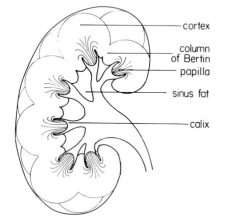

cortex

column of Bertin

papilla

sinus fat

calix

Fig. 3.12. The kidney is formed of a collection of renal pyramids, each draining its collecting ducts into a papilla. Where the pyramids come together they merge into a column of Bertin. A packing of fat separates the pyramids from the calices and pelvis.

Chapter 3/*The Kidney—Structure and Function*

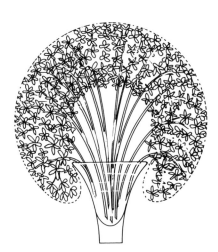

Fig. 3.13. Each pyramid has the structure of a bunch of flowers in a vase: the stems are the ducts of Bellini, the flowers the glomeruli, and the vase the papilla.

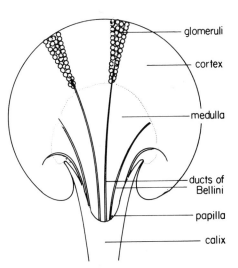

Fig. 3.14. The collection of glomeruli form the 'cortex', the collecting tubes the medulla. The collecting tubes open onto the papilla obliquely so that increased pressure inside the calix will close them by valve action.

'compound' or elongated mounds, many of the collecting ducts open not on the side of the papilla but into a kind of crater on its top, and so are unprovided with protecting valves (Fig. 3.15). In such *compound papillae* an increase of pressure (e.g. in reflux from the bladder) allows infected urine to flow back up the collecting tubes to extravasate and damage the renal parenchyma.

Smaller collecting tubes open into the main ducts of Bellini and these fan out into the renal cortex. Into each of these ducts open myriads of straight connecting segments from the nephrons which are arranged rather like clusters of flowers or corn on the cob (Fig. 3.16).

Each *nephron* consists of a filtering plant and a processing tube. The filtering plant is the glomerulus, the processing system the proximal and distal convoluted tubules and the loop of Henle.

The glomerulus

Each *glomerulus* is made up of a knot of capillaries invaginated inside a hollow sphere—*Bowman's capsule*—out of which leads the proximal tubule (Fig. 3.17). These capillaries are unusually permeable for their endothelial walls are punched with innumerable dimples to increase their porosity. The capillary endothelium rests on a thicker glomerular basement membrane which serves the function of filter paper in the laboratory. Like filter paper, it is supported on a grid which is formed by comb-like feet of the epithelial cells of Bowman's capsule. These cells (Fig. 3.18) resemble little octopuses, whose tentacles

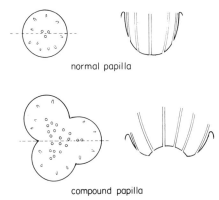

normal papilla

compound papilla

Fig. 3.15. In a normal papilla (above) most of the ducts of Bellini will be closed when the pressure inside the calix is increased, but in a compound papilla (below) those that open into the hollow of the crater, formed where the papillae fuse together, have no protective valves.

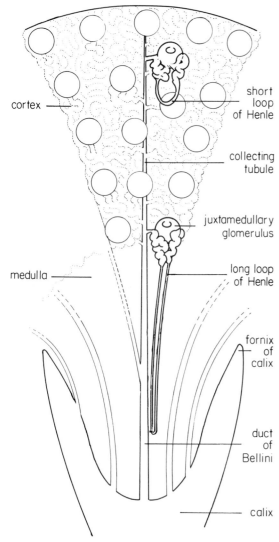

cortex

short loop of Henle

collecting tubule

juxtamedullary glomerulus

medulla

long loop of Henle

fornix of calix

duct of Bellini

calix

Fig. 3.16. The nephrons are arranged on their collecting tubes like corn on the cob. Those nearest to the medulla have long, hairpin loops of Henle.

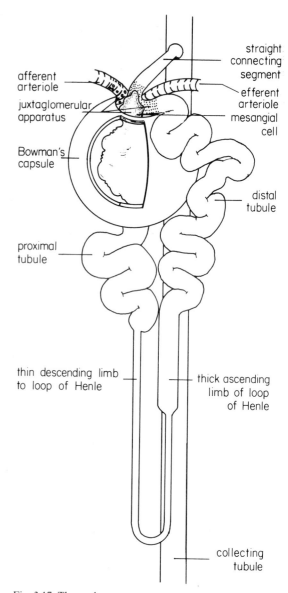

afferent arteriole

juxtaglomerular apparatus

Bowman's capsule

proximal tubule

thin descending limb to loop of Henle

straight connecting segment

efferent arteriole

mesangial cell

distal tubule

thick ascending limb of loop of Henle

collecting tubule

Fig. 3.17. The nephron.

interlock like a zip-fastener. The spaces between the tentacles are the 'slit pores' (Fig. 3.19) and each slit pore is bridged over by a thin 'slit-pore-membrane'. Using peroxidases of known molecular size it is possible to measure the size of the proteins that can pass through these slit pores: protein molecules of 40 000 mol wt can go through, but those of 160 000 mol wt are too big. However, filtration is not merely a matter of the size of the molecule: the proteins that go to make the glomerular basement membrane are negatively charged, and repel

Chapter 3/*The Kidney—Structure and Function*

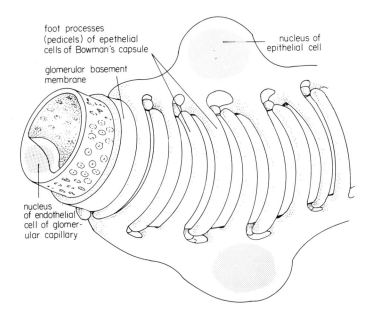

Fig. 3.18. Structure of the glomerular filter.

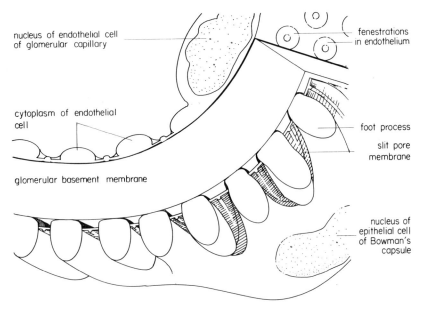

Fig. 3.19. A closer view of the glomerular filter.

protein molecules (e.g. albumen) with the same negative charge, while attracting or accepting positively charged ones.

The glomerular capillaries are enormously permeable, some 50 times more permeable, say, than capillaries elsewhere, e.g. muscle. As a result enormous volumes of fluid pass through the basement membrane every day. It is estimated that the whole body water is thus 'processed' four times over every day, and that the entire plasma volume is filtered every half-hour.

The pressure inside the glomerular capillary is about 60 mm Hg and plasma oncotic pressure about 25 mm Hg, providing a filtration pressure of about 35 mm Hg to push against the pressure inside Bowman's capsule of about 10 mm Hg. The first task in the processing plant is to recapture the excessive and wasteful amount of water that is squeezed out in the glomerulus.

The proximal tubule

Seventy-five per cent of the reabsorption of water from the glomerular filtrate takes place in the proximal convoluted tubule. This is formed of thick active cells with their surface area immeasurably increased by being provided with numerous bristles—the brush border. Along with water, these actively metabolic cells also recover most of the amino acids lost in the glomerular filtrate, as well as glucose and phosphate.

The loop of Henle

The more concentrated filtrate now passes through the loop of Henle which in seven out of eight nephrons is quite short. Only those nephrons lying in the inner part of the kidney have a long loop of Henle and this dips down like a hairpin towards the tip of the renal papilla. The loops of Henle are made up of thin rather functionless-looking cells. This allows osmosis to act on the glomerular filtrate and salt and water to be withdrawn.

The distal tubule

Rising up into the distal convoluted tubule, whose cells are again thick and metabolically active, but without a brush border, sodium is exchanged for potassium and hydrogen in order to regulate the body's acid-base balance. Defects in this distal convoluted tubule may result in an inability for the kidney to form an acid urine—so-called renal tubular acidosis.

Connecting and collecting tubules

Finally the processed and concentrated filtrate reaches the straight connecting tubule and thence flows into the collecting tubule and passes down the papilla to enter the calix. During its passage in the collecting tubule it has once more to run the gauntlet of the concentrated tissue in the renal papilla and more water is reabsorbed, probably under the influence of the antidiuretic hormone in this part of the tubule.

BLOOD SUPPLY OF THE KIDNEY

No surgeon who has ever had to operate on the renal parenchyma can ever forget how rich is its blood-supply. Between them the kidneys receive one-fifth of the entire cardiac output, and an essential preliminary to almost any operation on the kidney is to make sure that one has access to and control of the renal artery.

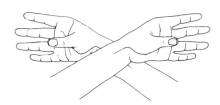

Fig. 3.20. To remember the branches of the renal arteries cross your hands in front of you: the thumbs remind you of the single posterior segmental branch, the four fingers represent the four main arterior segmental arteries.

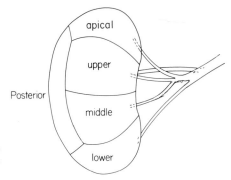

Fig. 3.21. Arrangement of the segments of the kidney, each one is supplied by one of the five main segmental arteries.

Renal arteries

As a rule there is only one *renal artery* on each side, but it is not at all uncommon for one or more of the main branches of the renal artery to take origin independently from the aorta. There are five main branches of each renal artery, arranged like the thumb and fingers of your hand (Fig. 3.20). Each segmental artery supplies its own geographical part of the parenchyma, and there is no anastomosis between them (Figs 3.21, 3.22). Unfortunately there is no neat anatomical correspondence between the segmental arterial territories and the drainage system of collecting tubules and calices. However, when planning an operation that requires cutting into the renal parenchyma, e.g. to remove a stone, one makes one's incision parallel to, and in between, the main segmental vessels. (They can in fact be mapped at the time of operation very easily by using a Doppler probe.)

Entering its proper territory, each segmental artery divides into smaller 'arcuate' arteries, which curve out in the line that divides 'cortex' from 'medulla'. From each arcuate artery spring scores of radially directed branches along the stems of the bunches of collecting tubules that make up each papillary system (Fig. 3.23).

From these radially running branches go individual afferent arteries to each glomerulus. Just before the afferent artery enters the glomerulus it runs close up against the junction of the loop of Henle and the distal convoluted tubule. At this part the cells of the tubule are darkly stained ('macula densa'), and here also some of the muscle cells in the wall of the afferent artery contain conspicuous cytoplasmic granules that are believed to be the precursors of renin. These juxtaglomerular cells and the macula densa of the tubule are together termed the *juxtaglomerular apparatus*. It is believed that if there is a diminution of blood volume or a fall in blood pressure, the juxtaglomerular cells respond by releasing renin. *Renin* is an enzyme that splits one of the plasma proteins to form *Angiotensin I*. Reaching the lung, Angiotensin I is further modified to

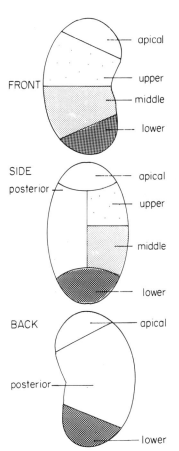

Fig. 3.22. Diagrammatic representation of the five segments of the kidney.

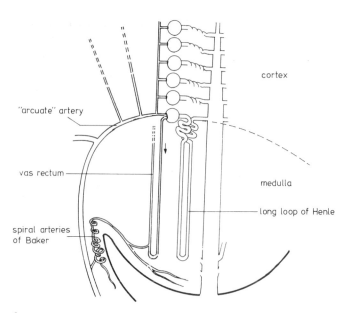

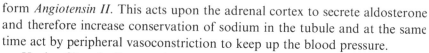

cortex

"arcuate" artery

vas rectum

medulla

long loop of Henle

spiral arteries
of Baker

Fig. 3.23. Blood-supply of the renal papilla.

form *Angiotensin II*. This acts upon the adrenal cortex to secrete aldosterone and therefore increase conservation of sodium in the tubule and at the same time act by peripheral vasoconstriction to keep up the blood pressure.

Having filtered off so much water, the blood leaving the glomerulus in the efferent arteriole is immediately brought into close contact again with the proximal and distal tubules in a second capillary plexus. In the special case of the nephrons lying in the inner part of the kidney, near to the medulla, which have the long, hair-pin loops of Henle, special offshoots from the efferent arterioles accompany these long loops down into the papilla and up again (vasa recta).

Renal veins

Unlike the neatly compartmented system of the renal arteries the veins all communicate together (Fig. 3.24). This has the advantage that one can safely ligate several venous branches without risking infarction of the kidney. Not uncommonly the main left renal vein splits into two before entering the vena cava, one part passing in front of the aorta and the other behind it. This can be dangerous if the operator is unaware of the possibility. On the left side the renal vein is long but on the right it is often right up against the vena cava. For this reason it is usual to use the left kidney for living donor transplantation.

In patients with hypertension suspected of having a renal cause, it is possible to obtain blood from each renal vein and have it measured for renin.

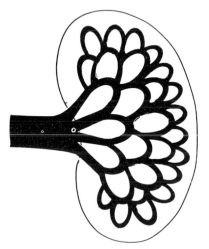

Fig. 3.24. The veins of the kidney are arranged in arcades which communicate freely with each other.

STRUCTURE OF THE COLLECTING SYSTEM

The renal papillae are covered with a thin cubical epithelium perforated by the openings of the ducts of Bellini, but the whole of the rest of the pelvis and calices

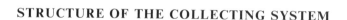

Chapter 3/*The Kidney—Structure and Function*

are lined by transitional epithelium indistinguishable from that which lines the bladder and ureters. The transitional epithelium is surrounded by a strong and supple muscular wall made up of smooth muscle cells that are intimately joined to each other by jig-saw type connections ('nexuses') which allow contraction to pass in waves down the calices and into the renal pelvis so actively pumping urine out of the kidney. This peristaltic activity is relatively slow, compared with that of the bowel, but it is very efficient, and it manages to go on without needing a nerve supply (Fig. 3.25).

To allow the calices to move freely and perform their peristaltic work, they are separated from the parenchyma by a packing of fat (the 'sinus fat') which is fluid at body temperature. In practice this sinus fat also contains the larger veins and arteries of the kidney, but fortunately there is a thin layer of connective tissue between the muscle and the sinus fat, which is easily opened up at surgical operations to provide virtually bloodless access right up to the necks of the calices.

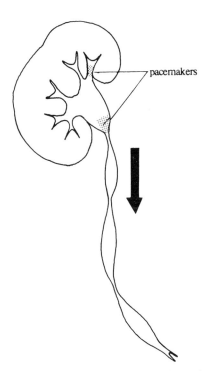

Fig. 3.25. Co-ordinated peristalsis passing discrete compartments full of urine down the ureter.

FURTHER READING

Baker S.B. de C. (1959) The blood supply of the renal papilla. *British Journal of Urology*, **41,** 53.
Graves F.T. (1971) *The Arterial Anatomy of the Kidney*. Wright, Bristol.
Ransley P.G. (1978) Vesicoureteric reflux: continuing surgical dilemma. *Urology*, **12,** 246.
Weiss R.M. (1976) Initiation and organisation of ureteral peristalsis. *Urological Survey*, **26,** 2.

EMBRYOLOGY

In primitive vertebrates there is one set of nephrons for every somite of the body. They fall into three groups. Most cranial of all—the *pronephros*—never appears in man's embryological recapitulation of his family tree. The next set—*the mesonephros*—also disappears. It is only the most caudal set of nephrons—*the metanephros*—that persists and turns into the adult kidney of man today. However their excretory ducts still remember the vanished pronephros and mesonephros of times past (Fig. 4.1).

The excretory duct of the most primitive nephrons of all ran the length of the body—the *Wolffian duct*—but we retain only the part of it belonging to the mesonephros, hence its name—*mesonephric duct*. The duct is important in the subsequent development of the kidney. Occasionally it fails to develop, and then there is no kidney on that side at all—*renal agenesis* (Fig. 4.2).

Not content with its section of the Wolffian duct, the mesonephros does not disappear before it has led to the formation of a second duct, this time called the

Fig. 4.1. Embryological development of the kidney.

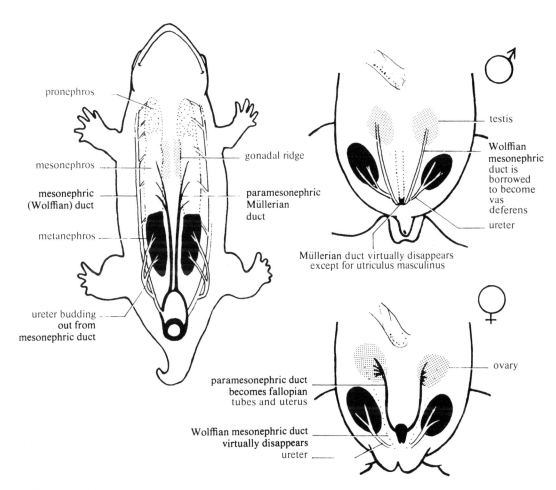

pronephros

mesonephros

mesonephric (Wolffian) duct

metanephros

ureter budding out from mesonephric duct

gonadal ridge

paramesonephric Müllerian duct

testis

Wolffian mesonephric duct is borrowed to become vas deferens

ureter

Müllerian duct virtually disappears except for utriculus masculinus

ovary

paramesonephric duct becomes fallopian tubes and uterus

Wolffian mesonephric duct virtually disappears

ureter

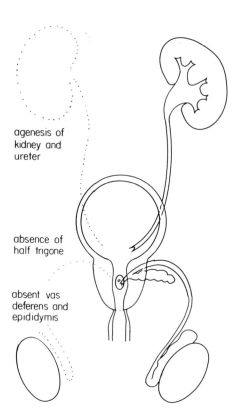

agenesis of
kidney and
ureter

absence of
half trigone

absent vas
deferens and
epididymis

Fig. 4.2. Agenesis of the kidney.

para-mesonephric or *Müllerian duct*. This is of some interest because it is taken over in the females by the gonad to develop into the uterus and the Falloppian tube. In males, all that lingers of the paramesonephric Müllerian duct is the little pit on the verumontanum sometimes called the 'utriculus masculinus' and a tiresome little cyst which occasionally undergoes torsion where it sits on the head of the epididymis.

The most caudal group of nephrons, the metanephros, develops into the adult kidney. A large branch grows towards them out of the mesonephric Wolffian duct and forms the adult ureter. In the female the rest of the mesonephric Wolffian duct is discarded, except for some minute tubules that can only be distinguished in the broad ligament with a strong light. In the male the mesonephric Wolffian duct is adapted to form the vas deferens and seminal vesicle: it therefore not too surprising that from time to time a boy is born whose ureter drains into the seminal vesicle.

Duplex kidney and ureter

The ureter usually begins to branch where it approaches the metanephros. If it divides some distance caudal to the metanephros one may see the adult kidney divided into two hemi-kidneys, usually fused together with a kind of waist. If

Chapter 4/*The Kidney—Congenital Disorders*

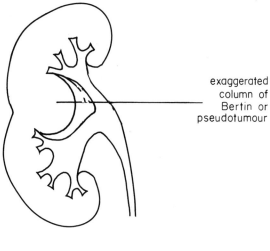

exaggerated
column of
Bertin or
pseudotumour

Fig. 4.3. Pseudotumour of the kidney—a particularly big column of Bertin.

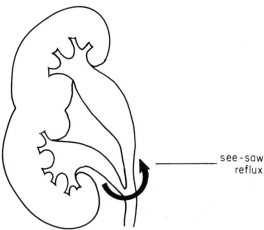

see-saw
reflux

Fig. 4.4. See-saw reflux.

the fusion is almost complete it gives rise to a bulge in the parenchyma that can be mistaken for a soft tissue tumour—it is merely the exaggerated appearance of the fused adjacent columns of Bertin. It is sometimes called a *pseudotumour* (Fig. 4.3).

Usually the upper hemi-kidney has two main calices, the lower one usually has three—but the numbers are variable. The ureters may divide anywhere between the bladder and the kidney. When they join in between, urine may be forced from one ureter up the other—the so-called see-saw reflux. Because the lower hemi-kidney is the bigger one, it usually squeezes the urine up to the upper hemi-kidney (Fig. 4.4).

In the adult with a duplex kidney and ureter, the ureter from the lower half-kidney enters the bladder superior (cephalad) to the ureter from the upper half-kidney (the Weigert–Meyer law). The explanation lies in the embryology of the tail end of the fetus. Just as the tubes connecting the mesonephros to its duct

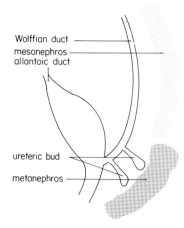

Fig. 4.5. Duplex kidney: two ureteric buds sprout from the Wolffian duct towards the metanephros.

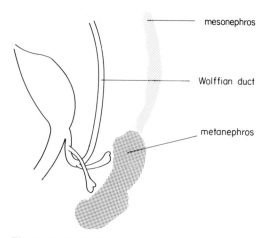

Fig. 4.6. As the Wolffian duct forms its hairpin bend, the ureteric buds are carried with it.

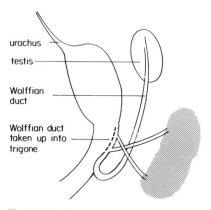

Fig. 4.7. The inner wall of the Wolffian duct is taken up into the developing trigone. The upper part of the Wolffian mesonephric duct is borrowed by the testis.

Fig. 4.8. In the end, the ureter from the upper half of the kidney comes to enter the trigone below that belonging to the lower half, and the entry of the Wolffian duct that is now borrowed to form the vas deferens, is even further caudal.

sprout out from the duct, so the ureter buds out from the Wolffian duct towards the metanephros. It usually postpones branching until it gets near the metanephros, but quite commonly it branches early, or even buds out as two parallel sprouts from the lower end of the Wolffian duct (Fig. 4.5). But with the overgrowth of the tail-end of the fetus, the Wolffian duct forms a loop downwards towards the tail (Fig. 4.6) and carries with it the ureteric buds. This loop becomes quite exaggerated (Fig. 4.7), and now a second change takes place, in that the anterior part of the loop of the Wolffian duct becomes absorbed into, and contributes towards, what is to become the trigone of the adult (Figs 4.7, 4.8). By the time the loop of the Wolffian duct has become taken up entirely into the trigone, the ureter from the upper part of the metanephros finds itself opening into the trigone, caudal to that from the lower half-metanephros, and both ureters come to lie cephalad to the opening of the

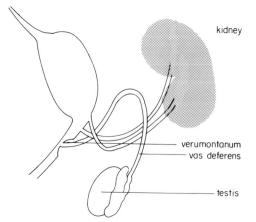

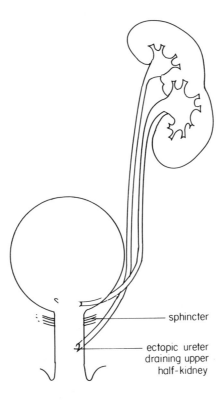

sphincter

ectopic ureter
draining upper
half-kidney

Fig. 4.9. If the more caudally opening ureter is placed downstream of the sphincter it causes incontinence.

Wolffian duct. Since, in the boy, the Wolffian duct gets borrowed to form the vas deferens, it follows that the opening of the vasa through the ejaculatory ducts must be caudal to those of the ureters (Fig. 4.8). In the majority of patients with this anomaly, duplex causes no symptoms and is entirely safe. It is, however, occasionally associated with three important additional complications—ectopic entry of the ureteric orifice, reflux up the ureter, and/or ureterocele. These complications may occur on one or both sides, and singly or together, in any permutation.

1. ECTOPIC URETER

The most caudal ureter draining the upper half-kidney may open well caudal to the sphincter, and in girls, into the vagina, and so urine constantly dribbles from the ectopic ureteric orifice and they are wet, day and night (Fig. 4.9).

2. REFLUX

Because the upper ureteric orifice draining the lower hemi-kidney has a relatively short course through the muscle of the bladder wall (Fig. 4.10) it has a less effective flap-valve, and reflux of urine may occur from bladder to kidney (Fig. 4.11). (Reflux may, one must note, also take place up the ectopic or lower ureteric orifice.)

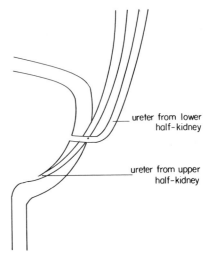

ureter from lower
half-kidney

ureter from upper
half-kidney

Fig. 4.10. The ureter draining the lower half-kidney may have such a short tunnel through the bladder that it has no protective valve and permits reflux of urine from the bladder to the lower half-kidney.

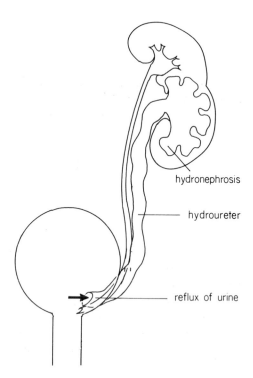

hydronephrosis

hydroureter

reflux of urine

Fig. 4.11. Reflux giving rise to hydronephrosis in the lower half-kidney.

3. URETEROCELE

When the inner part of the Wolffian duct is incompletely absorbed into the trigone it may form a kind of balloon where the ureter enters the trigone. This most often occurs at the lowermost ureteric orifice in duplex (Fig. 4.12) and if it is found in an ectopic ureter, may pout down through the external urinary meatus in a girl as a pale translucent 'cyst' (Fig. 4.13).

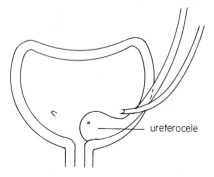

ureterocele

Fig. 4.12. The upper half-kidney draining into the lower of the two ureteric orifices may open into a ureterocele where the inner wall of the Wolffian duct has not been completely absorbed.

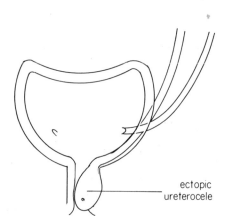

ectopic ureterocele

Fig. 4.13. The ureterocele may occur in an ectopic ureter, and so present as a 'cyst' near the external meatus in a girl.

Errors of position of the kidney

ROTATED KIDNEY

It is not at all unusual to see a kidney which faces forwards instead of sideways. In such a case the outline is that of an ellipse and some of the calices point medially. The condition is of no consequence, but it presents an unusual radiographic appearance that may deceive the unwary (Fig. 4.14).

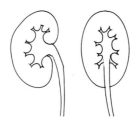

Fig. 4.14. Diagram of a rotated kidney: note the medially pointing calices.

Fusion of the kidneys

HORSESHOE KIDNEY

Sometimes both kidneys are rotated, and their lower poles fused together in front of the aorta. This is called a horseshoe kidney. It is important because it offers an obstacle in surgery of the aorta, the isthmus joining the two kidneys having to be divided in order to get at the aorta (Fig. 4.15).

Horseshoe kidneys are often found in association with other congenital anomalies of the urinary tract such as ureterocele and reflux, and they also occur in association with congenital narrowing at the pelvi–ureteric junction leading to hydronephrosis. The isthmus joining the two parts of the horseshoe has nothing whatever to do with the hydronephrosis. Horseshoe kidney is quite often detected by accident when the abdomen is palpated in a lean patient. Unless there is some associated pathology, it does not require any surgical intervention.

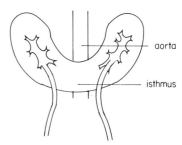

Fig. 4.15. Two rotated kidneys may fuse together in the midline in front of the aorta to form a 'horseshoe kidney'.

CROSSED RENAL ECTOPIA

Instead of the two kidneys being joined in the midline as in the horseshoe kidney, here one kidney is stuck to the other on the opposite side. The ureters arise in the proper way from the right place in the trigone. As in the horseshoe kidneys, it is thought that the two metanephroi have fused when they were in the pelvis of the fetus, and the one drags the other up as it rises in the course of the development of the hind part of the fetus. Again, on its own, it is of no consequence, but it often is associated with other congenital oddities needing treatment such as hydronephrosis or reflux (Fig. 4.16).

PELVIC KIDNEY

These represent persistent failure of the metanephros to rise up in the fetal body. The kidney remains in the pelvis. One would expect it to get in the way of the baby during childbirth, but it hardly ever does. Perhaps these kidneys are more likely to get infected than normal ones. The real hazard is that they may be encountered in the course of an operation and not be recognized. Since these pelvic kidneys have to have their proper number of five segmental arteries, and

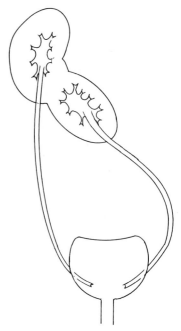

Fig. 4.16. Crossed renal ectopia. Note that the ureter enters the trigone in the right place but the metanephros has crossed over to become stuck to the other side.

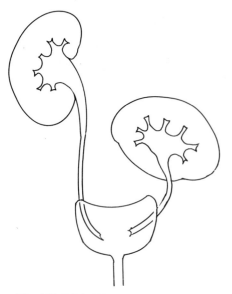

since these are supplied from the aorta, common, external and internal iliac arteries in a most astonishing and confusing pattern, the unwary surgeon who finds one of these lumps at operation and does not recognize it, is in for a sanguinary operation if he tries to remove it. Usually they need no treatment at all (Fig. 4.17).

THORACIC KIDNEY

This is not a proper error of development of the kidney at all. If a baby is born with a congenital failure of development of the diaphragm, one kidney may find itself in the chest within a hernia along with other viscera and such a 'thoracic kidney' is detected in a routine chest radiograph. The kidney is not really in the thorax—it is separated by the thin layer of diaphragm and pleura. Again, it does not need to be meddled with, but can be occasionally mistaken for a tumour in the lung and so give rise to trouble and an (unnecessary) operation (Fig. 4.18).

Fig. 4.17. Pelvic kidney. Lying in front of the sacrum the contrast in the IVU may easily be overlooked.

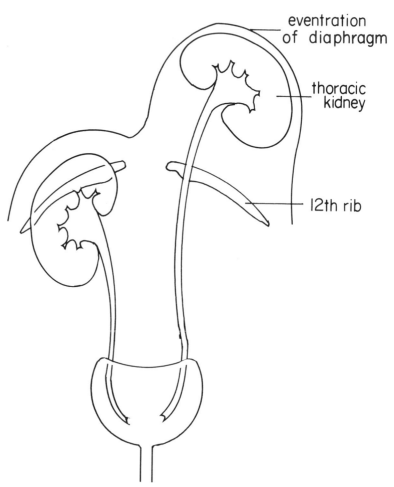

Fig. 4.18. When the diaphragm fails to develop properly the kidney, along with other viscera, may be displaced into the thorax.

Chapter 4/*The Kidney—Congenital Disorders*

Errors of development of the kidney

If the mesonephric Wolffian duct fails to develop at all, then there can be no trigone, no ureter, and no kidney induced in the metanephros by the ureteric bud. This is called *agenesis*. As one might expect, there is usually no seminal vesicle or vas deferens on that side in the male (Fig. 4.19).

If the ureteric bud has begun to develop, but something goes wrong with it, then nephrons may not be properly caused to form in the metanephros. There may be a trigone and a ureteric orifice, but the ureter is likely to be very thin and irregular, and it may end in a minute nubbin of tissue that may or may not contain a few poorly-formed glomeruli and often contains other odd-looking tissue including cartilage, tubules like those in the epididymis and so on. If one cannot identify any real kidney-like tissue the condition is named *aplasia* (Fig. 4.20); if it seems like a kidney here and there, it is called *dysplasia* (Fig. 4.21). In dysplastic kidneys one often sees little cysts where the nephrons form urine but it cannot get out down the poorly-formed ureter. *Hypoplasia* is a term you should avoid: it implies that the kidney is small but otherwise normal. Such a condition is very rare—there is usually something wrong with a very small kidney, either it is dysplastic or it is scarred from acquired disease.

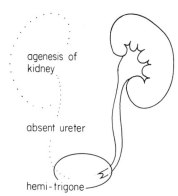

Fig. 4.19. Agenesis.

CYSTIC DISORDERS OF THE KIDNEY

Not all these are of congenital origin, but this is a good place to consider them. They are very common, and they can arise in one of three ways—from *dilatation* of the collecting tubules (of unknown cause) seen in medullary sponge kidney, from *obstruction* of the collecting tubules (of various causes), and from *diverticula* pouching out from the collecting tubules. Some of these are seen in new-born infants, others occur as the kidneys grow older.

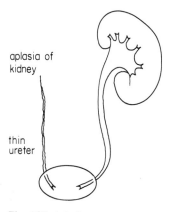

Fig. 4.20. Aplasia.

Medullary sponge kidney (Fig. 4.22)

In this condition either part or the entire kidney may be affected, and it may be unilateral or bilateral. It is usually only noticed in young adults, and then gradually gets worse. Nobody knows why it happens. It is sometimes familial, and it is associated with hemihypertrophy (lop-sidedness, where people have one arm or leg bigger than the other). In the kidney the trouble lies in the collecting tubules which become large and dilated: there is stasis of the urine in them, and sooner or later little stones form in the stagnant urine. Along with the stones they often become infected. In time the affected parts of the kidneys, or the entire kidney itself, becomes swollen, the swelling being formed by the medulla, which on cut section looked like a sponge filled with bits of grit—hence the term medullary sponge kidney. The radiographic appearance is typical. If the patient is lucky, and the disorder limited to one part of the kidney, this can be removed by partial nephrectomy and the patient saved the misery of

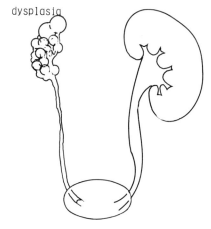

Fig. 4.21 Dysplasia.

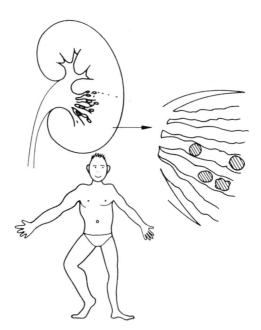

Fig. 4.22. Medullary sponge kidney. Congenital 'ectasis' of the collecting tubules which lead to stone formation and eventually to renal failure. This is associated with unilateral hemihypertrophy of the limbs—so ask about odd sizes of shoes and gloves!

repeated episodes of passage of stones down the ureter—a painful business. Infection and scarring in the tubules upstream of the big floppy tubules in the medulla gives rise to failure of acidification and concentrating power.

Obstruction cysts

If the metanephros has developed, and then something goes wrong with the ureter in fetal life so that it becomes narrowed and dysplastic, urine is secreted by the metanephros and cannot get out. The tubules and nephrons are

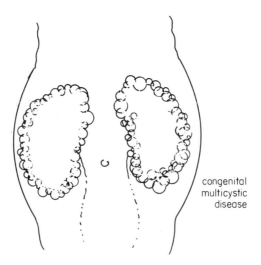

congenital multicystic disease

Fig. 4.23. Congenital multicystic disease. The ureters are blocked or absent. There is hydramnios and the condition is incompatible with survival.

Chapter 4/*The Kidney—Congenital Disorders*

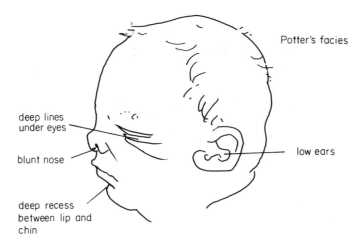

Fig. 4.24. Potter's facies, from lack of amniotic fluid.

distended and the kidney on that side becomes more or less full of cysts. Seen on one side, this is included in the general category of dysplastic kidneys, but when it is found on both sides, the baby is born with giant *congenital multicystic kidneys* resembling bunches of tiny grapes (Fig. 4.23). The condition is incompatible with life, and just as well. The babies nearly always have ugly squashed-flat faces (for there is no amniotic fluid) (Fig. 4.24) and have other congenital anomalies such as congenital holes in the heart.

Occasionally the *calix* alone is obstructed: there may be a congenital narrowing of the neck of the calix, or perhaps the neck may become narrowed from scarring caused by undetected previous inflammation. The calix is distended, and gives rise to infection or calculi (Fig. 4.25).

In *pyelonephritic scarring* of the kidney, the collecting tubules may become obliterated, and upstream the nephron is distended with fluid. As a rule this distension is not obvious to the naked eye, but appears in the microscopical section as the 'thyroid like' areas so characteristic of pyelonephritis. However, one occasionally sees quite large collections of cysts in small contracted scarred kidneys that are plainly caused by obstruction from the inflammatory disease (Fig. 4.26).

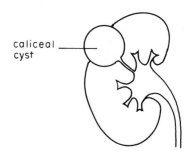

Fig. 4.25. Caliceal cyst.

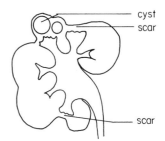

Fig. 4.26. Cysts formed as a result of obstruction to calices or collecting ducts by inflammatory scarring.

Diverticula of the collecting tubules

As the kidney grows older, it is not at all uncommon for one or two diverticula to grow out of the collecting tubules and give rise to cysts in the kidney. These may be solitary or multiple, and they may occur in one or both kidneys. Small renal cysts of this kind are nearly always found at post mortem in elderly people. In the course of an investigation for haematuria, it is again not at all uncommon to discover such simple cysts' (Fig. 4.27), and when they are large, they may pose a difficult diagnostic problem to distinguish them from renal cell carcinomas. Today, the diagnosis is usually settled by means of an ultrasound examination which shows no echoes in the fluid filled cyst, and confirmed by

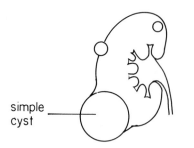

simple cyst

Fig. 4.27. Simple cysts—small ones are normal.

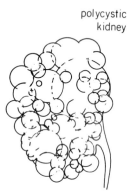

polycystic kidney

Fig. 4.28. Polycystic disease.

needle-aspiration of the clear fluid within it. If an angiogram is performed it will show a clear cavity without any vessels in it. The fluid within a cyst has a characteristic appearance in the CAT scan.

POLYCYSTIC DISEASE

Polycystic disease of the kidneys is a bizarre exaggeration of this process. The disease is inherited by a mendelian dominant gene which declares itself at different ages. Usually the process is detected in adult life, when it is noted as a lump on routine abdominal examination, or because the patient has developed haematuria, urinary infection, or hypertension. Instead of there being only one or two cysts, the kidney is riddled with them—usually on both sides (Fig. 4.28). There may be associated cysts in the liver and pancreas and in the cerebral vessels there are small berry aneurysms of the circle of Willis, which give rise to subarachnoid haemorrhage. One must always bear this association in mind when contemplating the removal of cadaver kidneys from a young patient who has died from such a cerebral haemorrhage.

Polycystic disease of the kidneys is important, because these patients slowly develop renal failure. Their progress is gradual, and they make a very rewarding group for conservative therapy. If their blood pressure is controlled, their urinary infection treated, and as uraemia unfolds, their protein intake is limited, it may be many years before they need dialysis or transplantation. In former times it was the custom to pop these cysts at open operation—so called Rovsing's operation. It has been shown repeatedly that this only makes the renal function worse, and the operation is now reserved for those rare cases in whom one or more cysts are kinking and obstructing the ureter or the renal calices. Infection occasionally takes place inside cysts. The diagnosis is usually obvious in the urogram, and can be simply confirmed with ultrasound scanning.

CONGENITAL DISORDERS OF FUNCTION OF THE RENAL TUBULES

Proximal tubular disorders

1. AMINO ACID TRANSPORT DEFECTS

As a rule there is a deficiency in the enzyme system transporting the amino acids back through the proximal tubule as well as in absorbing them in the bowel. Of these the most important is *cystinuria* (Fig. 4.29). Here there is a defect in the transport of four amino acids—'COAL'—cystine, ornithine, arginine and lysine. The disorder is inherited as a Mendelian autosomal recessive. About 3% of patients are homozygous. Unfortunately cystine is very poorly soluble in urine: heterozygous patients may lose as much as 500 mg/24 hours in their

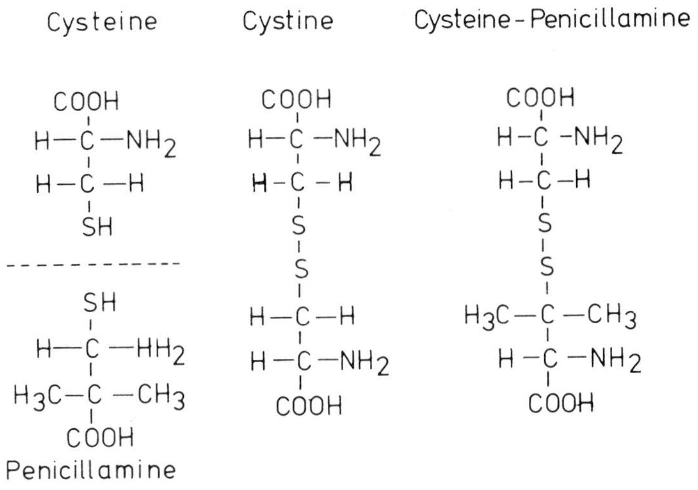

Cysteine Cystine Cysteine-Penicillamine

$$
\begin{array}{ccc}
\text{COOH} & \text{COOH} & \text{COOH} \\
\text{H}-\overset{|}{\text{C}}-\text{NH}_2 & \text{H}-\overset{|}{\text{C}}-\text{NH}_2 & \text{H}-\overset{|}{\text{C}}-\text{NH}_2 \\
\text{H}-\overset{|}{\text{C}}-\text{H} & \text{H}-\overset{|}{\text{C}}-\text{H} & \text{H}-\overset{|}{\text{C}}-\text{H} \\
\text{SH} & \text{S} & \text{S} \\
\text{- - - - - - -} & \text{S} & \text{S} \\
\text{SH} & \text{H}-\overset{|}{\text{C}}-\text{H} & \text{H}_3\text{C}-\overset{|}{\text{C}}-\text{CH}_3 \\
\text{H}-\overset{|}{\text{C}}-\text{HH}_2 & \text{H}-\overset{|}{\text{C}}-\text{NH}_2 & \text{H}-\overset{|}{\text{C}}-\text{NH}_2 \\
\text{H}_3\text{C}-\overset{|}{\text{C}}-\text{CH}_3 & \text{COOH} & \text{COOH} \\
\text{COOH} & &
\end{array}
$$

Penicillamine

Fig. 4.29. The relationship between cystine, cysteine and penicillamine.

urine, and homozygous patients more than 1 g. The homozygous patient is virtually bound to have urine that is supersaturated for cystine. The stones are radiodense, owing to their content of sulphur. By giving penicillamine (Fig. 4.29) the constituent cysteine halves of cystine are linked to penicillamine as a soluble molecule.

In *Hartnup disease* there is a transport defect involving tryptophane but the major burden of the illness does not concern the renal tubule, but follows from failure of uptake of tryptophane from the bowel. This results in nicotinamide deficiency which in turn leads to pellagra and cerebellar ataxia. In *Fanconi's syndrome* there is a complex failure of absorption of a cluster of amino acids along with failure to absorb phosphate, proteinuria and acidosis. Here microdissection reveals deformed proximal tubules.

2. RENAL GLYCOSURIA

Here the tubules fail to reabsorb glucose and it is found in the urine even when the blood sugar is normal: it needs to be distinguished from diabetes. It is harmless.

3. PHOSPHATURIA

Here the tubules fail to reabsorb phosphate from the glomerular filtrate. This results in so-called vitamin D resistant rickets.

Distal tubular disorders

A. RENAL TUBULAR ACIDOSIS

When the distal tubule is unable to pump out hydrogen ions the kidney cannot form an acid urine, and instead loses potassium, phosphate sulphate and organic acids. There is a metabolic acidosis with a low plasma bicarbonate. The acidosis leads to an increase in the amount of calcium not bound to protein, and so more calcium escapes in the glomerular filtrate, where, in presence of an alkaline urine, it tends to be precipitated in the tubules. This gives rise to speckled calcification in the renal medulla—one variant of 'nephrocalcinosis'. In these patients the glomerular function is good. The loss of calcium and phosphate may lead to osteomalacia. Such kidneys fail to make an acid urine when the patient is given an acid load. It may be remedied by giving the patient bicarbonate, potassium citrate, and perhaps, additional vitamin D.

B. NEPHROGENIC DIABETES INSIPIDUS

A sex-linked Mendelian recessive gene confined to males may cause their collecting tubules to fail to respond to anti-diuretic hormone. Profuse diuresis may lead to dehydration which may cause brain damage in the baby. A comparable condition may be acquired in hydronephrosis, obstructive atrophy, and pyelonephritic scarring.

FURTHER READING

Baert L. & Steg A. (1977) On the pathogenesis of simple renal cysts in the adult—a microdissection study. *Urological Research*, **5**, 103.

Crelin E.S. (1978) Normal and abnormal development of the ureter. *Urology*, **12**, 2.

Johnston J.H. (1976) Congenital anomalies of the calices, pelvis and ureter. In J.P. Blandy (ed.), *Urology*, p. 521. Blackwell Scientific Publications, Oxford.

Feldman A.E., Pollack H.M., Perri A.J., Karafin L. & Kendall A.R. (1978) Renal pseudotumors: an anatomic–radiologic classification. *Journal of Urology*, **120**, 133.

Mackie G.C. & Stephens F.D. (1975) Duplex kidneys: a correlation of renal dysplasia with position of the ureteral orifice. *Journal of Urology*, **114**, 274.

Pitts W.R. & Muecke E.C. (1975) Horseshoe kidneys: a 40 year experience. *Journal of Urology*, **113**, 743.

Potter E.L. (1973) *Normal and Abnormal Development of the Kidney*. Lloyd-Luke Medical Books, London.

Ransley P.G. (1976) The renal papilla and intrarenal reflux. In D.I. Williams & G.D. Chisholm (eds), *Scientific Foundations of Urology*, p. 79. Heinemann, London.

Spence H.M. & Singleton R. (1971) What is sponge kidney and where does it fit in the spectrum of cystic disorders? *Transactions of the American Association of Genitourinary Surgeons*, **63**, 37.

PENETRATING INJURIES

Penetrating injuries of the kidney may be caused by bullet or knife wounds. Low velocity bullet wounds will call for abdominal exploration and conservative management of the injury to the kidney and the other viscera injured in the track of the missile. High velocity injuries from modern weapons give rise to a huge cavity inside which everything is destroyed, and around which most of the tissues will be rendered devitalized. Military surgeons finding the kidney damaged in such lesions usually advise nephrectomy for fear of risking a fatal secondary haemorrhage a few days later.

CLOSED INJURIES

More common in civilian practice are the closed injuries of the kidney which result from accidental falls at work, or injuries received in sport. The cause of the renal injury often causes fracture of the lower ribs and may also shear off one or more of the tips of the transverse processes of the lumbar vertebrae (Fig. 5.1). To cause these bony injuries the initial blow must be very severe, and the pain and soft tissue contusion may be considerable.

One may distinguish three grades of renal injury: (a) where the parenchyma is split, giving rise to haematuria and surrounding haematoma, but usually self limiting, and followed by normal restoration of kidney anatomy and function (Fig. 5.2); (b) where the kidney is split into several fragments and continues to bleed; and (c) where there is a tear of the main renal artery or vein.

Management

The patient will give a history of having suffered a kick or an injury to the loin.

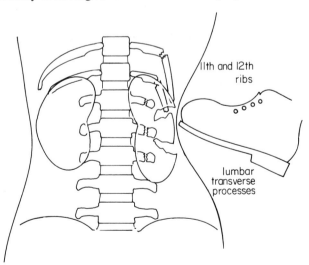

11th and 12th ribs

lumbar transverse processes

Fig. 5.1. Closed injury that damages the kidney often causes fracture of the lower ribs and lumbar transverse processes.

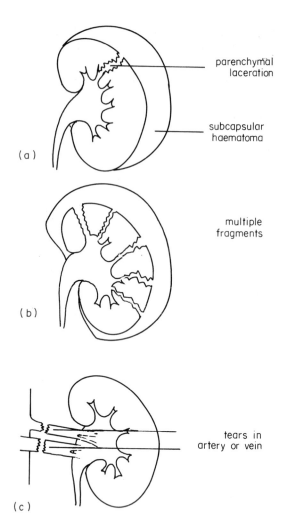

parenchymal
laceration

subcapsular
haematoma

(a)

multiple
fragments

(b)

tears in
artery or vein

(c)

Fig. 5.2. Three grades of renal injury: (a) laceration of the parenchyma with subcapsular haematoma; (b) fragmentation of the kidney; (c) tear of the renal artery or vein or both.

He may have other injuries, in particular those involving the ribs and these may be more important because of the risk of pneumothorax, or the spleen and/or liver, because of the associated internal haemorrhage. The most common symptom however is for the patient to notice blood in his urine soon after his injury.

At this stage there may be no physical signs other than vague tenderness in the loin, but every patient must be admitted for observation, because there is no means of telling (at this stage) how the injury to the kidney is going to develop.

On admission the patient is fully examined, with special regard to the chest. A chest X-ray is obtained, and an *emergency intravenous urogram* whatever the hour of day or night. The urogram is performed to make sure that there is another kidney on the other side. The patient is then kept under close observation: his pulse and blood pressure are measured at regular intervals, and every specimen of urine he passes is saved for comparison with the next.

One expects most of these patients to get steadily better: the colour of the blood in the urine gradually becomes more pale and less freshly pink. The vital signs stay stable.

The patient is frequently re-examined to note the pulse and blood pressure, and to watch for evidence of increasing dullness or a swelling in the loin, as well as for any sign of other intra or extra-peritoneal bleeding.

A *renal angiogram* should be obtained, as an emergency, when anything occurs that does not follow this normal tendency for the patient to stop bleeding and get better. If there is no excretion in the IVU an angiogram may reveal damage to the renal artery that might just be repaired in time if exploration is carried out immediately. If the falling blood pressure, rising pulse rate, or increasing swelling in the loin suggest continuing internal bleeding, an angiogram will give a good picture of the exact anatomy of the ruptured kidney, and help the surgeon plan his operative approach.

Nowadays the angiogram may actually show where the blood is issuing from a damaged segmental artery, and using gelfoam or minced muscle, the damaged vessel may be embolized from within, thus saving the patient an hazardous operation (Fig. 5.3).

In the patient who is getting steadily better, even though the urogram done as an emergency at the time of admission looks very strange, there is no need to interfere and no indication for an angiogram.

In the patient who needs to be explored the kidney is approached by the anterior transperitoneal route, so that the renal vessels can be secured before Gerota's fascia is opened. It has been found that in many patients Gerota's fascia will limit the haematoma and control loss of blood, but if opened early, one may be obliged to perform a nephrectomy in order to stop the haemorrhage. Once the renal vessels are controlled it may be possible to suture lacerated arteries and veins, repair lacerated renal parenchyma, or remove detached fragments of one or other pole.

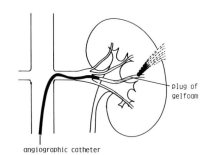

Fig. 5.3. Continuing haemorrhage from a torn segmental artery may be stopped by injecting the vessel with gelfoam or minced muscle under angiographic control.

Follow up

Five important complications (Figs 5.4, 5.5) have to be considered:

1. SECONDARY HAEMORRHAGE

Following any laceration of renal parenchyma there is a possibility that the clot sticking the pieces of kidney together may undergo lysis and permit bleeding to start again. For this reason in severe renal injuries it is usual to keep the patient in hospital and under observation for at least ten days.

2. LATE HYPERTENSION FROM RENAL ARTERY STENOSIS

The blood pressure should be monitored at regular intervals during the first few weeks after closed renal injury. Damage to the renal artery may be succeeded by

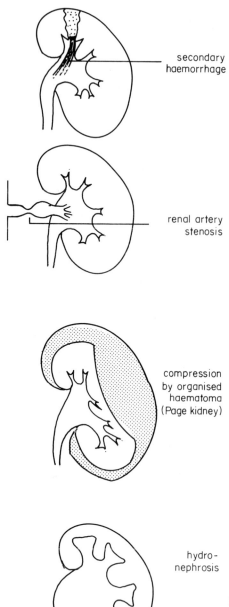

secondary
haemorrhage

renal artery
stenosis

compression
by organised
haematoma
(Page kidney)

hydro-
nephrosis

Fig. 5.4. Delayed complications of closed renal trauma—secondary haemorrhage, renal artery stenosis and compression by organized haematoma giving rise to hypertension and hydronephrosis.

Chapter 5/*The Kidney—Trauma*

hypertension, and is dramatically relieved by treating the narrow segment of artery.

3. HYPERTENSION FROM ORGANIZED HAEMATOMA AROUND THE KIDNEY (PAGE'S KIDNEY)

Occasionally haematoma forms a thick, tough rind around the kidney that compresses it and makes it ischaemic. This can be a remediable if unusual cause of hypertension.

4. HYDRONEPHROSIS

There seem to be a few well documented examples where hydronephrosis from injury to the renal pelvis or ureter was detected weeks or months after the accident. Far more often the hydronephrosis was present before the injury, and many surgeons believe that the hydronephrotic kidney is more prone to damage from closed trauma owing to its size, shape, and thin cortex.

5. PSEUDOCYST

A split in the renal pelvis may lead to loss of urine into the tissues around the kidney. Very occasionally this forms a 'urinoma' (Fig. 5.5) which may become infected and turn into an abscess that needs to be drained. Even more rarely, it forms a large cavity, communicating with the renal pelvis, lined by urothelium (and sometimes calcified), that must be carefully dissected out if it is to be cured.

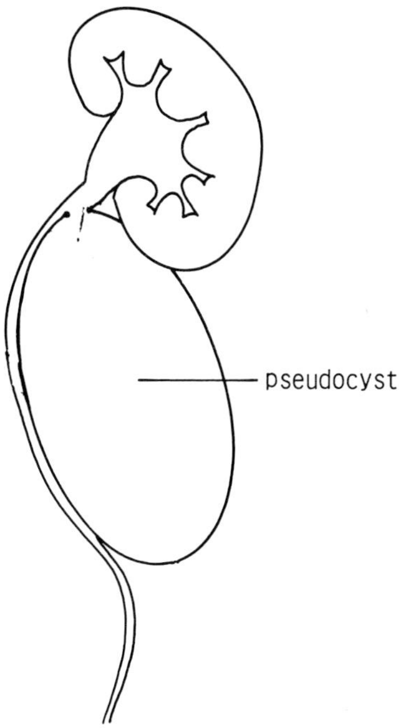

Fig. 5.5. Organization of granulation tissue around an extrarenal collection of urine—urinoma—leading to a pseudocyst.

FURTHER READING

Angorn I.B. (1977) Segmental dearteralization in penetrating renal trauma. *British Journal of Surgery*, **64**, 59.

Cocket A.T.K., Frank I.N., Davis R.S. & Linke C.A. (1975) Recent advances in the diagnosis and management of blunt renal trauma. *Journal of Urology*, **113**, 750.

Conrad M.R., Freedman M., Weiner C., Freeman C. & Sanders R.S. (1976) Sonography of the Page kidney. *Journal of Urology*, **116**, 293.

Pryor J.P. & Williams J.P. (1975) A study of 137 cases of renal trauma. *British Journal of Urology*, **47**, 45.

Selikowitz S.M. (1977) Penetrating high-velocity genitourinary injuries. *Urology*, **9**, 371.

Whitney R.F. & Peterson N.E. (1976) Penetrating renal injuries. *Urology*, **7**, 7.

Chapter 6
The Kidney—
Glomerulonephritis

Although by tradition the diseases to be described in this chapter are called *glomerulonephritis*, because the distinctive features of the inflammation are to be found in the glomerulus, it is probable that the entire nephron is also involved to some extent. The study of these disorders has become very complex, and advances are being made very rapidly, so that any account must necessarily be oversimplified. At the heart of the matter would seem to be a disorder of the immunological response of the patient. Again, at the cost of oversimplification, we can distinguish three elements in the pathology of these disorders: (a) a largely unknown process that causes hardly any detectable anatomical change in the glomerulus, but leads to an alteration in its permeability, and is possibly mediated by lymphocytes; (b) soluble complex disease—where the exact anatomical site of damage in the glomerulus depends upon the size of the complex; and (c) subsequent changes caused by the inflammatory response consequent upon fixation of complement by the soluble antigen–antibody complexes, and its aftermath, namely, scarring.

To keep the subject clear, it is also necessary to draw a distinction between the microscopical and electron-microscopical changes that are found in kidney biopsy material, and the clinical picture which depends upon the nature and extent of the damage done to the glomeruli.

CAUSES OF GLOMERULONEPHRITIS

Given the right circumstances almost any substance can act as an antigen, either alone or as a hapten in combination with peptides. In human glomerulonephritis antigens have included viruses and bacteria (especially Type A beta-haemolytic *streptococcus*), *Treponema pallidum*, and staphylococci. On a world-wide scale, perhaps the most common aetological agent must surely be *Plasmodium malariae*—cause of the dreaded 'blackwater fever', and the flatworm *Schistosoma mansoni* may cause it too. The list of drugs that have been incriminated is endless and ever-growing: it includes tridione, penicillamine, and butazolidine. In systemic lupus the patient's own DNA can act as the allergen.

Glomerulonephritis—the role of soluble complexes

In the healthy patient with enough antibodies the immune defences of the body respond to an unwanted antigen by smothering it with antibodies to form large insoluble complexes that are cleared away and dealt with by the reticuloendothelial system. If these large complexes appear in the kidney at all, they are soon got rid of; any illness that they give rise to is of brief duration and (usually) carries a good prognosis. Large complexes of this kind usually get stuck in the bigger capillaries of the mesangium rather than the smaller ones in the glomerular tuft.

In patients with a deficiency in their immune defence system there is not enough antibody to smother up the antigen so completely, and smaller *soluble complexes* are formed. Again, the larger of these tend to get stuck in the mesangium, but the smaller ones are held up in the glomerular filter. Some penetrate the basement membrane, but are trapped under and between the slit pores of the foot processes of the epithelial cells. Others only get as far as the space between the perforated and permeable glomerular capillary wall and the basement membrane.

As in any other inflammatory reaction, soluble complexes attract *complement*. It will be remembered that there are at least 11 different enzymes in the complement system. When the first of these (C1) is stuck to an antigen–immunoglobulin complex, a cascade of other complement factors are activated. These drill holes in cell membranes and result in their lysis, release histamine from leukocytes, mast cells, and platelets, and in turn the histamine dilates blood vessels and makes them more permeable. Other members of the complement system attract leukocytes.

Clearly the more complement fixation that occurs when these complexes are held up in the glomerular filter, the worse the structural damage that will take place, and the worse the long-term outlook.

TERMINOLOGY AND CLASSIFICATION OF GLOMERULONEPHRITIS

It is very easy to become confused and bewildered by the large number of terms that are used to describe the variations that are seen in this disease in its different degrees of severity and under different conditions. Recognizable histological and ultramicroscopical lesions may be *diffuse* or *focal* (according to whether they are only found here and there, or uniformly throughout the kidney). The changes may be found mainly in the glomerular *capillary* tuft or in the slightly larger capillaries of the *mesangium*. Sometimes there is very obvious extra *proliferation* of cells, sometimes in the capillary tuft, sometimes in the mesangium. In other varieties the principal change consists of a thickening of the wall of the capillary membrane—*membranous* glomerulonephritis—without very marked proliferation of cells. Finally, when there has been a tremendous amount of loss of protein through the damaged glomerular filter, the space of Bowman's capsule gets filled up by proliferation of its endothelial cells, together with macrophages from elsewhere. They form 'epithelial crescents' that actually block up the urine space—this is sometimes referred to as *extracapillary proliferative* glomerulonephritis.

Whether the glomerulonephritis is diffuse or focal seems in all probability to be a matter of the severity of the disease: focal lesions are in general less dangerous and carry a better prognosis.

Whether the membrane is affected primarily, or whether there is cellular proliferation, probably depends on how much complement has been fixed and how much inflammatory change has been added to the underlying clogging-up of soluble complex in the filter.

Where the soluble complexes fetch up, i.e. in the mesangium or the capillaries of the glomerular tuft, probably depends upon their size. With these variables, it is not surprising that the individual renal biopsy may show variations from one glomerulus to another, or that the observer interpretation of the electron and light microscope preparation is open to subjective variation.

In spite of all the variables certain histological patterns appear again and again and have been given an agreed terminology. It should be pointed out however that none of them signifies that any particular antigen is the culprit, and that (almost) any of the possible causative agents under the right circumstances can give rise to (almost) any of the following pictures.

Minimal change disease

Here light microscopy reveals nothing wrong with the glomerulus, and we still do not know what causes it. The most striking feature is an alteration in the permeability of the basement membrane (Fig. 6.1) which is thought to be due to an alteration in its negative charge, which permits albumen to escape, but retains other plasma proteins. Even with the magnification afforded by the electron microscope one cannot detect any abnormality in the glomerular basement membrane. However the supporting grid formed by the foot-processes of the epithelial cells of Bowman's capsule are sometimes seen to be fused together possibly as a response to the outpouring of plasma albumen.

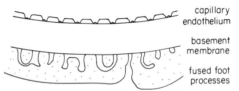

Fig. 6.1. Minimal change disease. There is an increase in the permeability of the basement membrane, probably through an alteration in its electrical charge. In response to the loss of protein, the epithelial foot-processes become fused together.

Although the exact nature of the immunological disorder that causes this alteration in electrical charge and permeability is still a mystery, it may well be cell mediated, for it responds to steroids and immunosuppressive medication.

Clinically the disease is mainly seen in children, and the clinical features all follow from the tremendous loss of albumen from the circulating plasma: with loss of albumen the plasma oncotic pressure falls, and plasma water leaks out, leading to widespread oedema. Along with the leakage of albumen is leakage of cholesterol, and the tubules do their best to reabsorb this, so that in turn there is hypercholesterolaemia and one may see streaks of surplus lipid in the parenchyma of the oedematous kidney. The oedematous swollen kidneys function poorly: there is uraemia and sometimes hypertension. Fortunately in most cases there is spontaneous recovery, and in most also one can hasten recovery by giving steroids or immunosuppressive therapy. In a few children there is a relapse as soon as the immunosuppressive medication is stopped, and in a few others the outcome is less favourable, usually because of more severe damage to the glomerulus and its mesangium.

Patterns of reversible damage in the glomerulus (diffuse)

1. MEMBRANOUS GLOMERULONEPHRITIS

All the capillaries here have thickened walls from deposits of (small) soluble complex that have got through the basement membrane but get trapped between and under the foot processes of the epithelial cells of Bowman's capsule (Fig. 6.2). The foot processes are even more jumbled and fused together than they were in the 'minimal change disease', and the accumulation of soluble complex forms 'lumps and bumps' between which the swollen basement membrane may protrude like teeth of a comb.

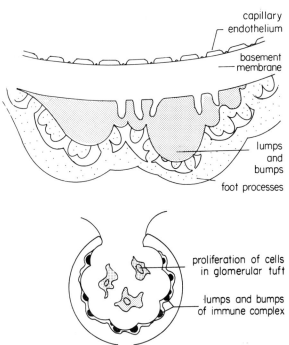

Fig. 6.2. Membranous glomerulonephritis. Lumps and bumps of soluble complex escape through the basement membrane but get trapped under the foot processes of the epithelial cells of Bowman's capsule.

Fig. 6.3. Endocapillary proliferative glomerulonephritis. Cells in the glomerular tuft are proliferated and swollen: there are big lumps and bumps of soluble complex.

2. ENDOCAPILLARY PROLIFERATIVE GLOMERULONEPHRITIS (Fig. 6.3)

Again, all the capillaries are very swollen, but now there is a proliferation of cells in the capillary tuft of the glomerulus where the small soluble complexes again form big lumps and bumps, mainly on the epithelial side of the basement membrane. The difference from (1) above is the proliferation of cells. The cells have mainly migrated down from the mesangium, but some of them are leukocytes attracted thither by activation of the complement cascade.

3. MESANGIAL PROLIFERATIVE GLOMERULONEPHRITIS (Fig. 6.4)

This differs from the endocapillary pattern in that the proliferation of cells is

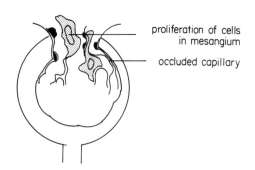

proliferation of cells
in mesangium

occluded capillary

Fig. 6.4. Mesangial proliferative glomerulo-nephritis. Proliferation of cells mainly in the mesangium, perhaps because the complexes are so large that they are held up here.

found mainly in the mesangium rather than the glomerular tuft, probably because the complexes are large ones and held up in the mesangial capillaries. When these patterns are seen the outlook is usually good, because like large complexes elsewhere in the body one expects them to be scavenged effectively by the reticuloendothelial system. However, the outlook is more grim when the renal biopsy shows either of the next two patterns.

Patterns of irreversible damage in the glomerulus (diffuse)

A. MESANGIOCAPILLARY GLOMERULONEPHRITIS (Fig. 6.5)

In all capillaries, both in the tuft and the mesangium, there is evidence of more severe damage resulting from the activation of the complement system. Especially in the capillaries one finds thickening of their walls, so much so that they may even be blocked off. Such a picture is commonly accompanied by an element of the next evil pattern as well.

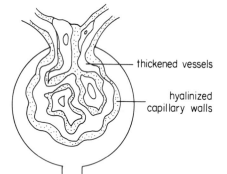

thickened vessels

hyalinized capillary walls

Fig. 6.5. Mesangiocapillary glomeruloneph-ritis. More sinister changes occur—thickened vessels and hyalinized capillaries.

B. EXTRACAPILLARY PROLIFERATIVE GLOMERULONEPHRITIS (Fig. 6.6)

In addition to all the changes described previously, in response to the outpouring of fibrin and other plasma proteins, cells begin to accumulate in the space of Bowman's capsule; some of them are derived from its epithelium and others are probably migrating macrophages. Bit by bit the space is all filled up until there is no more room for urine to get out. The glomerular tuft is squeezed. These epithelial 'crescents' carry a very poor prognosis. If detected early in the disease, occasional good results have been reported from the administration of anticoagulants and fibrinolytic medication.

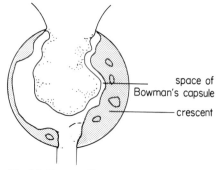

space of
Bowman's capsule

crescent

Fig. 6.6. Extracapillary proliferative glomeru-lonephritis. Bowman's capsule is beginning to fill up with 'crescents'.

C. END-STAGE KIDNEY

From now on the kidneys progressively get worse. Bit by bit more and more glomeruli become replaced by little spheres of hyalinized debris and fewer and fewer nephrons remain to do any useful work. Scarring begins to appear between the tubules and around the glomeruli, and in the end the shrunken scarred kidney presents the non-specific appearance of the *end-stage kidney*.

CLINICAL PICTURES OF GLOMERULONEPHRITIS

The nephrotic syndrome

Characteristically seen in the 'minimal change' lesion, where there is gross loss of albumen, the clinical picture is one of hypoproteinaemia with oedema, hypercholersterolaemia and renal failure. This may also be seen whenever the basement membrane has been damaged and can occur in a variety of histological pictures, and whether one should give immunosuppressive agents or not, and what will be the prognosis, can usefully be determined by a renal biopsy.

The nephritic syndrome

This is usually seen in consequence of more severe destruction of the glomerulus, but again, the clinical picture does not tell the clinician anything about the cause or the prognosis of the illness. As a rule there is a more rapid onset of illness. With complement fixation and damage going on in the kidney, there is haematuria and massive loss of protein and cells in the urine, so much so that one may find red cell and leucocyte casts in its deposit representing worm-casts from the collecting tubules. Hypertension is common in the acute phase and there may be oliguria and anuria. To begin with one cannot predict the outcome: this will depend on the size of the complexes, where they have become lodged, and whether the associated inflammation has got beyond the possibility of resolution.

Since the worst damage occurs with small-complex disease, and since this is thought to result from an inadequate immunological response on the part of the patient, it is not surprising that these cases seldom benefit from immunosuppression. Certain specific clinical syndromes are well-recognized, and deserve notice.

GOODPASTURE'S SYNDROMES

Although this is very rare, it is intensely interesting because here it seems as if the basement membrane itself is acting as an antigen. A patient begins with a pulmonary infection, and as a result, antigenic material is released from the basement membrane of the lung alveoli which apparently has much in common with that of the glomeruli. In consequence, antibodies to the lung material stick to the basement membrane in the glomeruli, attract complement, and cause inflammatory havoc. Clinically a rapid nephritic syndrome follows which is usually fatal.

HENOCH–SCHÖNLEIN NEPHRITIS

A sudden onset of abdominal and joint pains in a child is accompanied by purpura, and in some cases, by the nephritic syndrome. Usually the outlook is good, and the glomeruli show mesangial proliferative glomerulonephritis that will recover. However there may be focal crescents and in some patients the disease progresses.

POLYARTERITIS NODOSA

Along with focal necrotizing inflammation in the walls of other arteries all over the body, there may be similar changes in the arcuate branches of the segmental arteries of the kidney and in the glomeruli; some tufts are replaced by fibrinoid material, whilst others show extracapillary glomerulonephritis with prominent crescents reacting to the loss of fibrin in the urine.

LUPUS NEPHRITIS

This autoimmune disease is ten times more common in women than in men. The antigen is the patient's own DNA, and soluble complex may lodge in the glomeruli and give rise to the whole gamut of possible histological pictures. Clinically the picture is usually that of proteinuria and the nephrotic syndrome and only rarely that of acute nephritis. Fibrinoid necrosis is often found in the glomerular arteriole.

ALPORT'S SYNDROME

Here electron microscopy shows abnormalities in the basement membrane giving rise to proteinuria and eventually to the deposition of some crescents. It is inherited as an autosomal dominant, usually makes itself apparent in boys before puberty and is accompanied by deafness, ocular abnormalities, bony abnormalities and polyneuropathy. Not all members of the family will show the disorder whose inheritance is very complicated.

DIABETIC RENAL DISEASE

Although this is properly not a glomerulonephritis, and no immunological mechanisms are thought to be involved, it presents with the nephrotic syndrome and is marked by the presence of eosinophilic 'matrix' in the mesangium and glomerular capillary and severe hyaline thickening of the afferent and efferent arterioles. The basement membrane also is thickened. Its cause is not known.

AMYLOIDOSIS

Amyloid may be deposited in the kidney in both primary and secondary amyloidosis in between the basement membrane and the mesangium. It eventually goes on to form hyaline eosinophilic deposits which make the tufts less and less cellular, and fill up the space of Bowman's capsule. Along with these changes in the glomeruli the tubules are also under attack and the whole picture may be made catastrophically worse by the development of thrombosis of the renal vein.

MYELOMATOSIS

In multiple myeloma and its related disorders there is an excessive production of immunoglobulins. When the particular clones that are active in the patient are manufacturing light-chain immunoglobulins (as will be found in about half the sufferers) these will appear in the urine as a protein that coagulates at 45–55°C and then dissolves again in a higher temperature (Bence-Jones protein). Histologically the main finding is of dilated tubules (to accommodate the protein) and thickened capillary loops, perhaps caused by the need to filter so much protein. Myelomatosis often gives rise to osteolytic lesions and so there is hypercalciuria leading to deposition of calcium salts in and around the tubules.

FURTHER READING

Black D.A.K. (ed) (1973) *Renal Disease*, 3rd edn. Blackwell Scientific Publications, Oxford.
Cameron J.S. (1972) Bright's disease today—the pathogenesis and treatment of glomerulonephritis. *British Medical Journal*, **4,** 87, 160 and 217.
Kincaid-Smith P., Mathew T.H. & Lovell Becker E. (eds) (1973) *Glomerulonephritis: Morphology, Natural History and Treatment*. John Wiley & Sons, New York.
Risdon R.A. & Turner D.R. (1980) *Atlas of Renal Pathology*. MTP Press, Lancaster.

Chapter 7
The Kidney—
Interstitial
Nephritis

Almost as wide a spectrum of changes are seen in interstitial nephritis as we have encountered in glomerulonephritis, and in the same way, variations in the different varieties occur in the same patient and even in the same kidney. The common feature is that there is post-inflammatory scarring in the connective tissue surrounding the tubules rather than involving the glomeruli. The end result of the process, when it is long-continued and unrelieved, is to produce a small scarred kidney—the end-stage kidney.

SCARRING AND THE RENAL PYRAMID

It may be helpful to remind ourselves of the essential anatomical structure of the kidney (Fig. 7.1) each little unit consisting of an entire renal 'pyramid' or collection of nephrons draining into one papilla, arranged like a bunch of flowers in a vase. We can distinguish two main types of interstitial nephritis—medullar and cortical, and in each the lesion may be partial or complete.

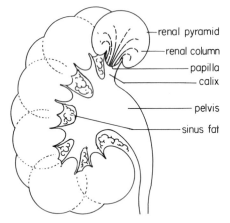

Fig. 7.1. The essential architecture of the kidney: it is made up of about a dozen pyramids fused together. In each pyramid the nephrons are arranged like a bunch of flowers, and the collecting ducts drain into the papillae. There is a packing of sinus fat between the pyramids and the calices.

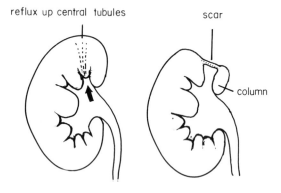

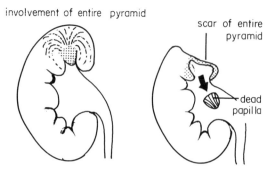

Fig. 7.2. Variations in the pattern of renal scarring depend upon whether only the middle tubules are affected, as in reflux (above) or whether the entire collection drains into the papilla (below) as in some forms of papillary necrosis.

Chapter 7/*The Kidney—Interstitial Nephritis*

Medullary interstitial nephritis

Whatever the cause of the inflammation, it seems to attack the medulla, and in most of its forms, its pattern of attack depends on the amount of the renal papilla that is involved (Fig. 7.2). In reflux uropathy for example, the defective papillary valves permit reflux of infected urine to pass up the most central of the ducts of Bellini into the inner portion of the renal pyramid, sparing the columns on either side. In more severe lesions, when the noxious agent leads to necrosis of the entire renal papilla, then there is scarring and shrinking of the whole of the pyramid that supplies the lost ducts of Bellini.

Cortical interstitial nephritis

Here the attack is upon the outer cortical part of the kidney and again it may be partial or complete: quite often only patches of cortex are affected, leading to patchy scars (Fig. 7.3). Other causes of scarring affect the whole of the kidney more or less uniformly, and the end-result is a contracted kidney without any lumps of healthy parenchyma spared from the disease process.

Given this background, it may be helpful to consider some of the more

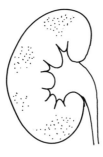
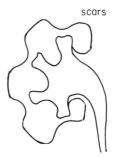

scars

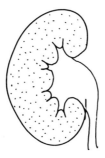
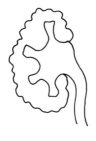

Fig. 7.3. Cortical interstitial nephritis. The cortex may be attacked in patches, or diffusely, with relatively little damage to the medulla.

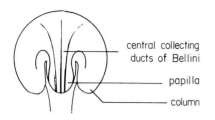

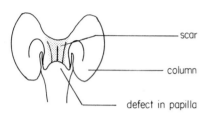

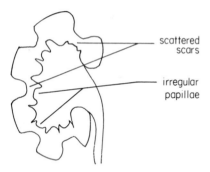

Fig. 7.4. Reflux nephropathy. Because of the lack of effective protective valves where the collecting ducts open onto the papilla, urine can be forced back up the ducts into the cortex. The ducts draining the columns on either side of the pyramid are less likely to be affected, and the typical scarring leaves bumps of healthy unscarred tissue in between.

common and important clinical pictures that occur as the kidney is involved in interstitial nephritis.

MEDULLARY INTERSTITIAL NEPHRITIS

Reflux nephropathy

Undoubtedly the most important cause of renal scarring and morbidity is the combination of a failure of development of valves to protect the lower end of the ureter from increase of pressure in the bladder, and of valves in compound papillae that allow reflux of urine to take place from the calices into the renal parenchyma. Since these deficient ducts of Bellini occur in the middle of the renal pyramid, this receives the worst of the attack and develops the most severe scarring, resulting in a characteristic pit in the contour of the renal cortex and a hollowed-out renal papilla (Fig. 7.4).

Papillary necrosis

A number of conditions may lead to death of the renal papilla, either partial or complete: they include reflux, obstruction, analgesic abuse, diabetes with infection, sickle cell disease and (rarely) Balkan nephropathy (Fig. 7.5). The occasional papilla may undergo necrosis while others remain unaffected, and the same agent may cause diffuse involvement of the renal cortex in one patient, and scattered papillary necrosis in another. Nevertheless, when papillary necrosis is seen, it causes scarring and obstruction to the ducts of Bellini and all the nephrons draining into them upstream of the dead papilla, resulting in a characteristic deeply pitted scar in the cortex. For a time one can identify the dead papilla before it separates, by a line of demarcation, like that which leads to the detachment of a gangrenous toe, which can be shown in the excretion urogram. Since many of the patients who get necrosis of their papillae also have infected urine, it is hardly surprising that stones form on the nidus offered by the dead papilla. These partly calcified, rather soft papillae may cause ureteric obstruction. Analgesic abuse is a common cause of severe and progressive

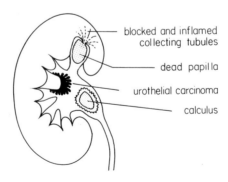

Fig. 7.5. Papillary necrosis. All the pyramid may be affected. The dead papilla may serve as the nucleus for stone formation. Some forms of papillary necrosis are followed by urothelial cancer.

Chapter 7/*The Kidney—Interstitial Nephritis*

interstitial nephritis as well as papillary necrosis. It may occur in endemic form, e.g. among the silly women in some Australian cities who regard analgesic tablets as an essential accompaniment to their morning coffee, and in the ill-fated town of Huskqvarna, where an entire population convinced itself that Dr Hjorten's phenacitin powder would protect it from influenza, etc. Unsuspected analgesic overconsumption is still common in Britain, and it is a common finding that these patients lie about their consumption of pain-killing tablets. Small wonder, when they are bombarded every day by advertisements promising fast, fast, fast pain relief, but omitting to add that slow papillary necrosis is the price one may pay.

Even more sinister is the long term consequence of analgesic nephropathy, a complication seen also in the unfortunate people who dwell along the Danube and suffer Balkan nephropathy: in time one may develop urothelial cancer in the lining of the calices and renal pelvis.

Obstruction

Persistent obstruction to the ureter and renal pelvis is followed by loss by atrophy and interstitial fibrosis of the papilla as a whole. This is followed in turn by progressive loss of the medulla and cortex until in the end each renal unit, each pyramid, is turned into a hollow balloon whose shell is no thicker than paper (Fig. 7.6).

CORTICAL INTERSTITIAL NEPHRITIS

Many different causes give rise to patchy changes in the parenchyma, and others to diffuse involvement of the entire renal cortex. In each case, there may be associated medullary scarring and in most examples, there may also be loss of the renal papillae. However, one can distinguish certain useful clinical patterns.

Patchy cortical interstitial nephritis occurs in analgesic abuse, in Balkan nephropathy, in haematogenous infection, in certain drug-induced interstitial nephritides, and in the metabolic illnesses seen in gout and nephrocalcinosis. Analgesic abuse causes slowly progressive interstitial nephritis in the cortex as well as the more dramatic loss of renal papillae. These patients, often denying a protracted over-consumption of aspirin, phenacitin and codeine tablets or similar medication, may turn up with uraemia, proteinuria, and sterile pyuria of obscure origin. Their urograms show patchy scarring in the cortex.

In *Balkan nephropathy* people living along the Danube valley may get a very similar cortical scarring with occasional papillary necrosis complicated by a tragically high incidence of upper tract cancer of the urothelium. The cause is thought to be a fungus that attacks grain stored in damp barns.

Haematogenous infection leads to multiple small abscesses throughout the parenchyma that usually heal by complete resolution, but may end up with

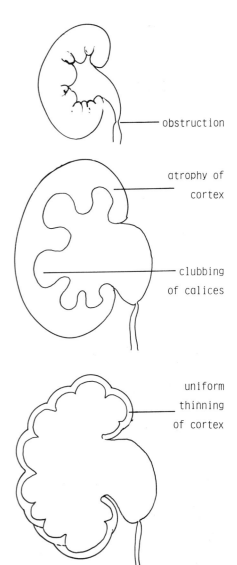

Fig. 7.6. Obstructive uropathy. Stages in the progressive atrophy of the renal parenchyma from continued obstruction.

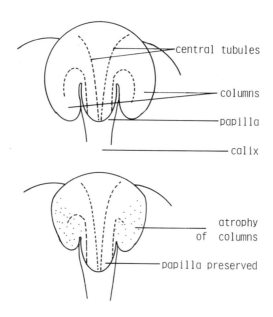

central tubules

columns

papilla

calix

atrophy
of columns

papilla preserved

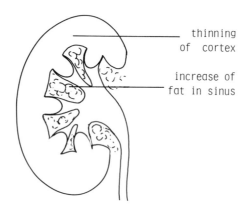

thinning
of cortex

increase of
fat in sinus

Fig. 7.7. Concealed cortical interstitial nephritis as seen in arteriosclerosis and old age. Wasting of the parenchyma is most marked in the columns at the edge of each pyramid; the space is taken up by an increase in the quantity of renal sinus fat—renal lipomatosis.

scattered patchy scars. In gout, sharp needles of urate are deposited in and around the tubules and set up a foreign body scar reaction: in nephrocalcinosis similar fibrosis is provoked by calcium deposits.

In certain *drug-induced conditions* there seems to be an allergic response to the tubular basement-membrane in a way that recalls the inflammatory response to glomerular basement membrane seen in some types of glomerulonephritis. This may occur with sulphonamides, ampicillin, penicillin, cephalothin and phenindione. It is seen with fever haematuria skin rashes and acute renal failure, and since the immune complexes occur in relationship to the tubules rather than the glomeruli, the inflammatory havoc that follows fixation of complement is seen around the tubules rather than the glomeruli.

Chapter 7/*The Kidney—Interstitial Nephritis*

Concealed cortical interstitial nephritis may occur in some patients, in whom the brunt of the change occurs not in the projecting part of the cortex, or the dome of the pyramids, but in the columns—the parts so often spared in reflux (Fig. 7.7). The result is to give a kidney that looks quite large and healthy, but its peripelvic fat is enormously increased to occupy the wasted renal columns—the so-called *lipomatosis* of the renal sinus. In some patients this change is seen without any obvious cause other than old age.

CLINICAL FEATURES OF INTERSTITIAL NEPHRITIS

Clearly the agent that leads to the condition will have its own particular symptoms in the case of diabetes, urinary infection, and urinary tract obstruction. In others the cause gives the clinician no hint of its action, and the patient presents with urinary infection in a scarred kidney, with a ureter obstructed by a dead and perhaps partly calcified papilla, or unexplained uraemia, often accompanied by proteinuria and an excessive amount of white cells in the urine. Haematuria must always be taken seriously, since it may well signify the complication of urothelial cancer. Analgesic abuse must never be forgotten, nor must the sad fact that our patients seldom admit to it.

FURTHER READING

Black D.A.K. (ed.) (1973) *Renal Disease*. Blackwell Scientific Publications, Oxford.
Freedman L.R. (1976) Pathophysiology of pyelonephritis. In D.I. Williams & G.D. Chisholm (eds), *Scientific Foundations of Urology*, p. 71. Heinemann, London.
Heptinstall R.H. (1976) Interstitial Nephritis. A brief review. *American Journal of Pathology*, **83,** 214.
Murray T.G. & Goldberg M. (1978) Analgesic-associated nephropathy in the USA: epidemiologic, clinical and pathogenetic features. *Kidney International*, **13,** 64.
Risdon R.A. & Turner D.R. (1980) *Atlas of Renal Pathology*. MTP Press, Lancaster.
Sherwood T. (1973) Ureteric reflux 1973: chronic pyelonephritis versus reflux nephropathy. *British Journal of Radiology*, **46,** 653.

Chapter 8
Urinary Tract Infection

Acute bacterial infection of the kidney is both common and important all over the world. In the West it attacks women many times more often than men: when they are toddlers, when they first attend school around the age of five, when they begin to menstruate, or when they get married. Later on it may make pregnancy miserable, and even after the menopause, a new set of urinary symptoms may succeed the previous ones. Exotic and interesting though many other aspects of urology may be, for the ordinary kind doctor, the proper understanding and effective control of common recurrent 'cystitis' is really a far more important lesson to learn.

PATHOLOGY OF URINARY INFECTION (Fig. 8.1)

Ascending

Bacteria may enter the urethra and gain entry to the bladder, from where reflux may carry them to the kidney. If the renal papillae are patent and the pressure inside the kidney is increased, they may be injected along with urine into the interstitium of the kidney to give rise to the train of events that ends up, as we have seen in the previous chapter, to *interstitial nephritis*. There is no doubt that many urinary infections in women are acquired in this way, and in either sex other organisms are inoculated into the urinary tract when any instrument is passed along the urethra into the bladder, or when a patient with an indwelling catheter is infected with airborne organisms that colonize the drainage system.

Anything which increases the pressure inside the urinary tract (e.g. reflux from bladder to kidney, build-up of pressure upstream of an obstructing calculus or a hydronephrosis) is likely to force urine into the kidney tissue, and if this urine is infected, it will give rise to acute inflammation, and this will be followed by scarring. Hence the particular importance, in all cases of urinary infection, of making sure that there is free drainage. Hence too the particular dread of leaving untreated any known obstruction.

Haematogenous

There is a second, no less important route of infection of the kidney, namely the bloodstream. *Haematogenous* infection of the kidney gives rise to multiple small abscesses scattered throughout the kidney. As a rule they are dealt with by the defence mechanisms of the body, but it is not at all uncommon to find them post mortem in patients who have suffered an episode of bacteraemia before death. In experimental animals most of these deliberately inoculated haematogenous organisms will also be dealt with, and the kidneys will heal up, unless there is some localized damage already present in the kidney. It is the same in man, a kidney that has previously been scarred, from whatever cause, is more susceptible to subsequent clinical infection from a haematogenous source.

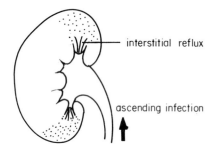

interstitial reflux

ascending infection

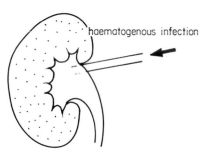

haematogenous infection

Fig. 8.1. Organisms may reach the kidney by reflux up the ureter or through the bloodstream.

Chapter 8/*Urinary Tract Infection*

Bacteriology of urinary infection

One commonly discovers in the urine, organisms that have originated in the patient's own bowel flora, e.g. *Escherichia coli, Klebsiella, Streptococcus faecalis,* and *Proteus mirabilis.* In a patient who has been given broad-spectrum antibiotics, or who has had the misfortune to sit around in hospital for any length of time, one is likely to discover hospital-acquired organisms, because her intestinal flora are likely to have been, at least in part, replaced by new strains often not very sensitive to antibiotics. (For this reason urologists are usually very cautious about using so-called prophylactic antibiotics.) In patients who get relapses of urinary tract infection, the new organism is usually a different strain picked up from their own bowel flora, and so not necessarily sensitive to the antibiotic that was last administered.

FACTORS PREDISPOSING TO URINARY INFECTION

1. Stagnant urine

Urine is a perfect culture medium (Fig. 8.2) for many organisms which will multiply very rapidly at normal body temperature if they once gain entry to a pool of urine that is not completely emptied out of the urinary tract (Fig. 8.3). These stagnant pools are seen under four circumstances:

A. Too infrequent voiding. Many women get into the habit of emptying their

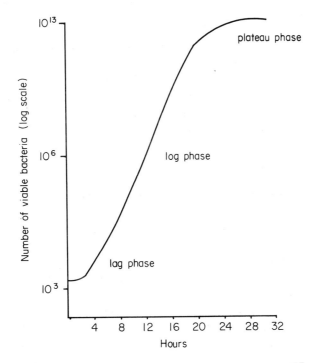

Fig. 8.2. Growth of micro-organisms in the urine.

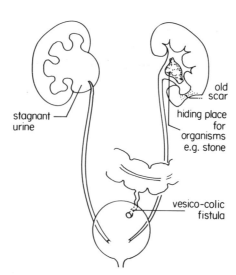

stagnant urine

old scar

hiding place for organisms e.g. stone

vesico-colic fistula

Fig. 8.3. Some of the common causes of persistent or relapsing urinary infection.

bladders only once or twice a day. By 12 hours a single organism that gains entry to the bladder may have multiplied to several million. One of the chief weapons in the therapy of urinary infection in women is to encourage frequent and complete emptying-out of the bladder so that organisms are never offered this opportunity to multiply.

B. Mechanical obstruction to the urinary tract. This results in incomplete emptying-out of the bladder, ureters or kidneys. It forms a major part of routine urological surgery. We see this presenting with urinary infection in hydronephrosis from obstruction at the pelviureteric junction, in dilatation of the ureter from obstruction by a stone, and in outflow obstruction to the bladder from obstruction from prostatic hypertrophy or a stricture in the urethra. Very similar infection is seen in people whose bladders do not empty because the detrusor does not contract effectively as a result of a disorder of innervation—the neuropathic bladder.

C. Undrained pockets of urine. These occur very commonly in the obstructed bladder where they are called diverticula; but they are also found in the kidney (caliceal diverticula) and in many other situations where parts of the urinary tract get filled with urine that does not empty out completely.

D. Dilated refluxing ureters—megaureter. There are a number of conditions that end up with the ureters becoming grossly dilated. In some of these the cause is an obstruction at the lower end, and in others there is free reflux of urine from the bladder up the ureter towards the kidney. In any event, once the system is inoculated with micro-organisms, the urine runs up the ureter in reflux, or remains in it when the ureter is obstructed, allowing organisms to breed.

2. Foreign bodies and hiding places for organisms

The most common hiding place for organisms are stones. They are usually crumbly and porous, and in between the little collections of crystals there is plenty of room for urine to enter and for organisms to hide. Hence one very often finds a stone sheltering organisms year after year, protecting them from antibiotics that might diffuse some way into the stone, but never in high enough concentration to kill off all the innermost micro-organisms.

Equally important as a cause of persistent infection though seen less often are other foreign or dead tissues. A carcinoma whose surface has begun to undergo necrosis will offer a good hiding place for organisms, sheltering them from antibiotics. A stitch or a piece of broken-off catheter will act in the same way.

3. Fistulae

Diverticulitis, Crohn's disease, or cancer may give rise to an abnormal hole that allows intestinal micro-organisms to enter the bladder.

4. Lowered resistance to infection

Many patients will tell you that their symptoms of urinary infection began a few days after an influenza-like illness. Though it is seldom possible to identify the virus that infects the urinary tract in the first few days, the clinical picture is so common, and so striking, that it leaves little room for doubt that (as elsewhere in the body) viraemia is followed by bacterial secondary infection.

No less important, if less common, are other causes of lowered host resistance. Never allow yourself to forget *Diabetes Mellitus*—so easy to detect—so shameful when you allow yourself to miss the diagnosis. Immuno-suppression for transplantation or in the course of chemotherapy for cancer lays the urinary tract open to acquired infection no less often than other systems.

Infection is also much more apt to attack tissues that have already been damaged. We see this in well-treated tuberculosis of the urinary tract, which leaves the patient with scars and calcified areas that are less able to resist ordinary haematogenous or urine-borne infection. The same applies to kidneys already damaged by interstitial nephritis—here the coincidence of bacterial infection may well deceive the clinician into concluding that the bacteria are the only pathological agency at work to damage the kidneys. For many years virtually all these scarred kidneys were assigned the label 'pyelonephritis' in the belief that bacterial infection was the common cause of all their destruction.

THE END RESULT OF URINARY INFECTION

Just like infection elsewhere in the body, infection in the urinary tract is followed by one of four processes (Fig. 8.4)—*resolution, suppuration, scarring* or *granuloma*. No doubt *resolution* is the common end-result. Most patients

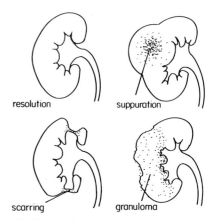

Fig. 8.4. The four possible results of infection in the kidney—resolution, suppuration, scarring, or chronic granuloma formation.

with common bacterial inflammation of the bladder (cystitis) end up with an absolutely normal bladder without any detectable evidence of previous inflammation. The same applies to the kidney. Most patients with clinical and radiological evidence of acute bacterial inflammation of the kidney end up with an absolutely normal kidney without scarring or shrinking.

Suppuration is seen in kidneys infected with staphylococcus, and in certain debilitated patients, and leads to a cortical abscess, a 'carbuncle' and sometimes to a perinephric abscess. It is seen upstream of obstruction, particularly by calculi. It is seen in the prostate (very rarely) and it is found as an occasional complication of infections of the wall of the urethra in men (urethritis).

Fibrosis and *scarring* in the kidney give rise to the many forms of interstitial nephritis which were described in the previous chapter. In the ureter they cause a stricture, since the scars in the wall of the ureter always shrink. In the bladder fibrosis is not common, but when it occurs it may cause interstitial cystitis, and a reduced bladder capacity. In the prostate it may be one of the many factors that cause a fibrous stenosis of the prostate and bladder neck, but this can seldom be proved with any degree of certainty. In the urethra the scarring is dreadfully important, since it causes urethral stricture—one of the most serious causes of urological disease.

Granulomata occur in kidneys infected by any of the organisms that are known elsewhere in the body to cause chronic inflammation. Thus we find chronic inflammatory granulomas in tuberculosis, brucellosis, and schistosomiasis. They are also seen in certain ill-understood reactions to ordinary urinary pathogens, perhaps as a result of some curious alteration in the inflammatory response, for instead of straightforward suppuration with the formation of an abscess and pus, or healing by fibrosis, there is a sinister, nasty, chronic, and ultimately fatal inflammatory disease (see malakoplakia and xanthogranuloma, page 86).

URINARY TRACT INFECTION AND VESICOURETERIC REFLUX

Many children are born with a defective valvular arrangement where the ureters enter the bladder. Sometimes (see page 47) this is associated with duplex ureter or ureterocele, but more often it occurs on its own in an otherwise normal child. Most of these children will grow out of it, as they get older and their trigone matures. Sometimes the reflux up the ureter is associated with the presence of compound renal papillae, so that when the urine squirts up the ureter, it passes straight through the top of the papillae and into the collecting tubules, rupturing their walls, and injecting urine into the interstitium (Fig. 8.5). It is not yet known for certain whether uninfected urine injected into the kidney tissue does any harm, but it is beyond doubt that *infected* urine does considerable harm, giving rise to acute inflammation, and being followed by scarring—the typical deeply pitted scars of 'reflux uropathy'. As the little child with these scars

Chapter 8/*Urinary Tract Infection*

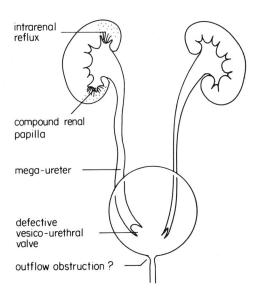

intrarenal reflux

compound renal papilla

mega-ureter

defective vesico-urethral valve

outflow obstruction ?

Fig. 8.5. Reflux uropathy.

continues to grow, and his kidneys grow with him, so the surrounding unaffected parts of the kidney appear to undergo hypertrophy, and the pits where the interstitial nephritis has occurred become deeper and more pronounced (Fig. 8.6). The necessary compound papillae with the necessary defective valve systems are most commonly to be found at the upper and lower poles of the kidney, so that the brunt of the scarring in reflux nephropathy is found here.

For this reason, when managing a child with urinary tract infection, the urologist has two questions to ask: (a) is there reflux? and (b) are there defective papillae to permit reflux into the interstitium? Both of these questions are answered, traditionally, by performing a *micturating cystogram* (see page 19). The child's bladder is filled with contrast medium, and he is told to pass urine while careful observations are made of the reflux of the contrast up to the kidney and into the renal parenchyma where it appears as a characteristic blush.

If there is no gross reflux, and if there is no intrarenal injection of contrast, many surgeons regard the condition as quite safe. Similarly, if the urine is sterile, even if there is gross reflux and interstitial injection of the contrast, many surgeons consider that this also is safe, and several series have been followed in which the affected children seem to have come to no harm.

On the other hand, if there is gross reflux with interstitial injection of urine as well as infection, most paediatric urologists would recommend an operation to refashion the vesicoureteric valve in such a way that reflux is prevented (see page 342). Unfortunately things even then are not so simple, for by the time the condition is first detected, there are rather few children who have not in fact developed their scars by the time the investigation is first performed. It has been argued that in these little patients any operation to correct reflux is like shutting the stable door after the horse has bolted. Any papillae that could allow

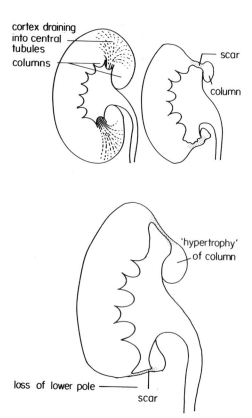

Fig. 8.6. Compound papillae that allow reflux to occur into the interstitium are usually found at the upper and lower poles. When these undergo scarring, the rest of the undamaged kidney continues to grow but the adult kidney continues to show the site of the scarring (below).

scarring to occur have already done so, and the others have proved that they can keep infection out of the parenchyma whether reflux is present or not. At the time of writing, this question is still hotly debated.

COMPLICATIONS OF URINARY TRACT INFECTION

1. Acute renal failure

Whether the infection is haematogenous, or comes up from the ureter, its immediate affect upon the parenchyma is like infection anywhere else i.e. there is *rubor calor* and *dolor* as well as *laesio functionis* ('lesson one' in surgery since the time of Hippocrates). The rubor and calor cannot be seen unless the kidney is explored at operation, when the acutely inflamed kidney is seen to be grossly enlarged, hot, and incredibly vascular (if one is obliged to operate upon it). If a urogram is performed at this stage the kidney outline is swollen, and surrounding oedema masks the otherwise clear edge of the kidney and the adjacent psoas muscle. Oedema also makes the necks of the calices seem narrow and drawn out (Fig. 8.7). Depending on the cause of the acute infection, these changes may be confined to segments of the kidney or may affect the entire organ. The acutely inflamed kidney works poorly, and may in fact become unable to form urine at all. When examined by isotopes (e.g. 99^{m}Tc dimercaptosuccinic acid DMSA) one may get a surprisingly poor uptake, and this may be falsely reported upon as showing a kidney with no useful function. With treatment, and when time has been given for the inflammation to resolve, function may return to normal.

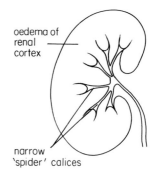

Fig. 8.7. Urography in acute infection—oedema makes the calices long and thin. Impaired filtration may (temporarily) give a very poor picture.

2. Septicaemia

The most sudden and perhaps the most serious of all the complications of urinary tract infection is septicaemia. One must never forget how huge is the blood supply of the kidney, or how thin are the linings of the renal collecting tubules, and how narrow an interval separates the urine space from the surrounding veins and lymphatics of the kidney. Given an increase in pressure within the kidney for whatever cause, and the presence of micro-organisms inside the urine, then there is a chance that micro-organisms will be injected directly into the veins and lymphatics issuing from the kidney into the cava or the cisterna chyli and thoracic duct. Many of the organisms that infect the urinary tract are Gram-negative. Gram-negative bacilli harbour a particularly potent 'lipid-A' endotoxin which stimulates the hypothalamus to cause fever and releases kinins that cause vasodilatation, increase capillary permeability, and inhibit cardiac muscular function (Fig. 8.8). Gram-negative septicaemia may occur after almost any urological operation, usually without warning, but it is notoriously common when there is obstruction to the kidney or ureter as well as an infected urine.

One may detect the early phase of septicaemia, when the peripheral

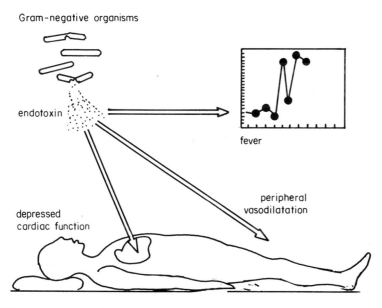

Fig. 8.8. Gram-negative septicaemia.

circulation is dilated, for the patient may have a rigor and fever, a bounding pulse, and his face and limbs may be vasodilated and warm. Within half an hour the picture changes dramatically: the blood pressure falls to unrecordable levels, the limbs are cold and clammy from vasoconstriction and the clinical appearance resembles that of a patient who has had a coronary thrombosis.

The first thing is to suspect the diagnosis. The next is to make sure. A needle must be got into a vein (not always easy), and blood sent for culture. Through the same needle an intravenous infusion is set up, at first with saline, later with a plasma-expander, while as soon as possible one should get a central venous cannula in position to monitor the pressure in the right heart. Then enough plasma-expander such as plasma or blood is given until the central venous pressure returns to normal. A massive dose of the most probably effective antibiotic is given intravenously with the first part of the infusion, and the patient is monitored at frequent intervals.

If there is anything which can be done to relieve urinary obstruction (if it is present) then this ought to be done without delay: if pus is present, particularly pus pent-up under tension inside an abscess, then it ought to be let out as soon as possible. But to start with, the first priority is to keep up the circulating fluid volume (by intravenous infusion, often of several litres of fluid), and give bactericidal antibiotics. Such a patient, whenever it is feasible, ought to be moved to an intensive-care unit where vital functions can be closely monitored, and where the often very rapid changes in physical and biochemical signs can be noted and responded to without delay. For in most patients improvement begins within one or two hours, and the lost fluid begins to return to the circulation, the central venous pressure rises, and unless the natural diuresis keeps pace with fluid overload, one may even have to perform venesection to keep the patient out of heart failure.

These are the emergency and urgent problems that may follow severe upper tract infection. The next groups are slower in onset but no less important.

3. Papillary necrosis and interstitial nephritis

Papillary necrosis has been mentioned along with interstitial nephritis as one of the sequelae of the inflammatory response to many different kinds of insult to the kidney, and acute infection is one of them. In diabetic patients especially, an acute upper tract infection is apt to lead on to sloughing of the renal papillae, and it is also seen in patients who have suffered an attack of infection complicating urinary obstruction. For the same reasons interstitial scarring is especially likely to follow infection that accompanies obstruction (Fig. 8.9).

4. Stone formation

Stones can often be seen to form some months after an attack of renal infection. It sometimes is obvious that they have formed around sloughed renal papillae, but in many patients one cannot identify a missing papilla, and it must be

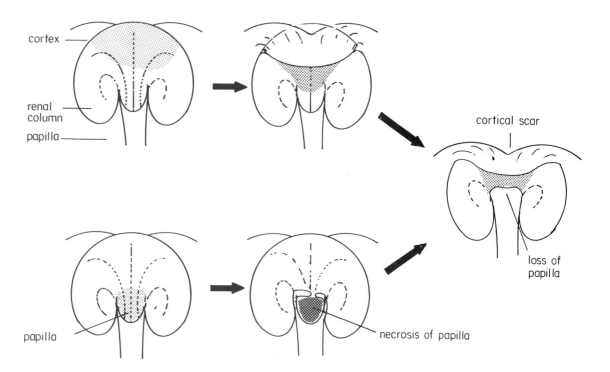

cortex

renal column

papilla

cortical scar

loss of papilla

papilla

necrosis of papilla

Fig. 8.9. Damage mainly in the cortex, or in the papilla, may end up with the same deeply pitted cortical scar and blunted calix.

assumed that the stone has formed around bacteria or bacterial debris in the urinary tract (Fig. 8.10). They are most commonly seen in patients with an urea-splitting infection e.g. *Proteus mirabilis* which metabolizes urea to ammonia, makes the urine alkaline, and precipitates calcium phosphates.

5. Suppuration

If the infection has been haematogenous, and begins in the renal parenchyma as an abscess or a series of little abscesses which later coalesce, one can get at first a large inflammatory lump in the parenchyma of the kidney which is followed by a large abscess. This was not uncommon in the days before antibiotics, when bacteraemia following a staphylococcal boil in the skin would lead to a *renal carbuncle* (Fig. 8.11). Today one sees the same kind of lesion in people who are ill for other reasons (such as diabetes). It is also seen occasionally in patients whose initial attack of renal infection has been half-treated with too brief and too small a dose of antibiotics. In some countries parenchymal haematogenous renal carbuncles are found amongst drug addicts, injecting themselves with infected equipment. When the infection is confined to the parenchyma there need be no pus in the urine. The kidney is swollen and tender. The radiographic features are those of a soft-tissue mass. Ultrasound shows it to contain echoes suggestive of a neoplasm rather than a cyst. If one keeps a high index of suspicion one can sometimes make the right diagnosis, confirm it by aspiration of pus, and cure the patient with a vigorous and protracted course of

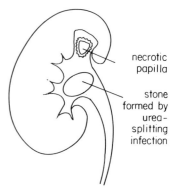

necrotic papilla

stone formed by urea- splitting infection

Fig. 8.10. Infection causes stones either by causing necrosis of a papilla or by precipitating matrix directly.

Chapter 8/*Urinary Tract Infection*   85

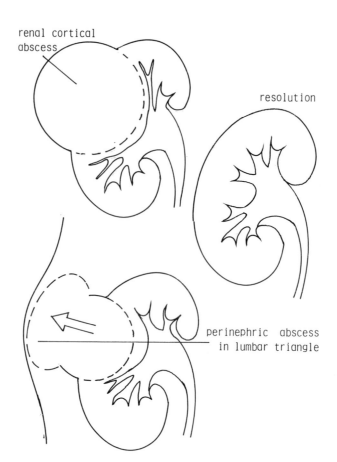

renal cortical
abscess

resolution

perinephric abscess
in lumbar triangle

Fig. 8.11. Suppuration in the cortex forms an abscess (renal carbuncle) which usually resolves with treatment, but may rupture into the perinephric fat and even point in the lumbar triangle.

antibiotics. Occasionally the 'carbuncle' will form a *perinephric abscess* that will point and call for drainage, but nephrectomy should not be necessary. When in doubt an angiogram may be performed, but it can be difficult to interpret with certainty from tumour.

6. Granuloma

When there is a continuing cause for urinary infection, for example when a stone is left untouched year after year, then the interstitial inflammation continues, and changes its character.

XANTHOGRANULOMATOUS PYELONEPHRITIS

Here the interstitial inflammation becomes transformed by the infiltration of histiocytes which become laden with lipid, yellow in colour (resembling that of an adenocarcinoma of the kidney), and spreads into the tissues surrounding the kidney (Fig. 8.12). In amongst the stiff and adherent yellow tissue are many small abscesses, some of them invading the liver, or burrowing under the fascia

Chapter 8/*Urinary Tract Infection*

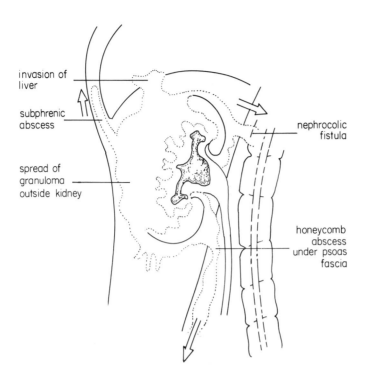

invasion of liver

subphrenic abscess

spread of granuloma outside kidney

nephrocolic fistula

honeycomb abscess under psoas fascia

Fig. 8.12. Chronic granulomas usually occur where there are neglected stones. They track all round, burrow under the psoas, and cause fistulae into the bowel.

of the psoas muscle to form a honeycomb of sinuses, or invading the wall of the colon to form a nephrocolic fistula. Unless this entire mass is removed, the patient loses weight and progressively deteriorates. Clinically there is often a palpable lump, and the radiological features resemble those of any other solid space-occupying lump in the kidney, so that it may be impossible to distinguish the xanthogranuloma from a renal carcinoma. At operation the densely adherent, brilliantly yellow mass may seem to be inoperable. One needs to remember the existence of this condition, for it is important to remove the mass if possible, for it does not respond to more conservative measures, and will not resolve with antibiotic treatment.

MALAKOPLAKIA

A very similar non-specific granuloma that occurs in the kidney, and elsewhere in the urinary tract such as the bladder, ureter and testis, is malakoplakia. Multiple abscesses occur in the kidney with dense fibrosis around them, and in the bladder and ureter, heaped-up brownish plaques are found that may bleed or cause obstruction. The specific feature that makes the diagnosis is the finding of *Michaelis–Guttman bodies* (peculiar calcified spherules) in and around the chronic inflammatory cells. Again, this condition, though only an inflammation, is a clinician's nightmare, for unless it is removed, it persists, invades, and ultimately may kill the patient.

Chapter 8/*Urinary Tract Infection*   87

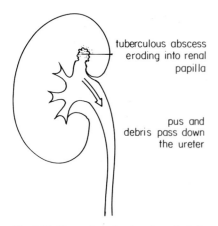

Fig. 8.13. The early lesion in tuberculosis is a small abscess that erodes a renal papilla.

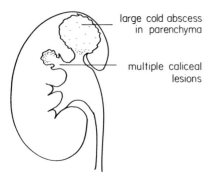

Fig. 8.14. In later stages, large, cold abscesses destroy the entire pyramid and more and more papillae are affected.

Generally fungus infections occur only in the kidney of the severely debilitated patient, or the patient given long courses of antibiotics and immunosuppressives. Here one encounters *blastomycosis, aspergillosis, coccidiomycosis* and *mucormycosis*. One may also find (rarely) *actinomycosis*, causing a chronic invasive granuloma of the kidney. The origin of the actinomycosis is usually in a rotten tooth or periodontal disease. The lump is detected in a urogram which shows a space occupying mass, and the diagnosis is only made after nephrectomy.

GENITOURINARY TUBERCULOSIS

Properly speaking this falls into the group of granulomas of the kidney, but it is such an important entity that it deserves a section to itself. Nowadays tuberculosis is not common in the United Kingdom, but it is frequently met with overseas.

Pathology

Today the offending organism is usually the human variety of *Mycobacterium tuberculosis*. In Britain this is usually Phage Type B but in immigrants from India mainly Phage Type I. Only 2–3% of patients with pulmonary tuberculosis go on to develop genitourinary tuberculosis. It reaches the kidney by haematogenous spread, and no doubt in most instances there is complete resolution of the tiny miliary tubercles that form in the renal cortex.

In the earliest cases that are detected, one finds a small focus in one or other of the renal papillae (Fig. 8.13). At this stage the patient may notice frequency of urination, and perhaps a little haematuria. The excretion urogram will show a barely-detectable irregularity in one or more renal papillae.

In later stages the little tuberculoma in the papilla has enlarged and grown out towards the cortex forming a larger abscess, often partially calcified (Fig. 8.14). Still later, active granulomas cause the necks of the calices to become narrowed, giving rise to infected dilated calices upstream of the narrowing (Fig. 8.15). Left unchecked, the entire kidney may be converted into a bag of

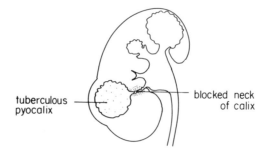

Fig. 8.15. Granulation tissue obstructs some caliceal necks, giving pyocalices upstream of them.

Chapter 8/*Urinary Tract Infection*

more-or-less calcified, tuberculous, caseation tissue (Fig. 8.16). This gives a striking appearance in the plain abdominal radiograph—the so-called cement kidney.

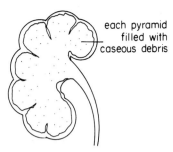

each pyramid filled with caseous debris

Fig. 8.16. Eventually the kidney is converted into a calcified bag of caseous debris—the cement kidney.

SPREAD TO THE URETER AND BLADDER

In the beginning the infection is confined to the kidney, but soon active tuberculous granulation tissue is found in the ureter and active inflammation in the wall of the bladder. In the ureter the oedema and inflammation makes the ureter thicker and shorter, so that the ureteric orifice is drawn up, giving a typical appearance on cystoscopy of a 'golf-hole' ureter (Fig. 8.17). Under the healing influence of anti-tuberculous therapy, the active granulomas in the wall of the ureter heal with fibrosis, causing a stricture and giving rise to hydronephrosis upstream of the healing area (Fig. 8.18).

In the bladder the early phase of tuberculosis may cause such gross oedema that it may look like a tumour on cystoscopy. Actual little tubercles, such as one might expect, are almost never seen. Biopsy of the oedematous mass, or of the merely rather red bladder that is seen at this stage may reveal acid-fast bacilli and characteristic tubercles. Again, as the disease progresses or as the granulomas heal up thanks to treatment, the wall of the bladder is replaced by fibrous tissue, its volume is much reduced, and the patient begins to experience very severe frequency of micturition.

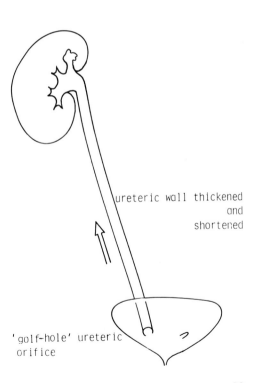

ureteric wall thickened and shortened

'golf-hole' ureteric orifice

Fig. 8.17. The ureter in tuberculosis is oedematous and shortened, pulling out the ureteric orifice.

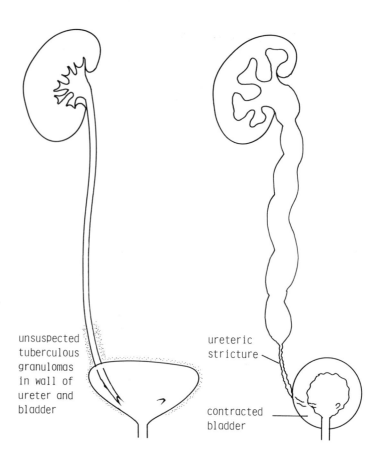

unsuspected
tuberculous
granulomas
in wall of
ureter and
bladder

ureteric
stricture

contracted
bladder

Fig. 8.18. Unsuspected tuberculous granulation tissue in the wall of the ureter will undergo fibrosis and shrinkage with treatment and so gives rise to obstruction. Similar scarring makes the bladder shrink down.

Diagnosis

In the early case diagnosis calls for a highly suspicious mind. Every patient with pus in the urine that cannot be explained by associated bacterial infection must have tuberculosis excluded by examination of early morning specimens of urine for acid-fast bacilli in the deposit (with the *Ziehl–Neelsen* stain), and on culture (using the *Loewenstein–Jensen* medium). This is a culture medium containing a detergent that inhibits growth of other contaminant organisms during the six weeks that it may take the tubercle bacilli to appear on the slope. A negative result is declared after six weeks. In cases of doubt at least six specimens should be examined in this way. Guinea-pig inoculation offers an additional test for detection of tuberculosis, but carries hazards of transmitting infection to laboratory staff and has been largely given up.

UROGRAPHY

In the earliest cases the IVU may show an eroded papilla, in later instances, traces of calcification and larger hollow areas in the cortex, with more or less narrowing of calices and perhaps of the ureter. In late examples large parts of

Chapter 8/*Urinary Tract Infection*

the kidney, involving several complete renal pyramids, may be replaced by calcified caseating tissue. Secondary infection may give rise to stone formation on previously damaged tissue. (Beware of African patients who may not show much calcification in their otherwise classical tuberculous lesions—remember that they are also relatively free from stone formation as well).

CYSTOSCOPY

Unless there has been haematuria it is not always necessary to perform cystoscopy. It may show uniform inflammation of the mucosa of the bladder. Occasionally shallow ulcers may be seen, and from time to time the characteristic deformed ureteric orifice of the golf-hole ureter will be noticed. Biopsy of the wall of the bladder may give the diagnosis. When in doubt, a catheter is passed up to the suspected kidney, and the irrigations sent for culture and search for acid-fast bacilli.

CONSIDER THE WHOLE PATIENT

One must never forget the rest of the patient. Many of these unfortunates will have active tuberculosis elsewhere in the body, particularly active pulmonary disease. Since the detection and therapy of these other types of tuberculosis is best left to experts in that field, the wise urologist should call in an expert to advise him.

Treatment

Today (after appropriate consultation) the patient is started off on Rifampicin 450 mg, INAH 300 mg and Ethambutol 800 mg daily for the first three months, after which treatment is continued with Rifampicin and INAH in the same dose for another three to six months. In patients with resistance to the first-line medication other regimes may have to be used.

In the *early case* with only the small lesion in one or more renal papillae, one expects to see complete resolution of the disease with perhaps, at worst, a little fleck of calcification to mark the place where the tuberculous granuloma was active in the first weeks.

However, in the early case, one does not know for certain whether there are silent but active tuberculous granulomas in the wall of the ureter or the bladder. With treatment these heal up so very rapidly, that unless one is particularly vigilant, one may fail to detect stricture formation in the ureter before it has given rise to needless atrophy of the kidney upstream of the stricture. Hence the rule nowadays that the IVU is repeated after three and six weeks of commencing treatment. If the ureter is seen to be narrowed at this stage one may try the patient on a course of steroids (to overcome oedema), but if these do not rapidly (within two or three weeks) lead to a return to normal, then an operation to enlarge the narrow part of the ureter is necessary. Usually the

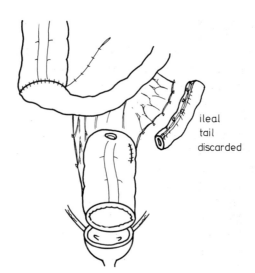

ileal
tail
discarded

Fig. 8.19. Caecocystoplasy enlarges the capacity of the contracted tuberculous bladder.

narrow part is at the pelviureteric junction, and calls for a pyeloplasty, but it may occur near the bladder and require reimplantation of the ureter.

In late cases, of patients whose kidneys, under treatment, shrink irreversibly, the kidney must be removed. In former times one had to remove the rest of the ureter as well (*nephroureterectomy*) but this is no longer considered to be necessary.

The patients must all be followed up for at least five years. During this time attention is paid to the development of hypertension and of renal calculi which might call for treatment on their own account. With modern regimens of therapy, relapse is very rare, but to make sure, annual examinations of the urine are carried out for acid-fast bacilli.

In patients in whom the bladder becomes exceedingly small as treatment leads to replacement of muscle by healing fibrous tissue, one may enlarge the capacity of the bladder by *cystoplasty*. There are several versions of this operation, but in general today the caecum is borrowed on its pedicle of ileocaecal artery, turned upside down and sewn onto the opened-out bladder. This results in a greatly enlarged capacity to the bladder and may allow the patient to return to a normal habit of micturition (Fig. 8.19).

Genital tuberculosis involving the prostate seminal vesicles vasa, epididymis and sometimes testis, may occur at the same time as renal tuberculosis, or out of the blue (see page 283).

BRUCELLA INFECTION OF THE KIDNEY

Although this is very rare, it is worth bearing in mind that *Brucella* can lead to a granuloma in the kidney almost indistinguishable from tuberculosis. It is worth remembering in communities where brucellosis is still rife amongst cattle.

Chapter 8/*Urinary Tract Infection*

HYDATID DISEASE OF THE KIDNEY

Even more rare in Britain is hydatid disease. It is caused by the larvae of the tapeworm *Taenia echinococcus* and is acquired by man from dogs who have been in contact with sheep. The hydatid cysts have their own polysaccharide wall, and around this the patient forms a second fibrous tissue wall. The fluid inside the cyst is highly antigenic and if spilt, can give rise to an anaphylactic reaction. It is usually clear, but microscopy shows the hooklets shed by the tiny tapeworm heads. If spilt, new cysts are formed. Today they present with vague loin pain and are detected with urography and ultrasound. In the host fibrous tissue wall one may see thin, calcified shadows, and on the ultrasound, one may detect the presence of 'cysts within cysts'. If these features are present, then the cysts should not be aspirated for fear of anaphylactic reaction, but the kidney should be removed with all due precautions to prevent spilling the contents of the cysts.

Hydatid fluid injected into the skin gives rise to a red wheal—the Casoni test: but this requires fresh fluid and is often not positive. More sensitive is the complement fixation test.

CHYLURIA AND FILARIASIS

In Burma, Malaysia and China a common problem is caused by a fistula between the perirenal lymphatics and the renal pelvis. Lymphangiography will show the communication between the two systems, and the patient suffers continual loss of the fat he has absorbed from his food into the urine. The urine may be like milk, from the fatty droplets leaking out of the cisterna chyli. More important, the patient becomes severely ill thanks to malabsorption. Although these patients can sometimes be shown to have suffered from *filariasis* this is by no means always the case—or at least—by no means always proven, and there may be some other as yet undiscovered cause for this strange fistula. *Wuchereria bancrofti* is a long, thin, hair-like roundworm about 10 cm in length and the thickness of a hair. It lives in lymphatics and lays little microfilariae that are sucked up by mosquitoes from the peripheral blood and carried to other victims. Around the living worm the body throws up a granulomatous reaction, and it is probably a result of this inflammation that the fistulae form, as a result of obstruction and dilatation of the affected lymph channels. Grotesque elephantiasis of the scrotum and lower limbs is one distressing consequence of similar lymphatic obstruction, and may require drastic, reductive, plastic surgery. Hydroceles are also found secondary to filariasis, containing thick milky fluid.

FURTHER READING

Asscher A.W. (1976) The natural history of urinary infection. In J.P. Blandy (ed.), *Urology*, Ch. 9. Blackwell Scientific Publications, Oxford.

Chapter 8/*Urinary Tract Infection*

Cameron D.D. & Azimi F. (1974) The value of excretory urography in the diagnosis of acute pyelonephritis. *Journal of Urology*, **112**, 546.

Edwards D., Normand I.C.S., Prescod N. & Smellie J.M. (1977) Disappearance of vesicoureteric reflux during long-term prophylaxis of urinary tract infection in children. *British Medical Journal*, **ii**, 285.

Flynn J.T., Molland E.A., Paris A.M.I. & Blandy J.P. (1979) The underestimated hazards of Xanthogranulomatous pyelonephritis. *British Journal of Urology*, **51**, 443.

Gow J.G. (1979) Genito-urinary tuberculosis. *British Journal of Hospital Medicine*, **22**, 556.

Marsh F.P. (1976) Natural and therapeutic defences against urinary infection. In J.P. Blandy (ed.), *Urology*, Ch. 10. Blackwell Scientific Publications, Oxford.

Michigan S. (1976) Genito-urinary fungal infections. *Journal of Urology*, **116**, 390.

Murray T.G. & Goldberg M. (1978) Analgesic-associated nephropathy in the USA: epidemiologic, clinical and pathogenetic features. *Kidney International*, **13**, 64.

Ramus N.I. & Mitchell J.P. (1974) Renal hydatid disease. *British Journal of Urology*, **61**, 402.

Ransley P.G. (1978) Vesico-ureteric reflux: continuing surgical dilemma. *Urology*, **12**, 246.

Yu H.Y., Ngan H. & Leong C.H. (1978) Chyluria—a 10 year follow up. *British Journal of Urology*, **50**, 126.

It is no exaggeration to say that surgery traces its origin to the ancient operation of 'cutting for the stone'. Even by the time of Hippocrates it was well recognized that this was a procedure that ought to be left to those specially trained to do it (advice which sometimes needs to be repeated even today). In the ancient world without postmortem dissection or X-rays, 'stone' meant stone in the urinary bladder. It took many years before it was recognized that most stones originated in the kidney.

Epidemiological studies show that the incidence of stones varies greatly in different populations, and that in the West there has been a stepwise increase in the incidence of calculi in the kidney and ureter, year by year, interrupted only by the two world wars. The inference is drawn that stone incidence reflects affluence and overfeeding, particularly with protein. To have a stone is not rare: nearly 20% of doctors are likely to have at least one episode of ureteric colic, and in other professions where dehydration is even more severe, the incidence can be higher.

STRUCTURE OF A STONE

It was recognized by Bowman (of the capsule) and Meckel (of the diverticulum) that stones did not consist only of crystalline material (like stones on the road). They had a structure. In each little stone there was an organic scaffold, clad in apatite (rather like the iron in ferroconcrete or the glass fibre in fibreglass, supporting a 'fill' of crystalline material (Fig. 9.1). In most stones the crystalline 'fill' was arranged in rings like the growth rings of a tree, but there is nothing to suggest that these measure episodes of precipitation of calculus or episodes of infection: similar growth rings can be produced artificially so long as crystals are deposited in media that contain an organic matrix-forming material as well. Nevertheless, we must always recognize that there are two elements in a stone, the matrix or scaffold and the 'fill' of crystalline precipitate. We know far more about the 'fill' than we do about the matrix, but this should never make us forget that it might be equally important. Nevertheless, no stones are known that do not contain some crystalline 'fill'.

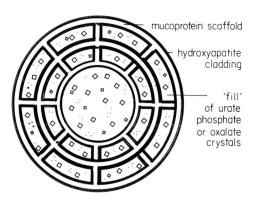

mucoprotein scaffold

hydroxyapatite cladding

'fill' of urate phosphate or oxalate crystals

Fig. 9.1. Diagrammatic representation of the structure of a stone.

Stone formation

If salt is added to a glass of water it continues to dissolve until a point is reached at which it will dissolve no further. This is the *saturation concentration*, well known to every schoolboy, who knows that it can be measured by the solubility product of the concentration of the ions making up the salt (Fig. 9.2).

However, under many conditions found in biological fluids, one can have a supersaturated solution which does not necessarily precipitate crystals—the *metastable* region—unless the solution is provided with a nucleus upon which stones can form, or unless the solution is allowed to remain stagnant and undisturbed for a considerable time.

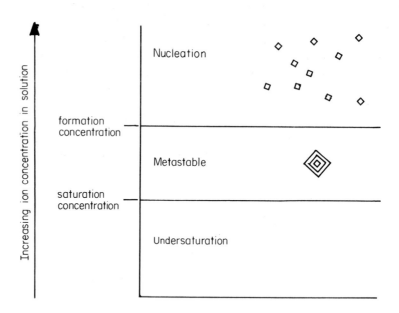

Fig. 9.2. Effects of increasing ion concentration in a solution such as urine.

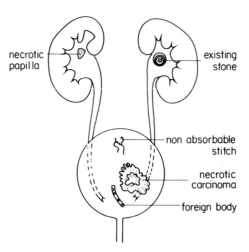

Fig. 9.3. Common conditions that act as nuclei for stone formation.

Chapter 9/*Urinary Calculi*

Above the metastable region is the concentration at which crystals will precipitate with or without a nucleus to form on: the crystals will be deposited on their own account. This is the range of *nucleation*.

Many factors influence the width of this 'metastable range': temperature, the presence or absence of colloids, the turbulence and rate of flow of the fluid. But above all, the concentration of the solute is of supreme importance. It will be influenced therefore by: (a) anything that gives rise to an excess of the solute in the urine, or (b) anything that makes the urine more concentrated.

Every schoolboy knows that to start a crystal growing, he must begin with something upon which the crystal can start—a nucleus. In the urinary tract many things will serve as a nucleus—dead papillae, dying fronds of cancer, foreign bodies such as sutures or the fragments of a burst catheter balloon. An existing stone is an ideal nucleus for the formation of more calculus (Fig. 9.3).

Many crystalline substances have a greatly different solubility in urine of different pH. Thus Magnesium ammonium phosphate is very insoluble in an alkaline urine (such as that provided by *Proteus mirabilis* which converts urea to ammonia), and urate is very insoluble in an acid urine (and can often be completely dissolved by making the urine alkaline with suitable medication).

All crystals like rest and quiet if they are to grow to any size, and there is a constant relationship between the presence of stagnant urine (e.g. in a ureterocele, a caliceal diverticulum, or in a hydronephrosis) and the formation of a stone.

SUPERSATURATION STONES

The purest example of the simple supersaturation stone is *cystine*. Here there is an inherited defect in the transport of cystine, ornithine, arginine and lysine ('coal') both in the renal tubule and in the gut (Fig. 9.4). Cystine is almost

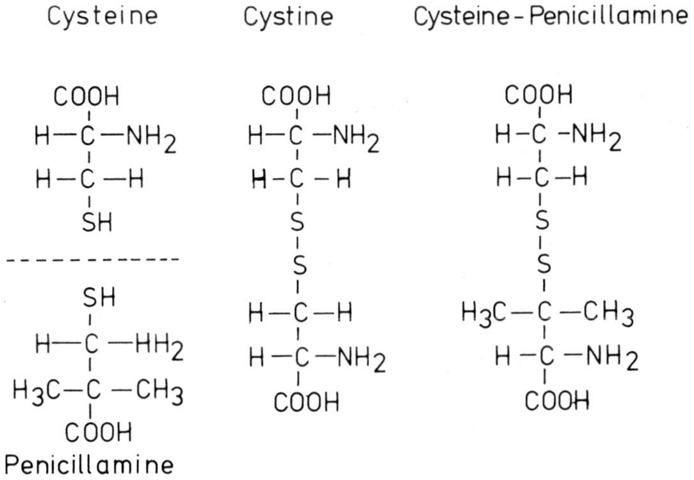

Fig. 9.4.

insoluble. If the patient is homozygous for cystinuria he or she may be passing almost 1 g/24 hours, and is almost certain to form stones. If heterozygous, the quantity of cystine is about half, and stone formation does not always occur. By giving cystinuric patients a very high fluid intake stones may be prevented and even dissolved. The cystine is more soluble in an alkaline urine.

Cystine is formed from two linked molecules of cysteine. By giving the patient penicillamine a soluble penicillamine–cysteine compound is formed that does not crystallize in the urine. In severe cases of cystinuria therefore penicillamine may be administered: but it does have side effects and must be used with care.

Another good example of a supersaturation stone is *uric acid*. Urates are soluble in alkaline urine with a pH greater than 6.8, but may precipitate in acid urine, especially when very concentrated as in the tropics. There is a congenital error in tubular function in which patients have difficulty in forming an alkaline urine, and tend to form urate stones unless given additional alkali such as bicarbonate. Others pass large amounts of uric acid in the urine because of gout or breaking-down of large volumes of protein, e.g. in the course of response of bulky tumours to chemotherapy. In such patients one can block the formation of uric acid by administering allopurinol (which inhibits xanthine oxidase) in addition to a high fluid input and alkalis.

Classical *calcium oxalate* or *calcium phosphate* stones are found when the urinary calcium concentration becomes excessive. This is seen in hyperpara-thyroidism (see page 99), as well as in patients losing calcium because of inactivity, e.g. when confined to bed with a fracture, or because of bony destruction by metastases. In these patients the ion in excess is calcium, but it is just as dangerous to have an excess of oxalate in the urine.

An excess of *oxalate* may occur in the rare congenital disease hyperoxaluria leading to formation of hundreds of little calculi in the collecting tubules of the kidneys. Fortunately many of these cases respond to treatment with large doses

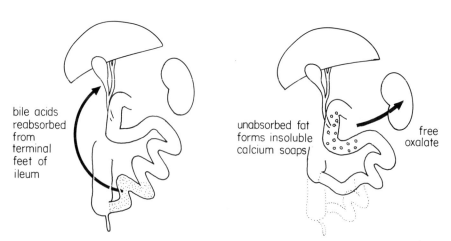

bile acids reabsorbed from terminal feet of ileum

unabsorbed fat forms insoluble calcium soaps

free oxalate

Fig. 9.5. Hyperoxaluria after disease or surgical removal of the last feet of the ileum.

Chapter 9/*Urinary Calculi*

of pyridoxine. Another form of hyperoxaluria occurs after illness or surgical removal of the last few feet of the ileum, e.g. in Crohn's disease. Bile acids are (Fig. 9.5) normally absorbed in this part of the bowel. If they are no longer absorbed, they are not available to be recycled in the liver, or excreted in the bile. Thus, fat in the diet is not emulsified and absorbed, but has to remain in the lumen of the bowel where it forms insoluble soaps with dietary calcium. This in turn leaves a relative excess of dietary oxalate available to be absorbed that in turn finds its way into the urine. This may be prevented by avoiding oxalate-containing food (e.g. tea, coffee, chocolate, spinach, rhubarb) and adding cholestyramine to the diet, which binds oxalate in the lumen of the bowel.

In *idiopathic hypercalciuria*, which is very common among stone formers, there is an excess of calcium in the 24 hour urine (in males more than 350 mg/24 hours, in females more than 300 mg/24 hours). It is not really certain that this matters in females, but it certainly is related to recurrent stone formation in a small group of males with a history of passing stone after stone. Its treatment is a matter for continuing argument. Basically one may try to limit the amount of calcium and oxalate in the diet, prevent it from being reabsorbed by giving something to keep it in an insoluble form in the bowel, or give something that finds its way into the urine and is believed to help keep the calcium oxalate crystals in suspension and stop them from sticking together to form an obstructive stone.

Three kinds of 'idiopathic hypercalciuria' are recognized:
1 *Renal*—in which there is a decreased tubular reabsorption of calcium.
2 *Resorptive*—in which there is an excessive mobilization of calcium salts from bone.
3 *Absorptive*—in which there is evidence of an increased intestinal absorption of calcium.

Logically one should adapt the form of treatment to the type of idiopathic hypercalciuria that one discovers. In practice however it must be pointed out that very few of the regimens now in use for this condition can be shown to do any good in prospective controlled studies.

Hyperparathyroidism

Perhaps the most important type of supersaturation stone is that seen in hyperparathyroidism. The parathyroid gland secretes a hormone that encourages osteoclasts to dissolve the bony skeleton and releases calcium into the bloodstream. Normally the secretion of the parathyroids are regulated by the level of calcium in the blood. Calcium in the blood exists, (a) as a large fraction bound to protein, and (b) a smaller fraction in solution of which only part is ionized. The product [CaxP] is kept constant. If the level of calcium is raised then that of phosphate falls and vice versa. We can distinguish three types of hyperparathyroidism.

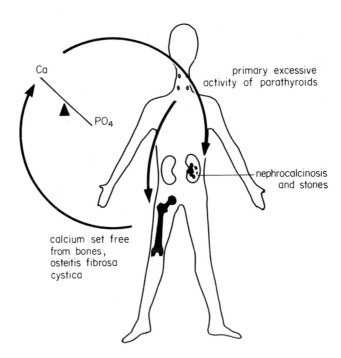

Fig. 9.6. Scheme of the sequence of events in primary hyperparathyroidism.

1. PRIMARY HYPERPARATHYROIDISM (Fig. 9.6)

For no very clear reason the parathyroid glands start to secrete more parathormone than is needed. More calcium salts are leached out of the skeleton and added to the blood to elevate the plasma [Ca]. In turn the plasma [PO$_4$] falls. (This fall in plasma phosphate may be related to compensatory slowing of reabsorption of phosphate in the proximal tubule; this formed the basis of a diagnostic test, now generally given up.) The superfluous calcium is filtered into the urine. In severe cases one may find precipitation of calcium containing stones in the renal tubules (a form of *nephrocalcinosis*). The more usual patients form stones downstream in the renal calices or pelvis. Occasionally the diagnosis is only made after discovering massive collections of over-active osteoclasts that lead to cystic areas in the bones—especially of the jaw (*osteitis fibrosa cystica*). In urological practice every patient with a stone should have his urinary calcium measured over a 24 hour period and his plasma calcium measured at least twice. If the plasma calcium is found to be elevated the diagnosis may be confirmed by measuring the plasma parathormone level using a radioimmunoassay.

2. SECONDARY HYPERPARATHYROIDISM

In renal failure among the metabolic products that cannot be excreted by the ailing kidney is phosphate and as the plasma [PO$_4$] rises so the plasma [Ca] must fall. The plasma [Ca] is sometimes precipitated in soft tissues (heterotopic

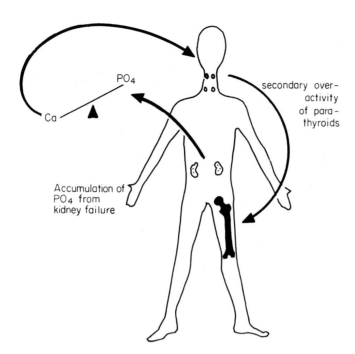

Fig. 9.7. Events in secondary hyperparathyroidism begin with the accumulation of phosphates along with other waste products as a result of renal insufficiency.

calcification) or put back into the bones. The parathyroids respond to the lowered plasma [Ca] by putting forth more parathormone, accomplishing this by hypertrophy of all four parathyroid glands. This secondary hyperparathyroidism is commonly encountered among patients on regular dialysis treatment for renal failure, and when detected, can largely be prevented by giving large doses of vitamin D to help absorption of calcium from the bowel. Occasionally it is necessary to remove the hyperplastic parathyroid glands (Fig. 9.7).

3. TERTIARY HYPERPARATHYROIDISM

There may come a time when the over-active hyperplastic parathyroid glands do not seem to know when to stop, and they keep on growing and overworking, and instead of secreting just as much parathormone as is needed to keep up the blood calcium, they put out an excess. Osteolysis proceeds apace while at the same time calcium is laid down in heterotopic soft tissues. This is not reversed by extra vitamin D and the parathyroid glands must be removed.

PARATHYROIDECTOMY (Fig. 9.8)

There are usually four parathyroid glands, normally about the size of a pea, and they lie behind or buried in the lateral lobes of the thyroid gland and are found by following along the superior and inferior thyroid arteries. Since many patients with parathyroid tumours also have small, benign nodules in the thyroid, the surgical discovery of any suspicious lump must always be checked

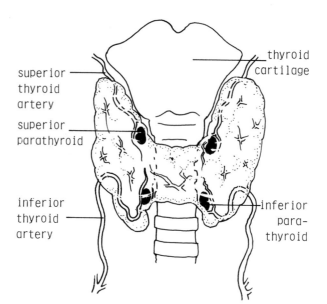

Fig. 9.8. Situation of the four parathyroid glands behind the thyroid, in close relationship to the thyroid arteries.

by careful frozen sections. Since primary hyperparathyroidism may be due either to an adenoma in one parathyroid gland, or to hyperplasia of all four glands, it is nowadays the rule to examine each parathyroid and take a biopsy of each one. The operation is technically difficult and calls for considerable experience of thyroid surgery if the results are to be good. Occasionally the offending parathyroid gland cannot be found and the plasma calcium remains elevated. It is then necessary to open and search the mediastinum—usually performed at a second operation through a median sternotomy incision.

HOW MOST STONES BEGIN AND GROW

Carr's concretions

In the kidneys of patients with recurrent calcium stones, tiny, spherical concretions can be found in and around the collecting ducts of the renal papilla. They are, at this stage very hard. They are made up of calcium phosphate and a mucoprotein, and it is possible that they actually originate inside tubular cells.

Randall's plaques

These little concretions accumulate under the epithelium at the tip of the renal papilla where they form shining plaques that can easily be seen with the nephroscope at operation. Randall observed them at postmortem and drew the inference that they would be likely to separate and form the nucleus of a small stone. When they separate they leave an irregularity in the papilla, in which

Chapter 9/*Urinary Calculi*

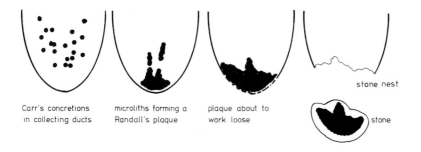

Carr's concretions in collecting ducts

microliths forming a Randall's plaque

plaque about to work loose

stone nest

stone

Fig. 9.9. How most stones begin in the renal papilla.

further stones may accumulate, just as they do in any irregular place offering a nucleus for precipitation (Fig. 9.9).

Papillary necrosis

Any of the many causes of papillary necrosis (p. 72) that lead to detachment of a little lump of dead tissue into a supersaturated urine may allow a stone to be deposited upon it. In some small calculi careful section and appropriate staining reveals the ghost of the original papillary tubules inside the middle of the stone.

Caliceal calculi

However they have been formed, the stone at this stage is usually quite small, and tends to take on a pyramidal shape, growing bit by bit until it forms a cast of the calix. Such caliceal calculi are very common. They may cause no symptoms year after year. Very exceptionally they are accompanied by severe pain, probably because they become jammed in the neck of the calix from time to time (Fig. 9.10). On other occasions the patient is troubled by recurrent

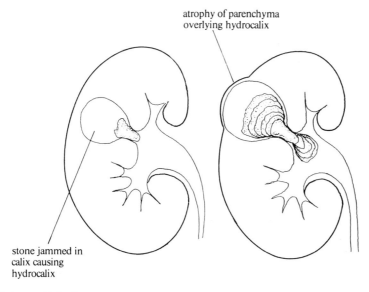

atrophy of parenchyma overlying hydrocalix

stone jammed in calix causing hydrocalix

Fig. 9.10. Stone in a calix.

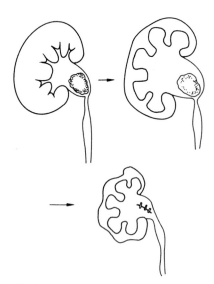

Fig. 9.11. Atrophy following obstruction from a stone impacted at the pelviureteric junction.

urinary infections that never clear up because the offending organisms can hide away from antibiotics in the porous crevices inside the stone. If such a caliceal stone is jammed in a caliceal neck, one may have an infected distended pyocalix upstream of the stone. In such a patient with persistent pain, persistent infection, or demonstrable pyocalix, the stone ought to be removed. In other patients a small caliceal stone can be safely observed.

Stone in the renal pelvis (Fig. 9.11)

Often a stone that has formed in a calix slips into the renal pelvis, but cannot get out down the ureter. It acts as a continuing nucleus for further stone formation, and inevitably grows. If one first discovers a pelvic stone that is less than 0.5 cm in diameter one can wait and hope that it might go down the ureter, but if it is larger than this, it ought to be removed before it gets jammed in the pelviureteric junction. If the stone is so jammed, and if the urine upstream of the stone is infected, then the patient runs a serious risk of bacteraemia. His kidney rapidly deteriorates from the combined attack of infection and obstruction—'pyonephrosis'.

Few of these stones do not give rise to pain, again usually fixed 'renal' pain in the loin, but sometimes, when they jam in the pelviureteric junction, they are accompanied by pain radiating towards the groin or vulva. Sometimes there is a paradoxical increased irritability of the bladder and the patient may experience frequency and discomfort on voiding. I have never understood this symptom, but have on several occasions been referred an elderly patient with supposed prostatism only to discover a stone in the kidney, removal of which entirely relieves the symptoms. Haematuria is often found in patients with stones in the renal pelvis.

Stone in the ureter (Fig. 9.12)

These give rise to pain often in inverse proportion to their size. 'The little dogs make the most noise'. The pain comes on suddenly and can be excruciating. Women who have experienced a difficult childbirth as well as a ureteric calculus say they would rather have another baby than another stone. The pain comes on in waves, makes the patient roll and twist in the attempt to get relief. Often there is an accompanying disturbance of intestinal transport and the patient frequently vomits. There is often gaseous distension of the small and large bowel and there may be constipation or sometimes diarrhoea. Even experienced surgeons may be misled into considering a diagnosis of intestinal obstruction when these bowel symptoms are particularly severe. On examination one may detect tenderness over the kidney or in the loin. Testing the patient's urine may reveal microscopic haematuria—indeed if the urine is examined soon after the colic, red cells are almost invariably present on microscopy.

Stones less than 0.5 cm in diameter can usually be passed down the ureter. They may have great difficulty in doing so, and the patient experiences very

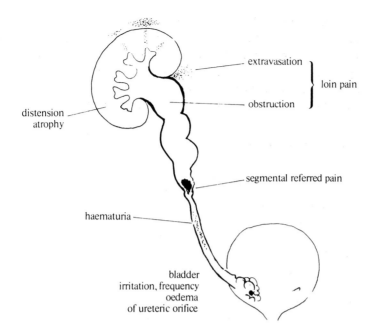

extravasation ⎤
              ⎬ loin pain
obstruction   ⎦

distension
atrophy

segmental referred pain

haematuria

bladder
irritation, frequency
oedema
of ureteric orifice

Fig. 9.12. Clinical features of a stone in the ureter.

severe pain, but so long as these stones make steady progress, and so long as there is no evidence of atrophy of the kidney parenchyma upstream of the stone, then it is safe to defer surgery. Again, the most dangerous situation is when obstruction upstream of the stone is accompanied by infection. Here there is a serious danger of septicaemia, and the obstructed, infected kidney is very likely to undergo serious inflammatory destruction.

Stone in the bladder (Fig. 9.13)

Many calculi end up in the bladder having safely gone right down the ureter. If there is some obstruction to the outflow from the bladder, the stones cannot get out. This is seen nowadays in the West almost exclusively in elderly men with prostatic outflow obstruction. In women, stones in the bladder are rare, except when they form on some other foreign material, such as a stitch or a fragment of catheter that serves as a nucleus for stone growth.

Many patients who are found today to have a calculus in the bladder have symptoms of outflow obstruction without pain or haematuria. But a few will still give the classical history of pain referred to the tip of the penis, which becomes worse on walking about and taking exercise, and is relieved by lying down. This is thought to be the result of the altered position of the stone, that gives most discomfort when it sits on the trigone in the standing position. Frequency, haematuria and painful voiding are often experienced, and many of the patients will also have symptoms of urinary infection.

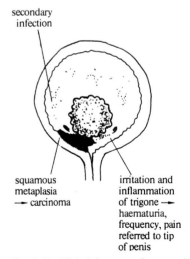

secondary
infection

squamous
metaplasia
→ carcinoma

irritation and
inflammation
of trigone →
haematuria,
frequency, pain
referred to tip
of penis

Fig. 9.13. Clinical features of a stone in the bladder.

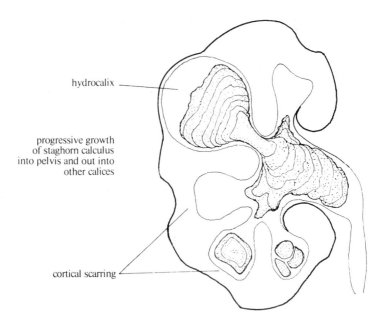

hydrocalix

progressive growth
of staghorn calculus
into pelvis and out into
other calices

cortical scarring

Fig. 9.14. Formation of a typical staghorn calculus.

Staghorn stones (Fig. 9.14)

Almost always as a result of infection of the urine with *Proteus mirabilis*, stones forming in the calices or the renal pelvis grow at a great rate until they fill almost the whole of the collecting system to produce a branched stone—the 'coral-like' stone or 'staghorn calculus'. The danger of these calculi is that they are nearly always infected and if they block the calices or the pelviureteric junction, as they quickly do, then the kidney turns into an obstructed and infected bag of pus. Septicaemia and pyonephrosis may be followed by perinephric abscess as an acute complication, or xanthogranuloma as a more chronic one (see page 86).

INVESTIGATION OF THE PATIENT WITH A URINARY CALCULUS

There are two jobs to be done: (a) to see if the stone is doing any harm and decide whether or not it needs to be removed, and (b) to find out, if possible, why the patient formed the stone so as to be able to help him avoid recurrences in future.

Should the stone be removed?

Of course if a stone is causing severe, unbearable and continuing pain, then it ought to be removed. But more often the reason why a stone must be removed is because it is threatening the kidney, or because there is a risk of bacteraemia. A

Chapter 9/*Urinary Calculi*

stone that is not causing obstruction, and is not likely to cause obstruction, may be safely watched. To decide, one needs to know the anatomical location of the stone and the state of the urinary collection system above and below it. Hence every patient with a calculus needs a urogram and urine culture. In many cases the decision is an easy one: the urogram reveals an obstructed system or the urine is infected. In many other instances one discovers a tiny stone that is making progress down the ureter, and will advise that it is safer to allow the stone to pass spontaneously than operate on it.

The chief difficulty arises in connection with stones in the ureter. In every case one must carefully weigh the risks of operation against the risks of allowing the stone to pass spontaneously. Very gross obstructive changes in a urogram performed at the height of the first attack of ureteric colic may resolve entirely within 24 hours. The indications for operating to remove a stone in the ureter require very careful thought and experience, but the following are useful guidelines:

1. STONE TOO BIG

Stones larger than 0.5 cm in diameter on the radiography may pass down a ureter without causing harm, particularly in a woman with a wide ureter, or in a patient who has previously passed such stones without endangering his kidney. But for most patients, one needs to seriously think about removing the stone if it is larger than 0.5 cm. The older generation of surgeons would advise operation if the stone was 'larger than a date stone'.

2. URINE INFECTED

Any stone with obstruction upstream of the stone and with infected urine means that there is a risk of septicaemia and the stone ought, almost certainly, to be removed without delay. Of course there are exceptions to this principle: many pelvic stones pose no emergency threat in spite of known urinary infection.

3. STONE MAKING NO PROGRESS

Despite several attacks of ureteric colic the little stone may not be moving down the ureter. To know how long such a stone can be safely left is extraordinarily difficult, and the decision must be tailored to the individual patient. No exact rules can be laid down.

4. KIDNEY AND URETER BECOMING OBSTRUCTED

As a rule when one is expecting a stone to pass safely down the ureter, its progress is monitored by repeating the intravenous urogram at intervals of, say, four to six weeks. If these show dilatation of the upper tract (not counting the initial obstructive urogram at the height of the first attack of colic) then probably the stone ought to be removed.

Why did the patient form the stone?

All patients with urinary calculi should be investigated to see whether there is some correctable disorder.

A. ANALYSIS OF THE STONE

No stone should ever be given to the patient as a trophy. (He can look at it and admire it, and, of course, your handiwork). It must be analysed principally to see if it contains cystine or uric acid. Appropriate medication must be called for if it is made of magnesium–ammonium–phosphate (and hence attributable to urea-splitting infection, usually with *Proteus mirabilis*) or calcium phosphate or oxalate.

B. BACTERIOLOGICAL STUDIES

Not only should the urine be carefully cultured, but so should the renal pelvis when it is opened at operation. In larger stones it can be very useful to have the calculus ground up and cultured: often one can discover the offending *Proteus* inside the stone when it has not been grown from the urine.

C. BLOOD CHEMISTRY

At least two samples of blood should be measured for calcium phosphate and urate. If the plasma calcium is found to be elevated on these, and repeated examinations, using a well-checked laboratory method, then it is wise to have the patient's plasma parathormone measured by radioimmunoassay.

D. URINE CHEMISTRY

A 24-hour specimen of urine should be measured for uric acid and calcium. When possible, in recurrent stone formers without any other obvious cause, it is wise to have the urinary oxalate measured as well. Unfortunately the technical method is at present not available in most laboratories. A qualitative test for cystine using nitroprusside should always be confirmed by quantitative measurement of cystine, lysine, arginine and ornithine in a 24-hour specimen.

FURTHER READING

Coe F.L., Keck J. & Norton E.R. (1977) The natural history of calcium urolithiasis. *Journal of the American Medical Association*, **238**, 1519.

Danielson B.G. (ed.) (1979) Proceedings of the Symposium on Urolithiasis. *Scandinavian Journal of Urology and Nephrology*, **Suppl. 53**.

Gardner G.L. & Doremus R.H. (1978) Crystal growth inhibitors in human urine: effect on calcium oxalate kinetics. *Investigative Urology*, **15,** 478.

Griffith D.P., Musher D.M. & Itin C. (1976) Urease; the primary cause of infection-induced urinary stones. *Investigative Urology*, **13,** 346.

Hautmann R., Lehmann A. & Komor S. (1980) Calcium and oxalate concentrations in human renal tissue: the key to the pathogenesis of stone formation? *Journal of Urology*, **123,** 317.

Malek R.S. & Boyce W.H. (1977) Observations on the ultrastructure and genesis of urinary calculi. *Journal of Urology*, **117,** 336.

Wickham J.E.A. (ed.) (1979) *Urinary Calculous Disease*. Churchill Livingstone, London.

Chapter 10 Neoplasms of the Kidney

Tumours may arise either from the parenchyma or the collecting system of the kidney. Of the parenchymal tumours one main variety is seen in children, the other in adults. Of the tumours of the collecting system most of the pathological features are identical with the tumours arising elsewhere in the urothelium.

RENAL PARENCHYMAL TUMOURS OF CHILDREN— EMBRYOMA, WILMS' TUMOUR

This tumour was described by Rance in 1814 before Wilms (1899) was born (such is the injustice of eponymous fame). It accounts for 10% of childhood malignancies and occurs in 1:13 000 live births. Odd genetic associations link Wilms' tumour with congenital aniridia, hemihypertrophy, exomphalos and macroglossia. Some family trees have an undue incidence of children with Wilms' tumour or multicystic disease and adults with renal cell (Grawitz) carcinoma, and neurofibromatosis.

Very few of these tumours are seen after the age of six (though rare examples occur, even in adults). In children there is a very important sub-group, found in the first few months of life, that behaves very differently from those found in older children.

The babies' tumour behaves almost as if it were benign: it is sometimes called a *mesoblastic nephroma* to distinguish it from the highly malignant tumour of older children.

Pathology

Mesoblastic nephromas are made up of diffuse mesenchymal proliferation between islands of healthy-looking, renal parenchyma. The ordinary *embryoma*, *Wilms' tumour*, shows no clear distinction between the healthy kidney and the malignant part. About one in ten are bilateral. Almost every tissue that could arise from mesoderm may be found in these tumours, and so one discovers bone, cartilage, smooth and striated muscle, nerve and connective tissue. The main (and the worst) parts are usually rhabdomyosarcomatous in appearance. They spread by direct invasion, boring into the psoas, the bowel and adjacent tissues. They spread by involvement of the renal vein and by haematogenous dissemination, usually to the lungs, via the lymphatics. If they get into the renal pelvis, it is relatively late, and haematuria is therefore a poor prognostic feature (Fig. 10.1).

Clinical features

'A big lump in a wasted baby' is the classical way in which these children are brought to your attention, but often these tumours cause pain, and are discovered at laparotomy. If haematuria occurs, as it does in a third of the babies, it is seldom found except when the urine is tested. Other features may

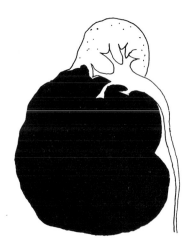

Fig. 10.1. Embryoma of the kidney (Wilms').

bring the patient to hospital: hypertension, fever and a raised red or white cell count may at first mislead the investigating team.

Investigations

The main differential diagnosis is from a *neuroblastoma*. The most useful investigation is the urogram, using, in the baby, a leg vein, and perhaps injecting the contrast straight into the vena cava so that a cavogram is obtained at the same time. Lateral radiographs are taken in order to be sure that the mass is not arising outside the kidney. Speckled calcification is more commonly seen in a neuroblastoma than in a Wilms' tumour, and the neuroblastoma usually shifts the kidney to one side or downwards rather than distorting the urogram. The other side is often involved. If the necessary skill is available, an arteriogram may help detect bilateral Wilms' tumour and so guide one in planning how best to treat the other side, e.g. by partial nephrectomy.

Management

Within the professional lifetime of many surgeons of today the outlook for the child with the Wilms' tumour has been completely transformed. Today more than 80% can be cured. But this is only accomplished by making sure that every example of this uncommon tumour is offered the very best and most up-to-date team management. There can be no doubt that the striking improvement in cure rate has only been obtained by close collaboration between surgeon, oncologist, and radiotherapist. No child with this disease should be treated except in a centre that is currently participating in studies to improve treatment. Your first duty therefore is to spot the tumour, and then to make sure the child is referred to an appropriate specialist centre: it is not a task for the occasional surgeon in a small hospital.

Treatment begins with a radical nephrectomy. The first step is transabdominal laparotomy at which the renal vessels are ligated early on before the kidney is handled and the malignant cells disseminated. A full exploration of the abdomen must be carried out, the liver and lymph nodes carefully palpated, and the other kidney minutely examined. Nephrectomy is preceded by the first of a five day course of *Actinomycin D*. After the kidney has been removed, *Vincristine* is added, and the bed of the kidney is treated with radiotherapy. To subject the little child to these severe drug regimens, such major surgery, and such a dose of radiotherapy, calls for the utmost skill in the day to day care of the child. Teamwork is essential. Experience is necessary. It is not a job for the amateur. Radiotherapy may be omitted for children in the first year of life.

The aftermath of this treatment may be complete cure. But a price may be paid. Some of the children given early types of radiation dosage were left with epiphyses that failed to grow, resulting in severe scoliosis.

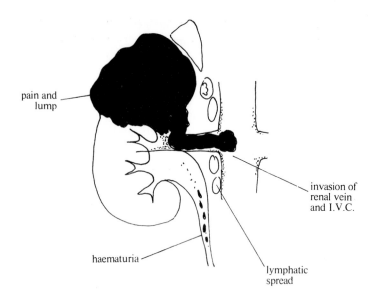

pain and
lump

invasion of
renal vein
and I.V.C.

haematuria

lymphatic
spread

Fig. 10.2. Adenocarcinoma of the kidney.

ADENOCARCINOMA OF THE ADULT KIDNEY— GRAWITZ TUMOUR, HYPERNEPHROMA (Fig. 10.2)

Grawitz has as little title to his eponym as Wilms to his, nevertheless he offers us a convenient shorthand for this tumour. Rare before puberty, more common in men, it is typically a cancer of elderly people. Like Wilms' tumour, there is an undue incidence of Grawitz' tumours in certain families, and in some it is associated with the von Hippel Lindau syndrome—cerebellar and retinal angiomas occurring with cysts in the liver and pancreas. It may perhaps be associated with cadmium pollution, possibly with oestrogen ingestion.

Pathology

Many healthy adults have tiny areas in their kidneys that resemble this tumour, and by convention, they are not called adenocarcinomas unless they are at least 3 cm in diameter (some pathologists say 4 cm). This is of course well within the size that can be detected by urography, ultrasound or angiography. Three grades of malignancy are recognized: a very well-differentiated papillary carcinoma, with an orderly arrangement of large, clear, lipid-packed cells; a moderately differentiated one; and an anaplastic type with a very poor prognosis. Macroscopically these tumours are usually blotchy, from breaking down of necrosed tissue, and bright yellow, from the lipid accumulated in the clear cells. They spread by direct invasion into the surrounding tissues, by invasion of the renal vein and so by haematogenous dissemination, and by lymphatic spread in the usual way of tumours elsewhere.

There is one interesting sub-group of these tumours that deserves to be remembered: it is rare, and almost certainly benign. Its cells are eosinophilic, they often present with hypertension, they have a characteristic angiographic 'spoke-wheel' picture, and they are usually called *oncocytoma*.

Clinical features

Haematuria, pain, and a lump are the three cardinal features of a Grawitz' tumour. Haematuria occurred in former times in most patients, but it was always a relatively late feature, since it meant that the cancer had eroded into the collecting system. Today it occurs in only 40% of patients, the others being diagnosed on the basis of other symptoms. Pain is quite common: it is difficult for the patient to describe and to localize. A vague pain in the loin is sometimes all he can say he has noticed. A lump may be felt by the examining doctor, but of equal importance is the feeling on the patient's part of a lump inside him. Always pay very careful attention to the patient who has noticed a lump—he is usually right.

Other curious symptoms seem to reflect an alteration in the immunological defences of the patient. One large group come to hospital for the investigation of loss of weight, illness, tiredness, unexplained fever and sweating, and are found to have pyrexia, raised sedimentation rate and wierd alterations in their blood count. Excess *erythropoietin* production by the renal cell carcinoma may send up the red cell count, but similar elevations may be seen in any or all of the white cell series and these may mimic leukaemia. On the other hand there may be marrow suppression, thrombocytopenia, clubbing and pulmonary osteo-dystrophy. Alas, many patients only appear in hospital because of symptoms arising in distant metastases, a lump in the chest wall, or a pathological fracture. It is worth remembering that the histological picture of the Grawitz' tumour is so characteristic that when your pathologist reports that a metastasis has arisen from a primary in the kidney he is usually right, even though the IVU may (then) seem to be normal.

Investigations (Fig. 10.3)

The first step is to have an *excretion urogram*. It will show a soft tissue mass (inevitably quite a large one). The mass may squeeze or displace the adjacent collecting system. At this stage one notes a 'space occupying lesion of the kidney'. What should be done then?

The next step is to get an *ultrasound* picture of the kidney. This will show whether or not there are echoes inside the mass. If there are no echoes, then a fine needle is passed into the cyst and it is aspirated, and the fluid is looked at, and sent for cytological examination. Turbid or blood-stained fluid suggests cancer. If there are echoes inside the mass, the kidney will have to be explored: echoes may be due to the presence of a multilocular cyst, to hydatid disease of the kidney, to thickened fibrin or pus inside a cyst, to the lump being an abscess, or a granuloma.

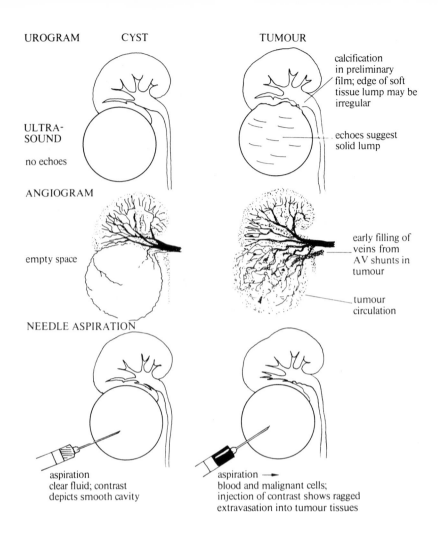

UROGRAM   CYST   TUMOUR

calcification in preliminary film; edge of soft tissue lump may be irregular

ULTRA-SOUND

no echoes

echoes suggest solid lump

ANGIOGRAM

empty space

early filling of veins from AV shunts in tumour

tumour circulation

NEEDLE ASPIRATION

aspiration clear fluid; contrast depicts smooth cavity

aspiration →
blood and malignant cells; injection of contrast shows ragged extravasation into tumour tissues

Fig. 10.3. Cyst or tumour in the kidney.

In many patients a correct diagnosis will be made by *angiography*, and if the diagnosis of cancer is made, then one may proceed to the first step in the operation to remove the cancer, by blocking the main renal artery with gelfoam or chopped muscle or oxycel (embolization). In some patients the diagnosis is so clear that there is no need to perform angiography.

Other methods of investigation are occasionally helpful. CAT scanning will confirm what the cheaper and quicker ultrasound has already revealed. Cavography will detect masses squashing or filling the inferior vena cava (but will not deter the surgeon from trying to get the lump out). Many of these patients are unwell and old, and one must be very careful not to do too many diagnostic investigations that will in fact not help the surgeon, or put off the essential decision, which is to operate or not to operate.

Management

The first step is to remove the lump. It is usually easier to perform the nephrectomy by a transabdominal approach (see page 325). If the inferior vena cava is invaded, it is carefully taped, opened and then closed after removing the tumour.

If there are multiple metastases, there is a chance, albeit a small one, that they will disappear if the main mass of tumour can be removed. It is a chance that most surgeons wish to offer their patients. No chemotherapy (at the time of writing) has been shown to offer any benefit, but there is an interesting suggestion that immunotherapy with BCG may help metastases disappear.

A lot of attention is given in recent years to 'bench surgery' for tumours arising in a solitary kidney, or in both kidneys at the same time. It is quite clear that partial nephrectomy is useful in such patients, but there is really no need to remove the kidney from the patient in order to do this.

Progestogens are sometimes given for cancer of the kidney. A controlled clinical trial is still in progress at the time of updating this edition. They can do no harm, but there is no sound evidence that they do any good.

Rare tumours that mimic renal adenocarcinoma

In practice one can never be certain that these rare forms of space occupying tumour in the kidney are not carcinoma unless they are removed. We have mentioned *oncocytoma*. There may also be unusual *benign multilocular cysts*, causing a smooth lump with multiple echoes and a puzzling angiogram, which are quite benign. There is a rare benign *angiomyolipoma* that originates probably in the renal sinus fat, and an equally rare *fibroxanthosarcoma*.

Secondary carcinoma in the renal parenchyma

As part of widespread metastatic spread, usually from a primary in the lung, one can have secondary carcinomas in the kidney. They are sometimes bilateral.

UROTHELIAL TUMOURS OF THE RENAL PELVIS AND CALICES

As with tumours of the bladder, these are usually of transitional cell (*urothelial*) origin. Sometimes however, the urothelium undergoes metaplasia and turns into squamous epithelium from which *squamous* cell carcinoma arises, or adenomatous epithelium that gives rise to *adenocarcinoma*. In most cases one cannot discover the aetiology, but they occur in association with papillary necrosis and interstitial nephritis in Balkan nephropathy and analgesic nephropathy (see page 73). There is always a risk of a patient with a bladder cancer developing other tumours in the kidney or ureter, but the risk is almost limited to patients who show very active bladders. As a general rule an excretion urogram should be performed every two years in such patients.

Pathology

This is identical to the tumour found in the bladder (see page 188). One recognizes three *grades* of histological malignancy G1, G2, and G3, for the urothelial tumours. Squamous cell carcinoma occurs in association with long standing stones of the renal pelvis; adenocarcinoma arises after prolonged infection, and is exceedingly rare. All these tumours spread directly through the muscle of the calices and pelvis, invading the fat of the sinus and the overlying parenchyma. They spread into surrounding tissues directly, seldom involve the renal veins, but in the later stages, metastasize by way of lymphatics. Sometimes one discovers 'daughter' tumours downstream in the ureter, but one has no way of knowing whether these have originated there or have been seeded down from the kidney.

Clinical features (Fig. 10.4)

Tumours arising from the urothelium of the kidney and calices give rise to haematuria or pain. Investigation reveals a filling defect in a calix, or a fuzziness that is difficult to make out. Further investigations to confirm the diagnosis include retrograde uretrography, the aspiration of urine for papanicolaou cytology and sometimes angiography. A long, flexible, fibre-optic ureteroscope is available. In the writer's hands, this has not yet given a picture sufficiently clear to be useful, though perhaps future technical improvements will cause him to change his mind.

These tumours are often multifocal, and arise all over the inside of the collecting system of the kidney. But occasionally they take the form of a well-localized, papillary tumour on an easily defined stalk. In such cases it is well worth attempting a local removal of the tumour.

Treatment

Except in the rare cases where a local removal is appropriate, the aim of the operation is to remove the entire kidney and ureter right down to and including the place where the ureter enters the bladder. The operation is called *nephroureterectomy* (see page 343).

If the tumour has been shown to invade the extrapelvic tissues or perinephric fat, then the excision is followed by postoperative radiotherapy.

Chemotherapy on the lines now being followed for bladder cancer offers a logical additional precaution for locally invasive tumours, and in some patients one may obtain reasonable control of renal superficial tumours by injecting chemotherapeutic agents up the ureter.

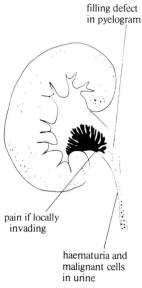

filling defect
in pyelogram

pain if locally
invading

haematuria and
malignant cells
in urine

Fig. 10.4. Salient features of a renal, papillary, transitional-cell carcinoma.

FURTHER READING

Clark P. & Anderson K. (1976) Tumours of the kidney and ureter. In J.P. Blandy (ed.), *Urology*. Blackwell Scientific Publications, Oxford.

Bengtsson U., Johansson S. & Angervall L. (1978) Malignancies of the upper urinary tract and their relation to analgesic abuse. *Kidney International*, **13**, 107.

Kantor A.F. (1977) Current concepts in the epidemiology and etiology of primary renal cell carcinoma. *Journal of Urology*, **117**, 415.

Mott M.G. (1975) Nephroblastoma (Wilms' Tumour). *British Journal of Hospital Medicine*, **13**, 161.

Harmer M.H. (ed.) (1978) *TNM Classification of Malignant Tumours*, 3rd edn. Union Internationale Contre le Cancer (UICC), Geneva.

Wallace D.M. (1976) Carcinoma of the urothelium. In J.P. Blandy (ed.), *Urology*. Blackwell Scientific Publications, Oxford.

Chapter 11
Vascular Disorders of the Kidney and Hypertension

INFARCTION

The renal arteries are end-arteries (Fig. 11.1) and so, if any of them are blocked, the entire territory supplied by them will become dead, with a thin rim of underoxygenated tissue around the necrotic zone. Infarcts of the kidney occur in old age, and give characteristic, deep, cortical scars. Others occur after operations on the heart in which clots are detached and plug one of the major segmental vessels. Clinically, such patients will have renal pain, sometimes have haematuria, and in subsequent urograms are noted to have loss of part of the cortex.

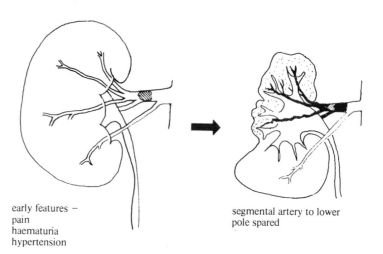

early features –
pain
haematuria
hypertension

segmental artery to lower
pole spared

Fig. 11.1. Infarct of the kidney.

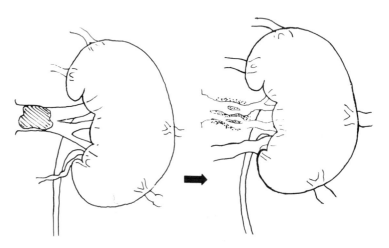

Fig. 11.2. Venous obstruction.

renal vein thrombosis may be followed by recovery thanks to alternative venous drainage – or may lead to atrophy

Chapter 11/*Vascular Disorders*

Venous thrombosis (Fig. 11.2)

Unlike the arteries, the veins of the kidney intercommunicate freely, and one expects complete occlusion of the main renal vein to be followed by recovery. Dehydrated children, ill from some other disorder, may develop pain and swelling in the kidney accompanied by haematuria. Urography shows no perfusion on the affected side. The treatment is to wait and see: most children will recover. The difficulty in practice is to make sure that the swelling is not a neoplasm. In adults the condition is very rare, and can be confirmed by means of a cavogram. It is sometimes seen as a sequel to acute glomerulonephritis. It is usually treated with intensive anticoagulant therapy, though sometimes success has been reported from open operation to remove the clot from the renal vein and cava.

ANEURYSM

One can recognize three types of renal artery aneurysm:
1 *Fusiform* aneurysm of the main renal artery, with or without extension to the origins of the main segmental arteries (Fig. 11.3).
2 *Saccular* aneurysm—sometimes of the main artery, sometimes of one of the major branches.
3 *Intra-renal arteriovenous fistulae*—sometimes these are congenital, more often they follow renal biopsy or operation, and most common of all, they

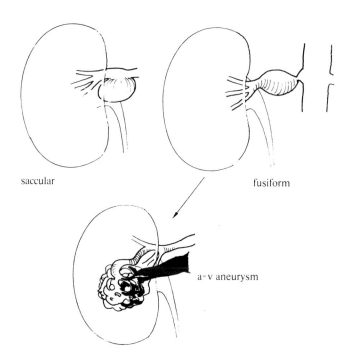

saccular

fusiform

a-v aneurysm

Fig. 11.3. Aneurysms of the renal artery.

Chapter 11/*Vascular Disorders*

occur in the middle of a *carcinoma* in which necrosis allows blood to pass from segmental artery branches into veins.

Clinically the saccular and fusiform aneurysms may go unnoticed unless the presence of calcification in their wall is detected in a plain radiograph, when it is easily mistaken for a stone. Sometimes ischaemia in the kidney parenchyma causes hypertension. Occasionally one can hear a bruit over the kidney. The arteriovenous shunt found in some malignant tumours may give rise to heart failure. Occasionally excess erythropoietin secretion by the affected kidney leads to polycythaemia.

Investigation of these cases depends essentially on good selective angiography.

Treatment of the malignant arteriovenous fistulae is of course by nephrectomy. In the unusual saccular aneurysms there is a great risk of spontaneous rupture, a risk estimated to be as high as 83%. If they do rupture, there is usually fatal, internal haemorrhage, so that unless the patient is already very ill from some other condition, it is much safer to explore to repair the aneurysm, when this is feasible, or remove both aneurysm and kidney, when it is not. Modern techniques involving cooling of the kidney, and perhaps 'bench surgery' using the operating microscope, may be used to facilitate reconstruction of the renal artery and its branches. 17% of aneurysms are intrarenal, 20% are bilateral and 50% involve the main artery or a major branch. Calcification is seen in 25%.

RENAL HYPERTENSION

Almost any disorder of the kidney may be complicated by hypertension; this includes pyelonephritic scarring, all forms of glomerulonephritis, tuberculosis, obstructive lesions of any kind, tumours, polycystic disease, and aneurysms. Hypertension itself may lead to damage to the renal arteries, and so make things worse by causing further ischaemia.

The renin–angiotensin mechanism

Renin is a proteolytic enzyme manufactured in the juxtaglomerular apparatus in response to a lowered pressure in the afferent arteriole of the glomerulus. Renin acts on *angiotensinogen*, one of the α_2-globulins in the plasma, to release *angiotensin I*, a decapeptide. Angiotensin I is further split by another enzyme in the lungs, to form *angiotensin II* (Fig. 11.4).

Angiotensin II has two effects: (a) it constricts peripheral blood vessels, and so raises peripheral resistance and helps maintain blood pressure, and (b) it stimulates the adrenal cortex to secrete *aldosterone*.

Aldosterone causes the renal tubules to conserve sodium and hence, results in water retention and an increase in circulating volume. Renin release is to some extent also governed by feed-back controls—thus an excess of aldosterone will inhibit release of renin, while on the other hand, low sodium in the

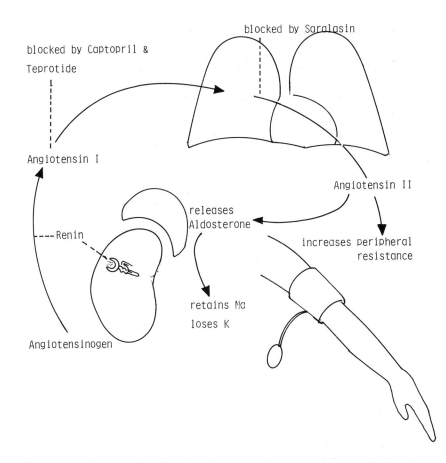

blocked by Captopril &
Teprotide

blocked by Saralasin

Angiotensin I

Renin

Angiotensin II

releases
Aldosterone

increases peripheral
resistance

retains Na
loses K

Angiotensinogen

Fig. 11.4. Train of events triggered off by the release of renin by the juxtaglomerular cells.

plasma promotes renin release. If the adrenals are diseased and there is a low output of aldosterone, then there may be compensatory release of renin. Conversely, in Conn's syndrome, an aldosterone-secreting tumour of the adrenal will inhibit renin production.

While many patients can be shown to have an increased renin secretion at a certain stage when renal lesions are initiating hypertension, a raised level of renin may not be found in a later stage.

Investigations for renal hypertension

Hypertension in young patients associated with a known disorder of the kidneys should always be investigated with a view to correcting the hypertension, by an appropriate operation. One may measure peripheral plasma renin, or pass catheters up the vena cava to take blood from the orifice of each renal vein and measure the renin content in them separately. Kidneys with an impaired arterial flow show a higher sodium concentration on the affected side, and one may collect urine from both kidneys with indwelling catheters (Howard–Stamey test). Renography will allow you to compare the blood flow to each kidney. All these investigations are more or less unreliable, and in the end, whether or not to operate on the kidney or the renal artery calls for the most careful consideration of each individual case.

In recent years chemical tests have been devised to check on the activity of the renin–angiotensin system. Saralasin blocks the action of angiotensin II, and when given, lowers the blood pressure if angiotensin II is responsible for keeping it up. Two other compounds Captopril and Teprotide stop angiotensin I from being turned into angiotensin II and have a comparable effect.

Above all, when one is looking for a disorder of the renal artery as a cause of the renin–angiotensin activity, it is necessary to obtain very good angiograms, and to be able to interpret them intelligently. Not every stenosis of the renal artery seen in the radiograph is accompanied by an impairment of renal blood flow. Several different types of vascular disorders are recognized as possible causes of renal hypertension.

1. ARTERIOSCLEROSIS (Fig. 11.5)

To some extent this is a normal concomitant of growing old. The atheroma may form a plaque at the origin of the main renal artery and partially or entirely block its lumen. In the smaller vessels the same process has a slightly different form—there is reduplication of the internal elastic lamina of the arterial wall

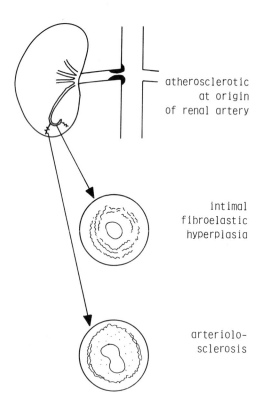

atherosclerotic
at origin
of renal artery

intimal
fibroelastic
hyperplasia

arteriolo-
sclerosis

Fig. 11.5. Variations on the theme of arterio-sclerosis. In the main renal artery and its major segmental branches, bulky plaques of ather-oma may block it. In middle-sized arteries, e.g. the arcuate vessels, there may be intimal fibroelastic hyperplasia. In the vessels of glo-merular afferent arteriole size, there is arterio-losclerosis, with hyaline material laid down directly under the intima.

Chapter 11/*Vascular Disorders*

and a narrowing of the lumen with fibrous tissue laid down in the intima. In the smallest vessels such as those entering the glomeruli, there is a third change in which eosinophilic hyaline material is accumulated under the endothelium.

All these changes are commonly seen in ordinary *benign hypertension*. As patients get older, there is some generalized shrinking of the kidney and occasional, obvious pits from old infarcts are seen.

In *malignant hypertension* the effect of the very high blood pressure on the smaller arterioles of the kidney is to damage their walls and lead to the deposition of eosinophilic material—so called fibrinoid necrosis.

2. RENAL ARTERY DYSPLASIA (Fig. 11.6)

This takes several forms according to whether the intima or the media of the artery is mainly affected. There may be thickening inside the internal elastic lamina (*intimal dysplasia*), or thickening in parts of the media with areas of thinning, leading to an angiographic appearance like a string of beads, the thin

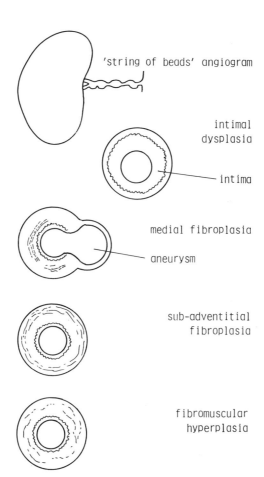

'string of beads' angiogram

intimal dysplasia

intima

medial fibroplasia

aneurysm

sub-adventitial fibroplasia

fibromuscular hyperplasia

Fig. 11.6. Renal arterial dysplasia may give a 'string of beads' appearance in the angiogram, and take several histological forms: intimal dysplasia, medial fibroplasia, sub-adventitial fibroplasia or fibromuscular hyperplasia.

places forming little aneurysmal balloons, the thick places causing stenosis. There may be fibrosis of the outer wall of the artery just under the adventitia (*sub-adventitial fibroplasia*) or the whole structure may be jumbled up with muscle and collagen of the media all being laid down in a disordered pattern (*fibromuscular hyperplasia*).

Treatment of renal hypertension (Fig. 11.7)

In many cases there is good reason for operating on the diseased kidney, e.g. where there is outflow obstruction from stenosis of the pelviureteric junction (see page 33), gross shrinking of the kidney from old interstitial nephritis, calculous disease, etc. Only in patients with a good kidney parenchyma and a localized disease of the main renal artery does the opportunity arise to carry out some form of renal arterial reconstruction. In such patients one may place a patch on the artery where it is narrowed, cut out the atheromatous segment and join the artery to the aorta again. Alternatively, one may replace the narrow part of the renal artery with a graft from the aorta, or an artery belonging elsewhere (either the splenic artery on the left side, or the internal iliac). Such operations give such poor results in patients over the age of 40 that nephrectomy is usually more likely to help them.

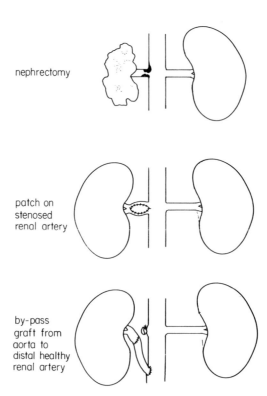

nephrectomy

patch on stenosed renal artery

by-pass graft from aorta to distal healthy renal artery

Fig. 11.7. Renal artery stenosis causing hypertension may be treated by nephrectomy if the other kidney is normal, by letting in a patch (from a vein) onto the stenosed vessel, or by means of an arterial graft, by-passing the narrowed segment.

FURTHER READING

Baum N.H., Moriel E. & Carlton C.E. Jr. (1978) Renal vein thrombosis. *Journal of Urology*, **119**, 443.

Fair W.R. (1976) Renovascular hypertension—assessment of functional disorders. In D.I. Williams & G.D. Chisholm (eds), *Scientific Foundations of Urology*, p. 117. Heinemann, London.

Lawson J.C., Boerth R., Dean R.H. & Foster J.H. (1977) Diagnosis and management of renovascular hypertension in children. *Archives of Surgery*, **112**, 1307.

Ledingham J.G.G. (1976) Renal disease and hypertension. In D.I. Williams & G.D. Chisholm (eds), *Scientific Foundations of Urology*, p. 113. Heinemann, London.

Marks L.S., Maxwell M.H., Gross C., Waks U. & Kaufman J.J. (1977) Angiotensin blockage in renovascular hypertension: a controlled prospective study. *British Journal of Urology*, **49**, 181.

McCarron J.P., Marshall V.F. & Whitsell J.C. (1975) Indications for surgery on renal artery aneurysms. *Journal of Urology*, **114**, 177.

Owen K. (1976) Renal hypertension. In J.P. Blandy (ed.), *Urology*, p. 375. Blackwell Scientific Publications, Oxford.

Stanley J.C. & Fry W.J. (1977) Surgical treatment of renovascular hypertension. *Archives of Surgery*, **112**, 1291.

Vandenburg M.J., Sharman V.L. & Marsh F.P. (1978) Prolonged treatment of high renin hypertension with a converting enzyme inhibitor. *British Medical Journal*, **2**, 866.

Wickham J.E.A. (1976) Diseases of the renal artery, veins and lymphatics. In J.P. Blandy (ed.), *Urology*, p. 348. Blackwell Scientific Publications, Oxford.

Chapter 12
The
Adrenal Gland

The surgery of the adrenal glands is mainly concerned with tumour formation in them. Endocrine control of cancer by adrenalectomy has been largely replaced by other techniques.

SURGICAL ANATOMY

Each adrenal gland lies medial and adjacent to the upper pole of each kidney. On the right the adrenal drains into the vena cava by an exceedingly short and delicate vein that is easily torn. On the left the adrenal vein enters the left renal vein, and must be carefully divided between ligatures during nephrectomy (Fig. 12.1). The arteries that supply the adrenal are all small, and they arise from the phrenic and the renal arteries as well as directly from the aorta. At operation the adrenal is easily torn, and there may be persistent bleeding from the rather vascular soft medulla.

PHAEOCHROMOCYTOMA

This is a tumour of the renal medulla, secreting catecholamines of which adrenaline and noradrenaline are the most important. Phaeochromocytomas may also arise in the para-aortic tissues, thorax or in the vicinity of the bladder.

Clinical features

These tumours secrete adrenaline and noradrenaline continuously or intermittently, and the patients have symptoms of paroxysmal or continued hypertension: they complain of headaches, palpitation, faintness and a sense of terror. Sometimes these episodes are precipitated by exertion, trauma, anaesthesia or

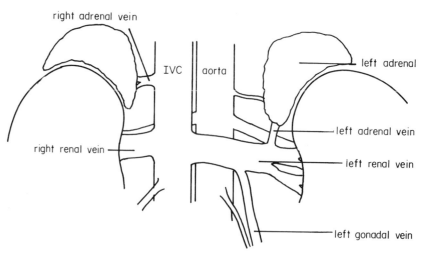

Fig. 12.1. Surgical anatomy of the adrenal glands.

childbirth. There may be excessive perspiration, and in an episode the patients may be seen to be very pale, from peripheral vasoconstriction.

Investigations

The most important thing is to be aware of the possibility of the condition. Elevated levels of catecholamines are found in the plasma or the urine by bioassay, or their breakdown products in the urine are measured—an easier and cheaper investigation. These breakdown products include *vanillyl-mandelic acid* (VMA) (Fig. 12.2). A positive VMA screening test implies a level in the 24 hour urine of $2 \times$ normal, and for this test to be useful the patient must be deprived of vanilla-containing products, bananas and coffee for 24 hours before the test is done.

Extra-adrenal tumours tend to make adrenaline rather than noradrenaline, and the measurement of these catecholamines in the urine or plasma may help localize the tumour. But in practice one relies on radiographic investigations.

A soft tissue mass may be revealed in tomographic cuts of the kidney region, but the best test is a good angiogram: phaeochromocytomas have a very rich blood supply and give a characteristic radiological appearance. The angiogram is also useful in that it will detect tumours arising outside the adrenal. Venograms are useful to show small tumours of the adrenal.

Treatment

In former times the surgery of these tumours was very dangerous because the slightest handling of the tissues around the tumour could provoke dangerous elevations of the blood pressure. Today the patient is thoroughly prepared by alpha- and beta-blocking agents. Phenoxybenzamine or phentolamine is used to block the alpha-receptors: propanolol is given to block the beta-receptors. Thus blocked, the patient is vulnerable to blood loss, and so through the operation blood loss is kept to the minimum, carefully measured step by step, and exactly replaced.

According to its situation and size, the adrenal is approached through the loin or through a transabdominal incision.

CONN'S TUMOUR—ALDOSTERONISM

There may be single or multiple small, aldosterone-secreting tumours in either or both adrenals. Usually they are benign, but as with most endocrine gland tumours, the occasional malignant one is seen. Aldosterone leads to hypertension, with sodium retention and loss of potassium, causing weakness and even paralysis. The symptoms are those of hypertension, to which are added those of polyuria, thirst and muscular weakness. The diagnosis depends upon discovering a high level of aldosterone in the plasma, demonstrating that this is reversed

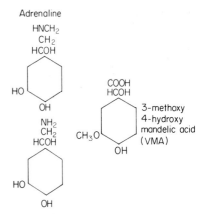

Fig. 12.2. Relationships between the structure of adrenaline, noradrenaline and their metabolic by-product, vanillyl-mandelic acid (VMA).

by giving spironolactone, and finding high plasma aldosterone levels associated with low levels of renin. Since these tumours are often small, detecting them may call for very skilful radiology, including very precise venography.

Spironolactone reverses the effect of the aldosterone excess, but has side effects (enlargement of the breasts, indigestion, constipation and perhaps impotence). Hence, if the tumour can be localized with precision and certainty, it is probably better to remove it. The patients are best prepared with a pre-operative course of spironolactone.

Operation for Conn's tumour may call for careful control by frozen section (as with the parathyroid glands). Many surgeons prefer to expose both adrenals at the same time, with the patient in the prone position, using the 12th rib approach. If a single adenoma is found the whole adrenal on that side is removed.

CUSHING'S DISEASE

Here the adrenals are secreting an excess of cortisol and the patient complains of the features of steroid overdosage—adiposity of the trunk and face, the buffalo hump of fat at the back of the neck, hirsutes and a red face, subcutaneous haemorrhages and cutaneous striae. There is usually some hypertension, steroid diabetes, and osteoporosis which may lead to pathological fractures.

There may be hyperplasia of one or both adrenals, or a single cortisol-secreting tumour. These are usually spontaneous, but very rarely they are secondary to overstimulation by ACTH from a basophil adenoma of the pituitary. A small number are due to ACTH release in carcinomatosis, usually from the bronchus.

The diagnosis is made by measuring an increase in the metabolites of cortisol in the urine—the *17-hydroxycorticosteroids*, to a level greater than 25 mg/24 hours. When the adrenal disease is secondary to ACTH stimulation, then an intravenous injection of ACTH will yield a rise in plasma cortisol level. This does not occur when there is a primary adrenal tumour. Similarly, when there is a tumour, the level of urinary 17-hydroxycorticosteroids does not fall after giving dexamethasone. If these investigations suggest that the adrenal is independent of ACTH stimulation, and therefore probably harbours a tumour rather than hyperplasia, then a careful search using angiography and cavography is made for the tumour.

If one can be fairly certain that the Cushing's syndrome is arising from a tumour, then only that adrenal needs to be explored and removed. However, when in doubt, or when the preliminary tests suggest hyperplasia, then it is usual to remove the entire gland on one side and about seven-eighths of the other one. These operations are necessarily done on very unfit, obese people, and carry a severe risk.

NON-SECRETING TUMOURS OF THE ADRENAL

Benign and malignant tumours may arise in the adrenal. The *neuroblastoma* of children is one of the more malignant of these, grows to a large size, and metastasizes early. It must be distinguished from Wilms' tumour (see page 111). Non-functioning adenomas, and sometimes carcinomas are also found. They may grow to a very large size. Some of them secrete large amounts of oestrogens and may give rise, in men, to gynaecomastia.

FURTHER READING

Dluhy R.G., Gittes R.F. & Hartwell Harrison J. (1978) The adrenals. In J. Hartwell Harrison *et al.* (eds), *Campbells Urology,* 4th edn, p. 2559. W.B. Saunders, Philadelphia.
Owen K. (1976) Adrenal Surgery. In J.P. Blandy (ed.), *Urology,* p. 1285. Blackwell Scientific Publications, Oxford.

Chapter 13
Renal
Failure

ACUTE RENAL FAILURE

Aetiology

There are many causes of acute renal failure (Table 13.1) and they fall into three main categories: (a) where there is under-perfusion of the kidney; (b) where the tubules are poisoned; and (c) where the tubules are blocked.

Table 13.1. Causes of acute renal failure.

1 *Poor renal perfusion*
    blood loss
    burns
    diarrhoea/vomiting
    bacteraemic shock
    coronary thrombosis
    ischaemia in transplanted kidney

2 *Renal tubular poisons*
    mercury
    phenol
    carbon tetrachloride
    glycol
    Clostridium welchii toxin

3 *Tubular blockage*
    myoglobin (in severe crush injury)
    porphyrins
    bilirubin
    haemoglobin (in mismatched transfusion)
    sulphonamide crystals
    hyperuricaemia

Pathology

The gross appearances of the kidney vary from one case to another. Usually the kidney is large, pale, and oedematous: the medulla is often congested, the cortex pale and ischaemic (Fig. 13.1). Microscopically the tubules are choked with debris that has accumulated from the drying up of the stream coming down from the glomeruli. Many of the different causes of poor renal perfusion can be prevented by early and adequate restoration of renal circulation, combined with administration, when appropriate, of an alpha-blocker. If unchecked, a shunting of blood occurs away from the cortex to the medulla due to the opening up of arteriovenous anastomoses, and this effect, if allowed to continue, leads to death of the full thickness of the renal cortex, from which there is no recovery. After a little while calcification is seen at the inner and outer limits of the dead cortex—the so-called tramline calcification. When this is seen, the kidney is dead.

Clinical features

In many patients the cause of the renal failure will be giving rise to its own

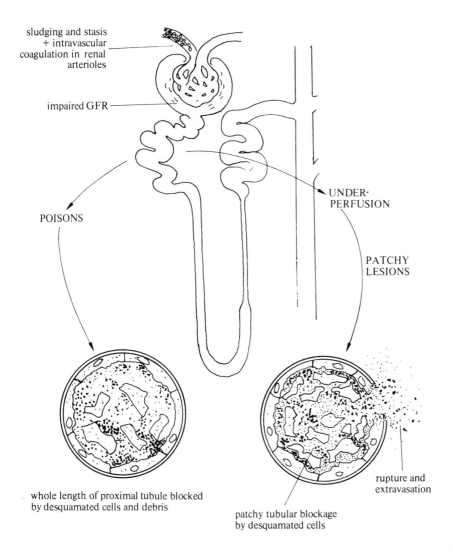

sludging and stasis + intravascular coagulation in renal arterioles

impaired GFR

POISONS

UNDER-PERFUSION

PATCHY LESIONS

whole length of proximal tubule blocked by desquamated cells and debris

patchy tubular blockage by desquamated cells

rupture and extravasation

POISONS   UNDER-PERFUSION

Fig. 13.1. Diagrammatic version of pathogenesis of acute renal failure.

particular symptoms, e.g. septic abortion, septicaemic shock, or multiple injuries with gross loss of blood. But in addition one can distinguish three phases—prodromal, anuria or oliguria, and recovery.

1. PRODROMAL PHASE

At first there is some glomerular filtration, and so some urine is usually formed, often heavily clouded with debris and casts. This initial prodromal phase is useful as a means of distinguishing the anuria of renal failure from that caused by accidental surgical obstruction to the ureters.

2. ANURIA OR OLIGURIA

After the prodromal phase comes a stage when there may be no urine at all, or a reasonable volume, but very dilute. Urea and creatinine and other toxic waste products are not got rid of and mount day by day as catabolism continues. The rate of accumulation of these waste products is much accelerated in patients with massive breakdown of tissue in sepsis or severe trauma.

3. RECOVERY

In most patients, unless the renal cortex has been rendered so ischaemic as to die, there is recovery. At first the urine that emerges from the damaged renal tubules is of low specific gravity and osmolarity, as if hardly processed in the tubules. Before long, a very large volume of this thin urine may be lost—obligatory diuresis—and many litres of fluid may have to be given, even intravenously, to keep the patient hydrated, and replenished with sodium.

Management of acute renal failure

The aim of management is to keep the patient alive until his kidneys reach and pass the phase of recovery. This may take two or three weeks. During this time there is continual breakdown of protein and accumulation of waste products, creatinine and potassium. During this phase he is in danger of being given too much water (which will lead to heart failure) and too much food (which will add to the burden of catabolism). He needs only as much water as he is losing each day in his sweat and respiration plus what little urine is formed. He needs only about 1000 calories/day to minimize unnecessary catabolism of his own proteins, and there is no point in giving more than this.

In a few patients recovery is reached before the level of creatinine or potassium have reached dangerous heights. More often it is necessary to remove these unwanted products. Unwanted potassium liberated in cell breakdown can be removed by the emergency administration of glucose and insulin followed by ion-exchange resins. Other waste products however have to be eliminated by dialysis (see below). The method of dialysis is often governed by the cause of the renal failure: often it is necessary to use haemodialysis when there is intra-abdominal sepsis or recent operations in the abdomen. In other cases it may be possible to keep the patient sufficiently well-dialysed using peritoneal dialysis. Haemodialysis may be needed because no other method of dialysis can cope with very large amounts of protein breakdown.

CHRONIC RENAL FAILURE

Acute renal failure may never reach the phase of recovery, and the end result of almost all other renal diseases may be renal failure. In some patients the rate of deterioration of renal function is very slow, as we see for example in patients with polycystic disease. In others the course is measured in weeks.

When the rate of deterioration is very slow one may be able to keep the patient relatively well by means of diet alone. Diet aims to limit the protein intake to the minimum, e.g. by restricting the protein in the diet to 20 g/day, a patient can be maintained with a creatinine clearance as low as 5 ml/minute. Diet is however most valuable in patients with not so severe renal impairment, e.g. a man with a creatinine clearance of 20 ml/minute can have his urea halved by the very modest restriction of his protein input to 40 g/day.

Clinical features of chronic renal failure

In addition to the signs and symptoms of the cause of the renal failure, patients develop certain important features as time passes: *itching* and *pigmentation* of the skin is a constant feature which is not prevented even by successful dialysis. It goes away with successful transplantation. *Anaemia* varies greatly with the amount of useful renal tissue that is left: it is hardly seen in polycystic disease, and can be very marked in glomerulonephritis and other types of end-stage renal failure where the kidneys have shrunk greatly. It is worst of all in patients in whom it has been necessary to remove the kidneys prior to transplantation because they are infected, or the cause of hypertension that is otherwise difficult to control.

Neuropathy is very variable. It seems to be caused by loss of myelin from peripheral nerves, resulting in weakness and loss of sensation, as well as distressing 'burning' paraesthesia in the feet.

Pericarditis is a sign that the patient is being underdialysed and that the urea has been allowed to rise too high.

Bone changes are important and common. There are two important factors. On the one hand, in renal failure the gut becomes insensitive to vitamin D, and less calcium is absorbed than normal. One consequence of this is that growing bone remains poorly calcified, osteoid being formed but not true bone. This is of course the same lesion as vitimin D deficiency and childhood rickets. In adults the result is *osteomalacia*: instead of the broad osteoid seams at the ends of growing bones so typical of childhood rickets, one finds microscopic evidence of broad osteoid around trabeculae in bone. The bones are nevertheless weak, prone to pathological fracture and deformity (Fig. 13.2).

The second and distinct pathological process is secondary hyperparathyroidism (see page 100). Because of renal failure, phosphates accumulate in the blood, and [Ca] falls. This lowered plasma calcium stimulates the parathyroids to secrete more parathormone. The result of this is to make osteoclasts dissolve bone and so one ends up with *osteoporosis*. In patients with renal failure one can have both processes going on at the same time (osteomalacia, with wide osteoid seams covering thinned-out osteoporotic trabeculae).

Thanks to secondary hyperparathyroidism, calcium salts are added to the blood from the bony trabeculae, However, because the plasma phosphate

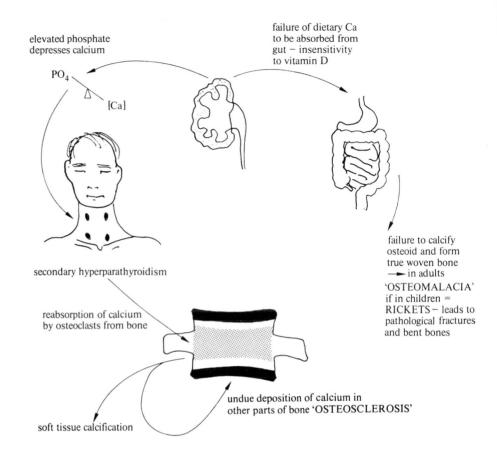

elevated phosphate
depresses calcium

failure of dietary Ca
to be absorbed from
gut – insensitivity
to vitamin D

PO_4

[Ca]

failure to calcify
osteoid and form
true woven bone
→ in adults
'OSTEOMALACIA'
if in children =
RICKETS – leads to
pathological fractures
and bent bones

secondary hyperparathyroidism

reabsorption of calcium
by osteoclasts from bone

undue deposition of calcium in
other parts of bone 'OSTEOSCLEROSIS'

soft tissue calcification

Fig. 13.2. Bone changes in renal failure.

remains high, these calcium salts cannot remain in solution, and are deposited as *heterotopic calcification* in soft tissues. One of these areas is at the junction of the vertebral body with the disk where the band of heterotopic calcification combined with osteoporosis gives a characteristic radiographic appearance called the 'rugger-jersey spine'. Other unwanted effects of this heterotopic calcification result in deafness.

Dialysis

PERITONEAL DIALYSIS

A silicone rubber catheter is inserted into the abdominal cavity and placed so that its end, provided with multiple side-holes, lies in the pelvis (Fig. 13.3). The dialysate fluid is allowed to run in to fill up the peritoneal cavity, left to equilibrate, and then allowed to run out. Formerly this procedure was done in bed, at daily or twice daily intervals. More recently improvements in the skill of managing these patients has led to the introduction of chronic ambulatory peritoneal dialysis. Here the fluid is allowed to run into the peritoneal cavity and

Chapter 13/*Renal Failure*

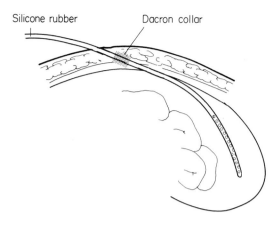

Fig. 13.3. Peritoneal dialysis by means of the Tenckhoff cannula.

is then left *in situ* for several hours before being allowed to drain out. Patients can walk around and look after the instillation and removal of the fluid themselves. There still remain however a number of important complications, of which the chief is, as one might expect, infection in the peritoneal cavity.

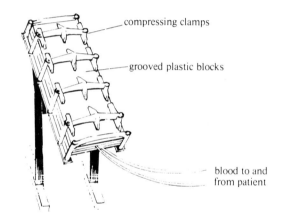

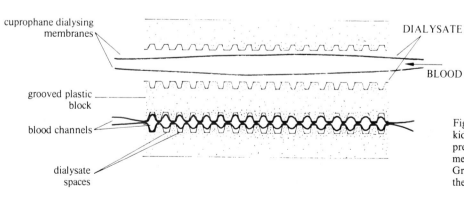

Fig. 13.4. Principle behind most 'artificial kidneys': blood circulates under its own blood pressure, or with the aid of a pump, over a thin membrane separating it from dialysate. Grooved plastic blocks form the channels in the Kiil design.

Chapter 13/*Renal Failure*

135

Blood is taken from the patient and allowed to flow over a thin membrane separating it from the dialysate. At first the blood was pumped out of the patient, through a long coil and back into the patient. In recent years these systems have been largely replaced by methods which allow the patient's own blood pressure to do the work. Several systems are in use, but all involve essentially the same principle—the blood is separated from the dialysis fluid by a thin membrane that allows unwanted waste products to escape from the blood, but retains proteins and red cells (Fig. 13.4).

One of the major difficulties with all forms of haemodialysis has always been vascular access i.e. how to get the blood out of the patient and put it back. In the early days we tied simple cannulae into the radial artery and vein, but these soon became blocked by thrombosis and inflammatory reaction around the ends of the plastic cannulae. Later these were replaced by implanting silicone rubber cannulae which emerged through little holes in the skin—the *Scribner shunt* (Fig. 13.5). Today, modifications of these indwelling shunts are still in use, but are largely replaced by methods in which a large hypertrophied vessel is formed by anastomosing a peripheral artery to a vein (Fig. 13.6). Just as in other arteriovenous anastomoses, huge veins form downstream of the anastomosis. In these deliberate *Cimino fistulae*, large veins form usually in the forearm, into which the patient is taught to place either two needles, or one with two channels, allowing blood to be drawn from the patient and returned after travelling through the dialysis machine. However the trauma of repeated needling, even of these giant veins, occasionally results in their becoming blocked by thrombosis, and as the years go by ever more ingenious techniques are introduced to provide suitable access for intermittent haemodialysis.

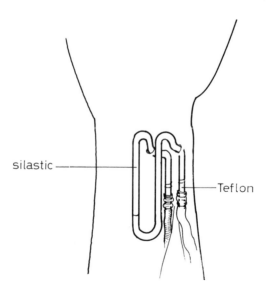

Fig. 13.5. Access to the blood stream may be obtained for short times using a Scribner shunt, where the cannulae are tied directly into (usually) the radial artery and cephalic vein.

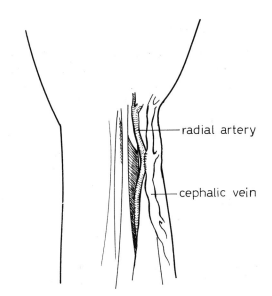

—radial artery

—cephalic vein

Fig. 13.6. Cimino fistula: the radial artery and the cephalic vein are anastomosed end-to-side or side-to-side.

Transplantation

The operative steps of renal transplantation are now standard and successful. A kidney is obtained either from a living related donor, or from a dead person. It is placed in one or other iliac fossae, extraperitoneally. The renal artery is anastomosed to the external or internal iliac artery and the vein to the external iliac vein. The ureter is led through a submucosal tunnel to the bladder, taking care to make a sufficiently long tunnel to prevent subsequent reflux (Fig. 13.7). As with any other operation in surgery, things may go wrong technically—but these are not the important problems in renal transplantation. Three major difficulties continue to dominate the field—rejection, preservation of the donor kidney, and obtaining enough donor kidneys.

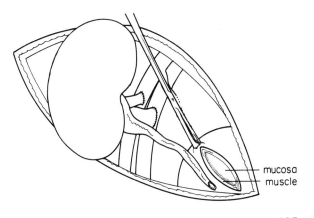

—mucosa
—muscle

Fig. 13.7. Transplantation of the left kidney from the donor to the right iliac fossa: the recipient artery is anastomosed to the right external iliac artery, the vein to the external iliac vein and the ureter is about to be anastomosed through the submucosal tunnel to the bladder.

When an unrelated transplant (allograft) is performed for the first time there is a latent period in which the anastomoses heal and the kidney perfuses and makes urine. But after 10–14 days lymphocytes in the regional lymph nodes enlarge, divide, show pyronin-staining deposits in their cytoplasm and begin to migrate towards the graft. Other lymphocytes are stimulated to produce immunoglobulins which are deposited on the intima of the vessels of the graft, there to attract platelets, fix complement, and lead to thrombosis and infarction of the kidney. This is the *first-set reaction*.

If a second graft is taken from the same donor and put into the same recipient, the same process is observed, but it happens much more quickly and much more severe inflammatory reaction is seen. This is the *second-set reaction*, and it signifies that the patient has become sensitized to antigens on the first graft. A graft from a different donor is handled in the sluggish manner of the 'first-set', i.e. the antigens are specific to the donor.

Grafts exchanged between *identical twins* provoke hardly any transplant rejection, nor is there of course any when tissue is transplanted from one part of the body to another in the same person. Antigens responsible for rejection are evidently inherited. We now believe that the most important of these antigens are to be found on the surface of the cell and that most cells in the body display them. They are the expression of a group of genes carried in the sixth pair of human chromosomes—the *Major Histocompatibility System* (MHS). The first of these antigens was discovered by the Nobel laureate Dausset as recently as 1958. Since then many others have been discovered. Some of them can be detected because the antigens they give rise to provoke serum antibodies that fix complement—Serum Detected (SDs). Others can only be detected in mixed lymphocyte culture, when lymphocytes of the host recognize foreign lymphocytes, swell, and undergo division (LAD or Lymphocyte-Activating-Determinants). Most recently these LADs have been further subdivided into those which provoke activity in the T-cells (thymus-derived lymphocytes) and those provoking activity in the B-cells (derived from the Bursa of Fabricius). Serologically Defined (SDs) antigens can be detected relatively quickly. To detect the LADs, however, requires two to three days of mixed lymphocyte culture, is technically exceedingly difficult, and therefore can only be done in living donor transplants, or in retrospect on cadaver transplants. It is increasingly exciting to realize that only some of the SDs and LADs are really important in human transplantation, while the others are relatively innoccuous. Each month, the Number 6 chromosome map becomes more and more completely filled in (Fig. 13.8).

Because of the way pairs of chromosomes are split up at meiosis and transmitted via the haploid gametes each child receives half its genetic programming from one parent and half from the other (Fig. 13.9). In a family of more than five children, there must always be a pair of siblings who are HLA-identical. When a parent gives a kidney to any of their children, one

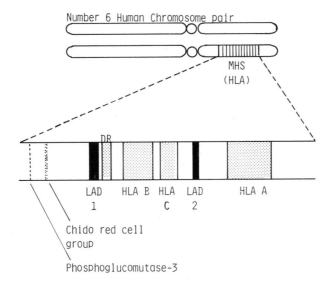

Fig. 13.8. Map of the Number 6 human chromosome pair showing the Major Histocompatibility System and where some of the genes are situated. (Modified from Festenstein & Démant 1979.)

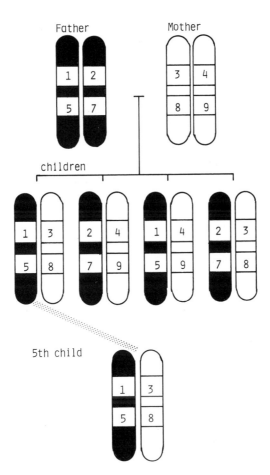

Fig. 13.9. Pattern of inheritance of the MHS. A fifth child must be HLA-identical with at least one of the other four siblings.

complete half-package of genetic information relevant to transplantation will be correct.

Cadaver kidneys, and kidneys from unrelated living donors cannot expect to do so well. There may be other and perhaps quite important antigens elsewhere on the Number 6 chromosome, other than those we can detect by HLA typing. That the MHS and the factors we can identify already are of great importance, if not perhaps the most important factors in graft survival, is shown in great collaborative experiments such as that undertaken by France Transplant and London Transplant a decade ago. Cadaveric transplants that were well matched for the (then known) serologically defined antigens did more than twice as well as those that were mismatched. Since then HLA typing has become more precise and more complex, it becomes even more important to ensure that the right kidney reaches the right recipient.

Unfortunately the chance of a given donor kidney finding a compatible recipient is only about 1:5000. This means that hospitals involved in renal transplantation must pool their resources and work together. They must share all the information about those patients who are waiting for a transplant, and be prepared when they have successfully obtained a pair of cadaver kidneys, to despatch them to the centres with the best matched would-be recipients. This requirement led to the setting up of large national and international kidney-sharing schemes. In turn, it demanded a way of keeping a kidney fresh and alive during the many hours that were needed in order to get a kidney from London to Stockholm, as well as to carry out the slow and laborious tests that were needed in order to establish the tissue type on the donor and recipient.

RENAL PRESERVATION

Over the last 10 years there have been steady improvements in the methods for preserving kidneys, improvements that make it now very simple and easy to keep a kidney in a viable state for 24 hours. Essentially the first step is to make sure that the donor kidney is not already badly damaged. Hence it is important not to use kidneys from severely shocked victims of road accidents, whose kidneys are already the seat of severe tubular damage. Kidney donors should be free from infection, with good blood pressure, and a good urinary output. This means, in practice, that suitable donors are restricted to patients who are dying in a very limited number of ways: trauma that involves decerebration and brain death, but leaves the heart beating so long as the lungs are kept ventilated, or patients with brain lesions, e.g. subarachnoid haemorrhage. Ideally the kidneys should be removed from the patient whose heart is still beating, and as the reader will know, there have been endless controversies about the ethics of this procedure. Today in Britain a strict code of practice has been generally accepted which makes it impossible for a prospective donor to be declared dead unless there is indisputable evidence of irreversible damage to the midbrain. The decision of death is one that the transplant team should have nothing to do with: it must be left to experienced and concerned doctors who are fully aware of all the pitfalls in the interpretation, say, of a flat electroencephalogram. Nor should the burden of responsibility be placed on one doctor's shoulders alone.

Once the donor is known to be dead, every effort compatible with observing the decencies should be made to ensure that the kidneys are maintained in as good a state as possible. The donor should be well hydrated. There is some evidence that the alpha-blocker, phenoxybenzamine, given before removal of the kidneys, may prevent vascular spasm in the donor renal artery.

Removal of the kidneys from the cadaver is a difficult operation: it must be done aseptically in an operating theatre with a complete team. A soon as each kidney is removed, the renal artery is cannulated and the organ irrigated with ice-cold fluid. The composition of the fluid has changed over the years, and today the best results are obtained using a fluid made up to resemble intracellular fluid as far as possible i.e. it is rich in potassium, isotonic, and low in sodium. In many centres sterile pumps are attached to the kidneys which keep the cold kidney slowly irrigated with sterile fluid, but the results of these storage methods seems to be no better than simple perfusion with ice cold Collins solution, followed by transport in a container packed with ice at $0°C$.

OBTAINING ENOUGH DONOR KIDNEYS

It is a tragedy when two lives could be saved by a pair of kidneys that are allowed to rot in a decaying body. Of course, proper safeguards must be provided to make sure that the religious or cultural rules of a patient or his family are not transgressed. Of course, whatever the law may state, it is only humane for a doctor to obtain the permission of the patient's relatives, and to respect their wishes without demur if they decline to allow kidneys or other organs to be removed from their loved-one. In practice, when the request is made tactfully and gently, very few relatives will refuse. This is not the difficulty. The shortage of cadaver donors for renal transplantation does not stem from the refusal of relatives to allow kidneys to be removed for transplantation, but from the failure of doctors and nurses to think about it. How easy is it to understand their feelings: they have worked hard, often for several days without rest, to save the life of their patient. How difficult is it for them not to feel that death, when it comes, is in some sense a failure.

IMMUNOSUPPRESSION

Azathioprine is the mainstay of immunosuppressive therapy today. It was a derivative of 6-mercaptopurine, and when used in combination with steroids, it led to a 45% 2-year success rate in unrelated cadaveric transplantation without any attempt at HLA matching. Other immunosuppressive agents have been tried from time to time down the years, but none has equalled Imuran (azathioprine) in safety or efficacy, until the most recent of them, *Cyclosporin A*, an 11-amino acid, fungal, cyclic polypeptide, currently under trial.

Most of these immunosuppressive agents have side effects. Bone marrow suppression is dose related, and seldom seen nowadays, but when severe, can result in such a low white cell and platelet count that the patient's resistance to infection is so impaired that he may perish. Peptic ulceration is a serious hazard in the early days after transplantation. Gastrin is normally largely destroyed in the healthy kidney, so that in renal failure it may rise anyway, and is not removed in dialysis. Steroids also tend to induce multiple peptic ulcers in the upper small intestine and duodenum. If there is a prolonged period of anuria after transplantation, in which steroids and immunosuppression are added to the existing high levels of gastrin, serious complications such as haematemesis and perforation may be seen. Cimetidine (to counter the high gastrin levels) and alkalis are given routinely. Mechanical failure of the vascular anastomosis leading to renal artery thrombosis or a false aneurysm at the site of the vascular suture is today exceedingly rare. However, the anastomosis may kink, or become narrowed, leading to renal artery stenosis, ischaemia and hypertension.

Reflux may occur if an inadequate tunnel is made between the ureter and the bladder, and be followed by hydronephrosis and renal atrophy, or be a factor in the perpetuation of urinary infection. The anastomosis between the bladder and the ureter may leak, often as a consequence of rejection and ischaemic necrosis of the lower end of the ureter. If so, urgent steps must be taken to put it right.

REJECTION OF THE TRANSPLANT

A recipient may have become sensitized to the donor's antigens in such a way that there may be an immediate 'cytotoxic' reaction. Within minutes of the recipient's blood passing through the donor kidney, it may become swollen, mottled, blue, and finally infarcted. This is hyperacute rejection, and can usually be prevented by preliminary testing of the recipient and donor lymphocytes before the transplant is done.

At any time thereafter one may see rejection. It comes on in 'episodes', manifested by local tenderness and swelling of the kidney, which is oedematous and red and tender to palpation because the surrounding tissues become involved in an inflammatory process. At the same time the function of the kidney falls off: there is an impairment in the glomerular filtration rate, the urine concentration and osmolarity is impaired and the patient's creatinine rises. There is a generalized response as well: usually the patient has a fever and sometimes a leucocytosis.

The distinction between local obstruction, infection, and rejection is often very difficult to make with precision, particularly in a kidney that is already somewhat damaged by those factors in the dying donor that would lead to underperfusion of the kidney, or that might have further damaged the kidney between the time of death and removal of the organs. In making this diagnosis many transplant units rely on isotope scanning (to show whether the kidney is being perfused or not), arteriography (to detect stenosis at the anastomosis), and needle biopsy of the kidney (to show early deposition of immunoglobulins and other evidence of graft rejection).

These 'rejection episodes' do not necessarily spell failure of the graft, indeed, they are almost the rule in transplantation. They are treated with massive 'pulses' of steroids, by pushing the dose of Imuran to the limits tolerated by the bone marrow, and in some centres, by giving anti-lymphocyte sera (globulins derived usually from the horse by repeated injection of human lymphocytes). Irradiation of the kidney was often used in the past, and is still employed in some units, as an adjuvant in the prevention or treatment of rejection. Its place is still a matter for controversy.

If the kidney fails utterly it is destroyed by becoming completely infarcted. The immunoglobulin laid down in its small vessels attracts complement and leads to occlusion with thrombus. The dead kidney is prone to become infected, and must be removed. Such a patient is then returned to the dialysis programme, usually for a time on haemodialysis, later perhaps on peritoneal dialysis.

Second and third transplants

Once the patient has got over the removal of the rejected kidney, he or she may be given another transplant. Equal care is taken to ensure that the second or third transplant is well matched and of good quality. The hazards of rejection are slightly increased and the technical difficulty a little worse because of previous scarring, nevertheless all is not lost if a transplant has become rejected, and there are many excellent results of 2nd and 3rd transplants.

Long term results of transplantation

Down the years there has been a steady improvement in transplantation results. Considering the risks and hazards of obtaining and inserting a donor kidney, and considering how unwell many of the recipients have been, it is amazing that the mortality today for unrelated donor transplantation is less than 5%, only 2% for related donor transplants and that at the end of one year one expects 80% of the living related transplants to be functioning well, as many as 50% of those obtained from unrelated cadavers. These figures could be improved still further if we had more cadaveric kidneys from which to select only those in very good condition and with a very good HLA match.

FURTHER READING

Brockis J.G., Hulbert J.C., Patel A.S., Golinger D., Hurst P., Sakar B., Haywood E.F., House A.K. & Van Merwyk (1978) The diagnosis and treatment of lymphoceles associated with renal transplantation. *British Journal of Urology*, **50**, 307.
Calne R.Y. (1980) Transplant surgery: current status. *British Journal of Surgery*, **67**, 765.

Evans D.B. (1976) Acute and chronic renal failure. In J.P. Blandy (ed.), *Urology*. Blackwell Scientific Publications, Oxford.

Festenstein H. & Demant P. (1979) *HLA and H-2: Basic Immunogenetics, Biology and Clinical Relevance*. Edward Arnold, London.

Lytton B., Finkelstein F.O., Schiff M. & Black H.R. (1976) Influence of rejection on graft survival after renal transplantation. *Journal of Urology*, **116,** 300.

Morton J.B. & Leonard D.R.A. (1979) Cadaver nephrectomy: an operation on the donor's family. *British Medical Journal*, **1,** 239.

Schiff M. (1978) Ureter in renal transplantation. *Urology*, **12,** 256.

ANATOMY

The anatomical situation of the renal pelvis has been described in the chapter on the kidney (see page 30). The ureter descends on each side, lying anterior to the psoas muscle, the iliohypogastric and ilioinguinal nerves, and behind the artery and veins going to and from the testis and ovary according to the sex of the patient. Each ureter is crossed anteriorly by a firm leash of vessels supplying the bladder and, in the female, the uterus—the superior vesical pedicle. This leash continues up into the so-called obliterated umbilical artery. In males it is crossed anteriorly by the vas deferens, just before the ureter enters the bladder. It then runs obliquely through the muscle of the wall of the bladder to open on the trigone (Fig. 14.1).

In women the ureter has an important surgical relationship with the cardinal ligament of Mackenrodt, a tough band of fibromuscular tissue which holds up the cervix like the guy rope of a tent (Fig. 14.2). The ureter passes through the middle of this ligament, and when the uterus descends, it drags the ureter down with it. In its tunnel in Mackenrodt's ligament the ureter lies just above the lateral fornix of the vagina, and if a stone is stuck there, it can be reached by an incision in the fornix—an operation seldom done today, but worth remembering. Of more importance is it to remember how vulnerable the

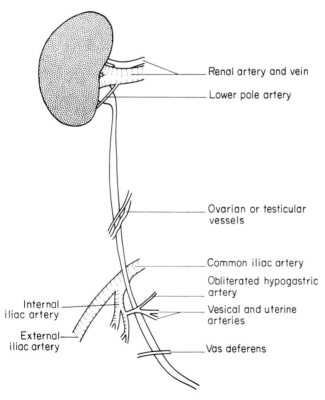

Renal artery and vein

Lower pole artery

Ovarian or testicular vessels

Common iliac artery

Obliterated hypogastric artery

Internal iliac artery

Vesical and uterine arteries

External iliac artery

Vas deferens

Fig. 14.1. Surgical relations of the right ureter.

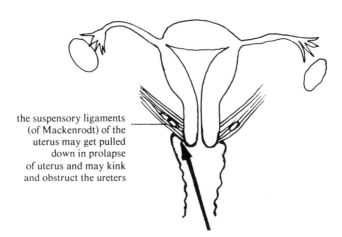

the suspensory ligaments (of Mackenrodt) of the uterus may get pulled down in prolapse of uterus and may kink and obstruct the ureters

Fig. 14.2. The close relationship of the ureter in its tunnel in Mackenrodt's ligament to the wall of the vaginal vault.

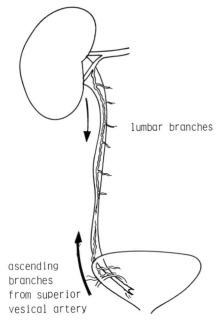

lumbar branches

ascending branches from superior vesical artery

Fig. 14.3. Most of the blood supply of the ureter comes down from the kidney. In its middle third it gets a useful additional arterial supply from the branches of the lumbar arteries. Its lower third has some blood coming to it from the vessels of the bladder and perhaps the vas—but they are not reliable.

ureter is in this situation to operations on the uterus performed via the vaginal approach.

Blood supply of the ureter

The renal pelvis has a wonderfully rich blood supply, which allows one to make long, thin flaps of almost any shape for the purposes of pyeloplasty. The ureter receives its main blood supply from the inferior segmental artery of the kidney (Fig. 14.3). This is reinforced at intervals by small branches of lumbar arteries, but its next important blood supply comes upwards from the superior vesical artery near the bladder. If the ureter is divided down near the bladder, this upwards supply is cut off. Hence the sinister reputation of attempts to join the ureter end to end near the bladder—the lower end may have a good blood supply, but the upper end often does not. Nevertheless the downwards-running artery of the ureter from the kidney is enough to preserve several centimetres of ureter in the operation of renal transplantation.

Nerve supply

The nerves supplying the ureter follow a segmental pattern: its upper part is supplied by T 10, hence pain in the ureter may be referred to the umbilicus; lower down it is felt at progressively lower levels until irritation of the lowest centimetre of the ureter may be experienced as pain referred to the tip of the penis or the vulva (Fig. 14.4).

PHYSIOLOGY OF THE URETER

Peristalsis

The muscle of the ureter is formed of long helices, one intertwined with another,

Chapter 14/*The Renal Pelvis and Ureter*

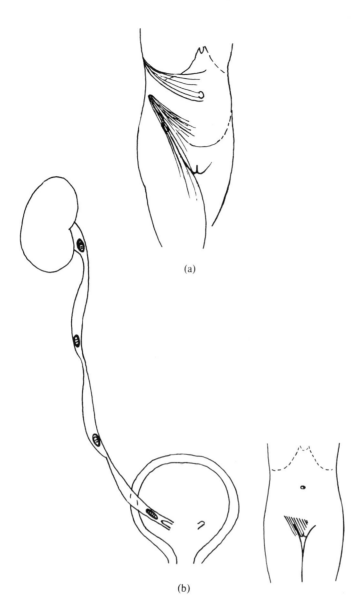

(a)

(b)

the whole tube being lined with urothelium on a thin layer of submucosa (Fig. 14.5). Each muscle bundle is composed of hundreds of smaller, smooth muscle cells, each one fitting into its neighbour by a jigsaw-like connection only visible with the electron microscope. These are called nexuses, and they allow a wave of electrical excitation to be transmitted from one muscle fibre to the next without the need for any nerves or ganglia in the ureter. The result is a slow, writhing, peristaltic motion of the ureter. It can be set off by distension or irritation (e.g. pinching with a forceps) and the wave of excitation passes up and down the ureter. Probably in normal life there is a kind of pacemaker which sets the

Chapter 14/*The Renal Pelvis and Ureter*   147

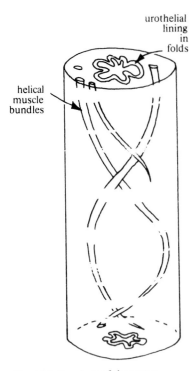

Fig. 14.5. Structure of the ureter.

rhythm of the peristalsis which is situated in the renal pelvis or perhaps in a calix (Fig. 14.6). Nerves are not involved at all in this peristaltic activity: just as well, because the denervated transplanted ureter works perfectly well.

Three things are known to affect this peristalsis. (1) The rate of urine flow makes the peristaltic waves go faster and faster until a point is reached at which the ureter remains open like a drainpipe. (2) Dilatation may reach a stage when

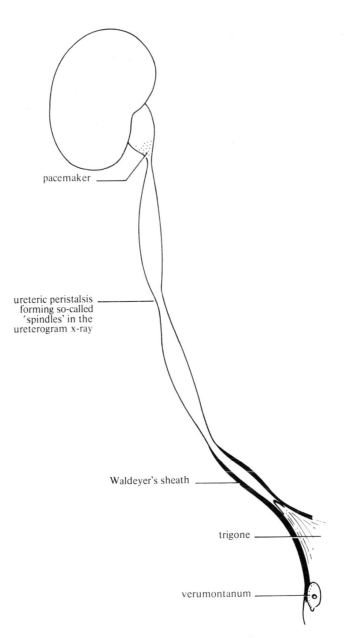

Fig. 14.6. Ureteric peristalsis probably originates in pacemakers in the calix or the renal pelvis.

Chapter 14/*The Renal Pelvis and Ureter*

the walls of the ureter no longer close together to form compartments. Peristalsis still works, even in non-compartmented tubes, but it is less efficient. (3) Periureteric fibrosis or inflammation, such as one sees in retroperitoneal fibrosis, may hold the ureter in a stiff envelope, even when it does not squeeze its lumen shut. This produces a very severe functional obstruction to ureteric peristalsis even though injected contrast medium or a catheter will run freely up and down the ureter.

INVESTIGATIONS OF URETERIC FUNCTION

When confronted with a dilated, 'wide' ureter in the radiograph one may not know whether it is obstructed or merely widened from some other reason. It is possible to introduce a cannula into the renal pelvis, run in contrast medium, measuring the pressure in the system at the same time, and so determine if there is any obstruction lower down the ureter. One chooses a rate of flow known to be as great as the most rapid rate of flow ever encountered in normal diuresis, and if the pressure rises then one knows there must be obstruction downsteam in the ureter. This forms the basis of Whitaker's test (Fig. 14.7).

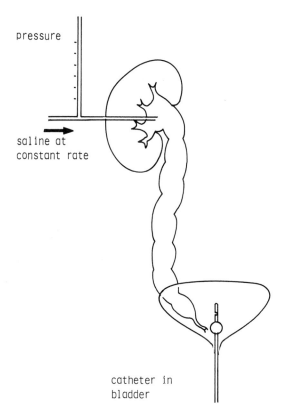

pressure

saline at
constant rate

catheter in
bladder

Fig. 14.7. Whitaker's test: to determine whether a wide ureter is obstructed or merely floppy, fluid is run into it at a constant rate and the pressure measured.

CONGENITAL LESIONS OF THE URETER

The embryology of the ureter has been described on page 43. It will be recalled that the ureter buds out as the ureteric process from the Wolffian mesonephric duct, and because of the sharp angle formed by the Wolffian duct as it enters the urogenital sinus, and the subsequent incorporation of the inner wall of the Wolffian duct into the developing trigone, the ureter comes to enter the bladder upsteam of the ejaculatory duct. When there is an early duplication of the ureteric bud, the ureter from the upper hemi-kidney enters the trigone downstream of the ureter from the lower hemi-kidney (the Weigert-Meyer law). A number of common congenital anomalies may arise, some of which have been mentioned earlier (see page 47).

Ectopic ureter

If the angle of the Wolffian duct is particularly long, low and acute, the opening of the ureteric bud may be situated downstream of the external sphincter (Fig. 14.8). This is seen in girls, where the ectopic ureter may be found just to one or other side of the external urinary meatus. It tends to occur when there is a duplex ureter, in which event it is the ureter draining the upper hemi-kidney that has the ectopic opening. The patient ought to complain of incontinence all her life, but curiously often the incontinence is not noticed until adolescence. The girl is wet during the day as well as at night. The little ectopic opening is often

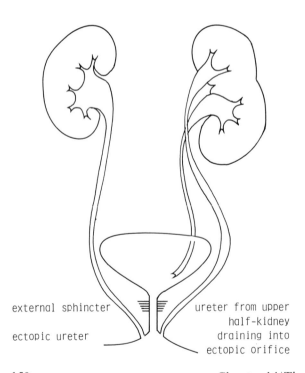

Fig. 14.8. The ectopic ureteric orifice that opens downstream of the external sphincter may give rise to persistent leak of urine.

external sphincter

ectopic ureter

ureter from upper
half-kidney
draining into
ectopic orifice

Chapter 14/*The Renal Pelvis and Ureter*

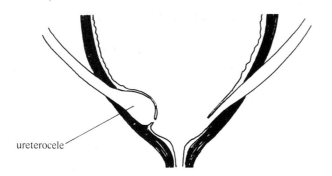

ureterocele

Fig. 14.9. Ureterocele.

very small and easily overlooked, but the kidney draining into the ectopic ureter is usually hydronephrotic.

Ureterocele

Sometimes the whole of the medial part of the Wolffian duct is not absorbed, and part of it remains as a kind of balloon-like covering for the ureter (Fig. 14.9). When these occur in the bladder, they obstruct the ureter, bulge into the bladder to give rise to a filling defect in the urogram and because they cause urinary stasis, one not uncommonly finds a calculus in them. Sometimes when they are very big, they prolapse through the urethra, and present at the external meatus as a large translucent balloon. Again, it is only to be expected that they are more common on the ureters draining the upper hemi-kidney of duplex systems.

They are treated in the first instance by incision of the little balloon. Sometimes this is followed by reflux up the ureter, and if in the course of the follow-up the ureter becomes dilated, then the ureter will have to be reimplanted with a tunnel to prevent reflux.

Reflux

Reflux probably occurs up ureters whenever the wall of the bladder around them becomes oedematous, and this is probably the mechanism whereby organisms reach the kidney as a later stage in urinary infection. Some children are born with short intramural tunnels for the ureter, and the openings of the ureteric orifices are somewhat widely set apart. In consequence, reflux of urine takes place during micturition. If the child is so unfortunate also as to have compound renal papillae, then reflux takes place not only up the ureter but also into the renal parenchyma and gives rise to interstitial nephritis (see page 80). Reflux must be sought for in any child with persistent or recurrent urinary infection. It can only be diagnosed by means of a micturating cystogram. One can recognize at least three grades of reflux: Grade 1 where only the lower 10 cm of the ureter are filled; Grade 2 where the contrast reaches the kidney but does

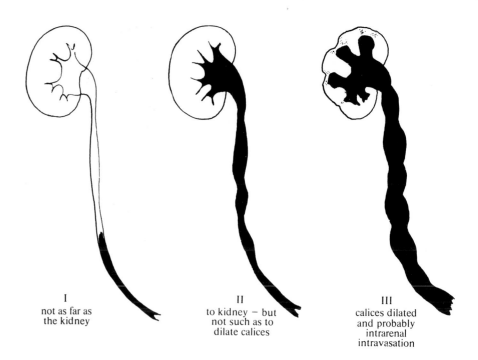

I
not as far as
the kidney

II
to kidney – but
not such as to
dilate calices

III
calices dilated
and probably
intrarenal
intravasation

Fig. 14.10. Grades of reflux.

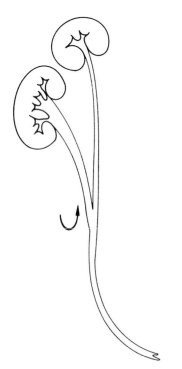

Fig. 14.11. See-saw reflux.

not distend it; and Grade 3 where in addition to filling the renal pelvis, it also distends it and probably enters the parenchyma as well (Fig. 14.10). Grades 1 and 2 usually get better with time, so long as urinary infection can be controlled with antibiotics. Grade 3 is much more serious: if the infection persists, and (some surgeons would add), if the reflux persists into the kidney even without infection, then the ureter ought to be reimplanted into the bladder.

Antireflux operations were very commonly performed a decade ago. Today the results of more conservative treatment seem to be no worse, and most paediatric urologists are inclined to give the child the benefit of a prolonged trial of antibiotics before recommending reimplantation of the ureters. In practice it is seldom that renal scarring is prevented by reimplantation of the ureters: one rarely comes across a child in whom severe reflux has not already damaged the kidneys by the time the diagnosis is made.

Simple duplex kidney

Duplex kidneys and ureters are very common and on their own, are of no account. Occasionally a patient is seen with severe intermittent pain, related to an odd disturbance of flow in the ureters—the see-saw reflux. The larger and more powerful pelvis of the lower hemi-kidney may squirt urine up the Y-junction and fill out the pelvis of the upper hemi-kidney (Fig. 14.11). This can be verified by ureterography and it can easily be put right by a suitable operation to throw both renal calices into one common system.

Chapter 14/*The Renal Pelvis and Ureter*

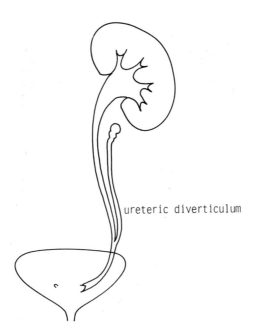

ureteric diverticulum

Fig. 14.12. Ureteric diverticulum.

BLIND-ENDING DUPLEX URETER

Rarely, the ureteric bud fails to induce a kidney from the metanephros and one has the curious oddity of a long ureteric 'diverticulum' (Fig. 14.12). Tiny ureteric diverticula near the lower end of the ureter are more common. None of them need any treatment unless they can be shown to be the cause of pain or persistent infection—and this is seldom the case.

Ureteric atresia

Ureteric atresia has been noted in association with congenital dysplasia of the kidney (see page 51).

Mega-ureter or wide ureters

Most wide ureters are dilated because they are obstructed. Some are wide because they are floppy and inert, thanks to some congenital defect in the muscle of their wall. Some of these are seen in association with absent development of the muscle of the abdominal wall (prune-belly). The prune-belly syndrome includes a congenital, big, floppy bladder and congenitally undescended testicles. Opinions differ as to the best way to treat either the undescended testicles or the wide ureters. Today most paediatric urologists believe in doing as little as possible.

Chapter 14/*The Renal Pelvis and Ureter*   153

To distinguish obstructed megaureters from floppy, inert megaureters one may need to use Whitaker's test (see page 149). Obstructed megaureters may be caused by a congenital narrowing of the part of the ureter that goes through the wall of the bladder, or they may be due to reflux, either on its own, or in association with some obstruction to urine flow further downstream, e.g. the bladder neck or congenital urethral valves.

Pelviureteric junction obstruction

Nobody knows what causes the very common congenital or acquired pelviureteric junction obstruction (Fig. 14.13). There is a narrow ring just where the renal pelvis joins onto the ureter. In the wall of the ureter there is a surplus of fibrous tissue. It may be that this represents the end result of inflammation, or, when the ring of fibrous tissue happens to be found next to the lower segmental artery, it may be that the presence of this vessel has something to do with the presence of the scarring in the wall of the ureter. The fact remains that the narrow zone is there. When the flow of urine exceeds the lumen of the narrow zone, then the pressure inside the renal pelvis rises and the kidney is subject to back pressure and so eventually to atrophy.

The narrow segment of the ureter is usually very short—1–2 mm in length, but occasionally it runs 3–4 cm down the ureter. Patients complain of pain in the loin, typically after a large intake of fluid. The pain may be colicky, and it often makes them vomit. It can be very severe. Later on infection may give rise to pyonephrosis, fevers and rigors. Calculi may complicate the picture.

In early cases the obstruction only comes on when there is a diuresis, and in between times the radiograph may look almost normal. A high fluid intake is

Fig. 14.13. Idiopathic hydronephrosis. Beginning with a stiff ring of fibrous tissue at the pelviureteric junction, the obstructed pelvis balloons out over the lower pole segmental artery.

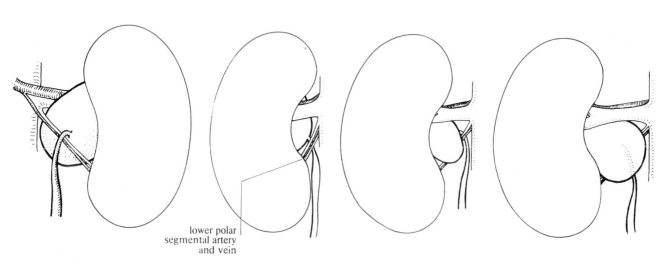

lower polar
segmental artery
and vein

Seen from behind the lower polar vessels appear to be causing the PUJ obstruction

Anterior view. With increasing enlargement the pelvis bulges forward over the lower pole segmental vessels

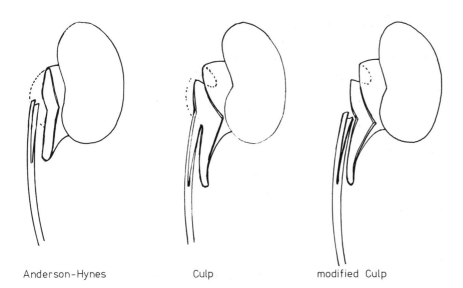

Anderson-Hynes   Culp   modified Culp

Fig. 14.14. The three standard pyeloplasty methods all have in common the insertion of a long, dependant, ∩-shaped flap into the spatulated, upper end of the ureter.

given at the time of the urogram (the stress urogram, or water-load urogram) to bring out the appearances. A similar answer may be obtained with an isotope renogram by giving a diuretic. To make the diagnosis one needs a high index of suspicion.

The lower part of the ureter ought to be defined before proceeding to an operation since often one discovers an additional source of obstruction further down the ureter and in planning the operation one ought to be prepared for it. Several technical methods of operating for hydronephrosis are available: all essentially consist of the widening of the narrow segment with a U-shaped gusset of the surplus renal pelvis (Fig. 14.14).

Retrocaval ureter

Rarest of all congenital oddities of the ureter is the retrocaval one, caused, it is said, by persistence of the postcardinal veins of the embryo. The ureter takes a course behind the vena cava (Fig. 14.15). The excretion urogram is characteristic. The part of the ureter behind the vena cava is useless and one should not waste time or court haemorrhage by following it there. Instead, the lower end of the ureter is anastomosed to the upper, baggy end with a long oblique anastomosis.

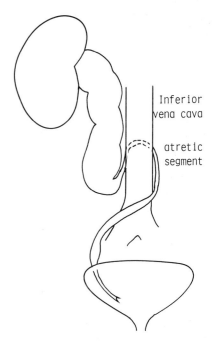

Inferior
vena cava

atretic
segment

TRAUMA TO THE URETER

Accidental injury to the ureter

The ureter is seldom injured in closed accidents except when the kidney is injured too (see page 57). In penetrating injuries with a knife or a gun-shot

Fig. 14.15. Retrocaval ureter.

wound, the ureter is so small and so easily overlooked that one may not notice that it has been injured until urine seeps out of the wound drain a few days later. If noticed at the time of injury the ureter may be joined together, so long as the suturing can be effected without tension. Otherwise the wise thing to do is to insert a tube and then plan a repair of the injured ureter at a later time.

Surgical injuries of the ureter

The ureter is at risk in any operation in the pelvis, notably for cancer of the uterus, rectum or ovary. It may also be injured during hysterectomy, particularly when the operating conditions are difficult and the landmarks obscured by carcinoma scarring or bleeding. Usually the ureter is injured near the place where it is crossed in front by the arteries of the bladder and uterus (Fig. 14.16).

If the injury to the ureter is noticed at operation, its ends may be sutured together over a protective splint, the splint being taken out via the bladder 10–14 days later. But often the injury is near the lower end of the ureter, where its blood supply is precarious and most surgeons feel that it is safer to reimplant such a ureter into the bladder as a primary procedure.

More often, unfortunately, the injury to the ureter is unnoticed at the time of operation. It may present in one of three ways:

1 The ureter may be obstructed. If only one ureter is obstructed, the patient

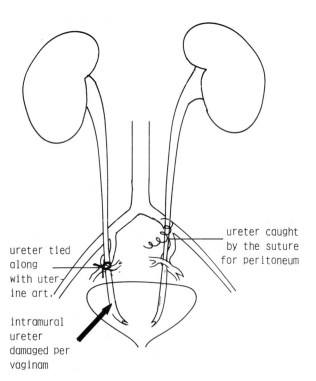

ureter tied along with uterine art.

intramural ureter damaged per vaginam

ureter caught by the suture for peritoneum

Fig. 14.16. Common site of ureteric injuries in pelvic surgery.

Chapter 14/*The Renal Pelvis and Ureter*

may have pain in the loin accompanied (if the urine is infected) by fever and rigors. The ureter in such a case has often been acutely kinked by the suture used to close the peritoneum, or has been inadvertently caught up in the ligature used to tie off the uterine artery.

2   If both ureters are obstructed the patient will be anuric. In such a case the difficulty at the time of operation that led to this unfortunate accident has often been accompanied by severe loss of blood, and perhaps other causes for primary surgical shock and poor renal perfusion. One may suspect renal failure. However, it is important to remember that renal failure in such patients comes on gradually, and so if the patient *suddenly* fails to make any urine, the cause is more likely to be surgical obstruction to both ureters. The diagnosis can be confirmed by an urgent high-dose urogram. In renal failure one may obtain a poor, faint nephrogram. In obstruction the nephrogram will be of distended, blown-up kidneys and after 12 hours the ureters will be filled as well.

3   The most common way in which this tragedy appears is for urine to trickle out via the vagina about four to five days after the hysterectomy. The ward nurse is dismayed to notice the fluid in the vaginal pack. One is dreadfully tempted to deceive oneself that the fluid is not urine, but only lymph or serous exudate. Never allow yourself to put off making the diagnosis. Get hold of some of the fluid. Have its urea measured. If it is urine, it will have a higher urea than that of the plasma. If the fluid is urine, the next investigation is to obtain an excretion urogram. This will almost always show which side has been damaged because the injured ureter will also be slightly obstructed. This diagnosis is then confirmed by retrograde ureterography on the operating table as an immediate precursor to the operation to reimplant the damaged ureter. In the writer's view the operation to mend the damage should be carried out as soon as possible, and there is no advantage in waiting and hoping for the fistula to close.

INFLAMMATION OF THE URETER

Acute ureteritis

Acute inflammation of the ureter is probably very common and accounts for much of the pain experienced by patients with acute urinary infections that are followed by rigors and pain in the loin and groin. It is accompanied by oedema of the wall of the ureter, and it permits reflux to take place from the bladder up to the kidney. It settles with time and antibiotics.

Chronic ureteritis

As a sequel of a severe acute inflammation of the lining of the ureter one not uncommonly finds the urogram showing odd lumps distorting its lumen: these little lumps are caused by *ureteritis cystica*, one of the variations on the theme of chronic inflammation of the urothelium. In ureteritis cystica little nests of urothelium are buried under the wall of the healing ureteric lining, roll up to form little hollow cysts and give rise to a characteristic series of tiny glistening bubbles in the mucosa. It gets well if left alone and needs no treatment. The important thing is to recognize ureteritis cystica and not to start over-investigating the patient on suspicion of cancer.

The ureter is almost always involved to some extent in *tuberculosis*. As we have seen (see page 89), in the early stages the tuberculous process may make the wall of the ureter oedematous, and may shorten it, so that the ureteric orifice is pulled up to resemble a golf-hole at cystoscopy. Later on, the healing of tuberculous granulations in the wall of the ureter leads to stenosis, usually at the pelviureteric junction, sometimes near the bladder. Both of these stenoses can be remedied by appropriate pyeloplasty or reimplantation of the ureter.

In *bilharziasis* (see page 182) the wall of the ureter is infested with copulating *Schistosoma* worms that inhabit its small submucosal veins and lay eggs which worm their way into the lumen of the ureter. The eggs provoke granuloma formation and scarring, and when they die, become calcified, and surrounded by fibrous tissue. In bilharziasis the ureter is characteristically dilated, but at the same time, obstructed. There is often secondary infection and frequently, this is complicated by calculi as well.

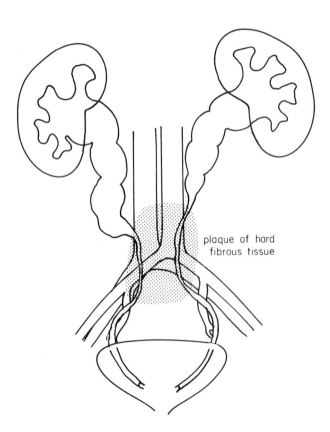

plaque of hard fibrous tissue

Fig. 14.17. Retroperitoneal fibrosis.

Chapter 14/*The Renal Pelvis and Ureter*

Retroperitoneal fibrosis

There is a little-understood condition in which a plaque of dense, white, fibrous tissue forms behind the peritoneum. It grips the ureters in a stiff corset, bringing them towards the midline and impairing their free peristaltic movement (Fig. 14.17). It squeezes the vena cava and it may obstruct the ureter. It may be associated with similar, bizarre, fibrous tissue formation in the palmar fascia (Dupuytren's contracture), in the fascia covering the penis (Peyronie's disease) and in the lobes of the ears. Occasionally retroperitoneal fibrosis is followed or accompanied by similar fibrous tissue in the mediastinum where it causes superior mediastinal obstruction, or in the porta hepatis, where it may give rise to intractable obstruction to the hepatic ducts.

When the ureters are involved the patients characteristically complain of a vague, ill-defined backache, accompanied by sweating and fever. Their sedimentation rate is very high, and they are often ill and have lost weight. There are no physical signs except when they are found to be uraemic or hypertensive. One or two of my patients with this condition were only diagnosed when retinal haemorrhages led to their hypertension being dis-covered, and in turn this led to an excretion urogram.

Investigations reveal more or less severe, upper tract obstruction with the ureters drawn in towards the midline, where under anaesthesia, one may sometimes feel a plaque of hard tissue. The differential diagnosis is from retroperitoneal spread from a carcinoma of the stomach, bowel or prostate. The ureters must be dissected out from their rigid tunnel of fibrous tissue (which must be sent for histological examination). The problem is to stop the fibrosis from coming back: the writer has had good results by wrapping the ureters up in omentum. Others rely on steroids to prevent the return of the fibrosis.

Other ureteric fibrosis

The ureters may become involved in scarring from other operative procedures in the pelvis, or after radiotherapy. One may sometimes find the ureter obstructed as a result of an inflammatory process, secondary to Crohn's disease or diverticular disease, or even appendicitis. In all these disorders the urogram shows a smooth wall to the ureter, and contrast easily runs up and down its lumen. The obstruction is, it seems, from the tethering of the ureter rather than from actual narrowing of its lumen.

NEOPLASMS OF THE URETER

Since the ureter is lined by urothelium, it forms transitional cell carcinomas in exactly the same way as those described for the renal pelvis (see page 115) and bladder (see page 188). They may be of three grades of malignancy—G1, 2 or 3—and they can be staged according to how far they have worked their way

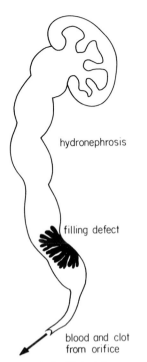

hydronephrosis

filling defect

blood and clot
from orifice

Fig. 14.18. Clinical features of carcinoma of
the ureter.

through the wall of the ureter. As we have already noted, carcinomas in the renal pelvis and ureter are common in the Balkan nephropathy and analgesic nephropathy syndromes, but they are rare otherwise, forming only about 3% of all urothelial cancers. There is a 0.3% chance that a patient with multiple bladder tumours will form a tumour in the ureter or kidney later on.

Clinically carcinomas in the ureter give rise to haematuria or pain from obstruction to the kidney and ureter on that side (Fig. 14.18). If they are near the ureteric orifice, one can sometimes see their fronds poking out of the ureter like the tentacles of a hermit-crab. The diagnosis rests on urography. Characteristically they give rise to dilatation of the ureter both upstream and downstream of the tumour (unlike a stone). Nowadays one attempts to conserve the ureter and kidney as far as possible though unfortunately all too often it is necessary to remove the kidney and ureter on the side of the tumour. What must never be done is to take away the kidney for a urothelial cancer and leave the ureter downstream, for a recurrent tumour often arises there and escapes detection until too late.

Secondary tumours in the ureter

The ureters are often invaded late in the course of cancers of the cervix of the uterus and of the prostate. In the former, it is usually unkind and unwise to do any operation to relieve the obstruction since in such patients the outlook is so grim, that all you achieve is to postpone an easy death from uraemia and permit the patient to die in agony from recurrent growth. In carcinoma of the prostate on the contrary, one may obtain prolonged remission by treating the tumour with stilboestrol or orchidectomy, and temporary control of obstruction is justified. In such cases a temporary 'medical nephrostomy' (see page 19) may be used to relieve uraemia. Occasionally silicone rubber splints may be inserted into the obstructed ureters to give prolonged relief of obstruction.

CALCULI IN THE URETER (see page 104)

Ureteric calculi are very common. From 10 to 20% of Europeans are likely to experience the pain of ureteric colic at some time in their lifetime. More than 90% of stones will pass spontaneously down the ureter without the need for any surgical intervention.

Clinical features

Patients with ureteric colic experience sudden onset of severe pain, making them vomit, roll about, and sweat. The pain comes in waves. It radiates to the umbilicus, to the groin, sometimes to the thigh or knee. There may be microscopical haematuria during the height of the colic. On examination, if the patient can be got to lie still, there may be tenderness along the line of the ureter

160

and in the loin over the kidney. There may be marked distension of the abdomen, enough to mimic intestinal obstruction.

Investigations

If the diagnosis is not obvious, (and it may resemble acute appendicitis, acute intestinal obstruction, or a ruptured ectopic pregnancy) then you should obtain an emergency urogram. A plain radiograph is performed to show a radio-opaque calculus. This is followed by a large dose of intravenous contrast medium, and a single 20 minute radiograph is usually all that is needed. If there is a stone, then there will be a delayed nephrogram, there may be extravasation of the contrast outside the kidney and renal pelvis, and the ureter dilated down to the site of the stone may be clearly visible. If none of these signs are present, then the pain can with some confidence be ascribed to some other cause.

An emergency urogram is not needed in the majority of patients. Particular care should be taken not to get frightened at the dreadful appearance that is seen in the acute radiographs taken during the height of the colic.

Management

The patient with acute ureteric colic needs relief of his pain. Give enough morphine or pethidine. Do not waste time with 'antispasmodics'. There is no evidence that any of them do the least good in ureteric colic, despite the claims of some pharmacologists. Put the patient to bed and give him or her a big dose of an opiate. Forget what you have been told about morphine causing smooth muscle spasm (this may apply to the guinea-pig's uterus—it has nothing whatever to do with the human ureter).

Do not encourage the patient to drink because (a) he feels dreadful enough anyway, and has probably vomited and (b) it may increase the dilatation upstream of the obstructing stone and may make the pain worse. It has been shown not to help stones pass, so why tease the patient?

Make sure he or she has no urinary infection. Monitor the temperature and have the urine examined for micro-organisms (with a gram stain) and for pus cells. If there is any doubt, administer the appropriate antibiotic. If you know for certain that there is infection, then you will probably be planning to remove the stone as an emergency.

If the stone is too large to go down the ureter safely, you may as well get ready to remove it within the next day or two. But if the stone is less than 0.5 cm in diameter, you can safely wait.

As soon as the acute pain has subsided, the patient may go home. Warn him or her that they may expect more attacks of pain, and supply them with some pain medication. Warn their doctor that they are passing a stone and may need help.

Another radiograph should be done in three to four weeks time. If the stone is making progress down the ureter, and if the kidney is unobstructed, the 'mini-IVU' (a plain and 20 minute film) is repeated after another four weeks, and so on until the stone has passed.

Indications for operation on ureteric stones

1. STONE TOO BIG

If the calculus if obviously far too large (clearly greater than 0.5 cm diameter) it should be removed, but one needs to temper the rules with a little common sense and experience. Many a patient has passed stones larger than this.

2. URINARY INFECTION

The presence of infection in the column of ureter above an obstructing stone invites bacteraemia. This is too dangerous a risk to permit your patient to run and you should arrange for the stone to be removed without delay.

3. PROGRESSIVE DILATATION OF THE URETER AND KIDNEY

So long as you are not misled by the initial disastrous appearance of the kidney in the first attack of colic, any subsequent increase in hydronephrosis or loss of renal parenchyma should force your hand and make you remove the stone.

4. FAILURE OF THE STONE TO MAKE PROGRESS DOWN THE URETER

This calls for judgement and experience and you must always temper the wind to the shorn lamb. Never be bullied by your patient into hasty operations. An urgent appointment to meet a client or to go on holiday is no justification for an operation which, from time to time, will be followed by loss of a kidney and threat to life.

5. SEVERE AND INTOLERABLE PAIN

Very much more judgement is needed here. It is seldom that one needs to remove a stone merely for pain, without there being at the same time infection or progressive dilatation or some other more respectable reason for operating.

Ureteric stones—choice of operation

In the upper third of the ureter there is a risk that the stone may slip back into the kidney, so that the incision has to be planned to allow you to expose the

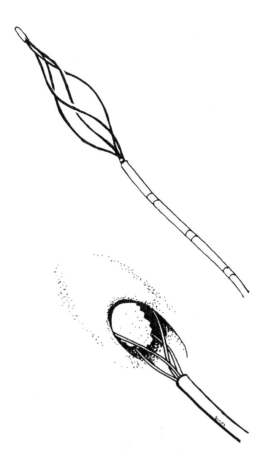

Fig. 14.19. Stones near the lower end of the ureter may sometimes be removable with the Dormia or Pfister 'basket'.

kidney if necessary. The patient is placed in the kidney lateral position and the incision is based on the 12th rib-tip approach (see page 337).

In the middle third of the ureter the ureter is approached by a short lateral incision in the loin. This is the easiest site (and the safest) for removal of stones in the ureter (see page 339).

In the lower third of the ureter a Pfannenstiel incision is used, and to get at the ureter the superior vesical vessels are divided between ligatures as the first step. The lower the stone is in the ureter the more difficult the dissection (see page 340).

Use of the Dormia, Pfister and other forms of basket (Fig. 14.19) is fraught with danger. They should only be used in stones less than 5 mm in diameter, within 5 cm of the ureteric orifice. Since these are just the very stones that are almost certainly going to pass spontaneously the use of the basket is very seldom indicated. Nevertheless it does have a distinct and genuine value. But it must never be used just to satisfy the whim of a spoiled and importunate patient who wants to go off on holiday in a hurry: these are just the patients who end up with a torn ureter and a lawsuit.

FURTHER READING

Gillenwater J. (1978) The pathophysiology of the urinary obstruction. In J.H. Harrison *et al.* (eds), *Campbell's Urology*, Vol. 1, p. 377. W.B. Saunders Co., Philadelphia.

Gosling J.A. & Dixon J.S. (1978) Functional obstruction of the ureter and renal pelvis. A histological and electron microscopic study. *British Journal of Urology*, **50,** 145.

Hanna M.K., Jeffs R.D., Sturgess J.M. & Barkin M. (1977) Ureteral structure and ultrastructure. Part III. The congenitally dilated ureter (megaureter). *Journal of Urology*, **117,** 24.

Johnston J.H. (1976) Congenital anomalies of the calices, pelvis and ureter. In J.P. Blandy (ed.), *Urology*, p. 521. Blackwell Scientific Publications, Oxford.

Lupton E.W., Testa H.J., Lawson R.S., Edwards E.C., Carroll R.N.P. & Barnard R.J. (1979) Diuresis renography and the results of pyeloplasty for idiopathic hydronephrosis. *British Journal of Urology*, **51,** 449.

Ransley P.G. (1976) The renal papilla and intrarenal reflux. In D.I. Williams & G.D. Chisholm (eds), *Scientific Foundations of Urology*, p. 79. Heinemann, London.

Roberts J.A. (1976) Hydronephrosis of pregnancy. *Urology*, **8,** 1.

Whitaker R.H. (1976) Pathophysiology of ureteric obstruction. In D.I. Williams & G.D. Chisholm (eds), *Scientific Foundations of Urology*, p. 18. Heinemann, London.

The anatomy of the bladder changes from childhood into adult life; in childhood the bladder is mainly an abdominal organ, easily felt, easily needled. In adult life the bladder is difficult to feel unless distended, and lies deep in the pelvis, well protected by the symphysis. Above, the bladder is covered by the peritoneum, against which rest loops of small bowel and the sigmoid colon. A long tail of urachus tethers the dome of the bladder to the umbilicus, representing the fetal allantois.

Anteriorly the empty bladder lies behind the symphysis, rising as it fills, usually in the midline, but sometimes bulging to one or other side. It may bulge out into a defect in the inguinal canal to form the 'bladder ears' so often seen in children's cystograms, and in adults, the bladder forms an important medial relation to an inguinal or a femoral hernial sac.

Posteriorly the bladder is separated from the rectum by the extraordinarily important, though very thin, fascia of Denonvilliers. This represents the fused recess of the peritoneum, but it is important because it offers a plane of cleavage for the surgeon setting out to remove the bladder, and an almost impenetrable barrier to the spread of cancer from the bladder or prostate into the rectum (Fig. 15.1).

Inferiorly the bladder rests in the male on the doughnut shaped prostate gland below which the pelvic diaphragm, (i.e. the levator ani muscle

Fig. 15.1. Surgical anatomy of the bladder: (a) in the male; (b) in the female.

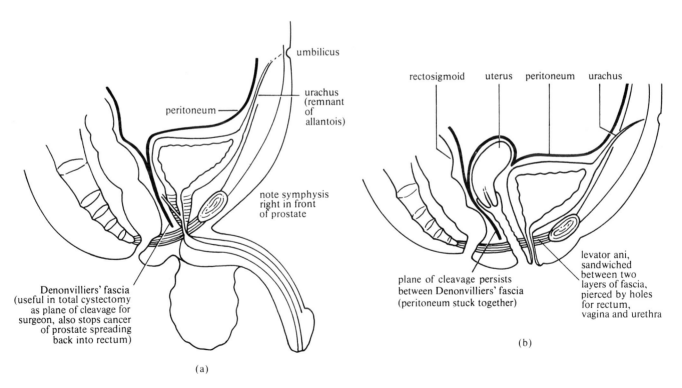

umbilicus

urachus (remnant of allantois)

peritoneum

note symphysis right in front of prostate

Denonvilliers' fascia (useful in total cystectomy as plane of cleavage for surgeon, also stops cancer of prostate spreading back into rectum)

(a)

rectosigmoid   uterus   peritoneum   urachus

plane of cleavage persists between Denonvilliers' fascia (peritoneum stuck together)

levator ani, sandwiched between two layers of fascia, pierced by holes for rectum, vagina and urethra

(b)

sandwiched in two layers of fascia) supports the entire contents of the pelvis.

In females the bladder really rests on the anterior wall of the vagina supported in turn by the levator ani shelf.

Structure of the bladder

The muscles of the bladder are arranged in the form of a felt or basketwork. The individual fibres sweep around the wall of the bladder and pass easily from the outer part of the wall into the innermost layer and back again. It is not arranged in layers, like the layers of muscle in the intestine. Outside the muscle there is no true 'capsule' of the bladder, but simply connective tissue and fat, rich in veins. Inside the muscular envelope of the bladder, is the urothelium supported by a thin layer of submucosa.

Blood supply

The bladder has a profuse arterial supply, richly interconnecting (Fig. 15.2), which allows one to fashion grafts and tubes from its wall with absurdly narrow bases (compared with the wide base needed by the plastic surgeon who has to work with human skin). This also means that it can bleed tremendously. The arterial supply comes into the bladder via three main branches of the internal iliac artery: the main supply comes in from the superior vesical pedicle, under which runs the ureter; lower down another leash of arteries supplies the base of the bladder and prostate; and there is a third leash which enters the system at the apex of the prostate.

From the bladder the *veins* pass as one might expect, to the internal iliac

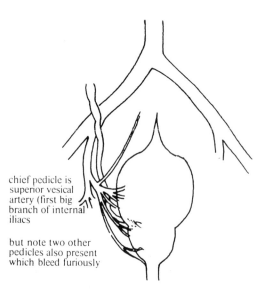

chief pedicle is superior vesical artery (first big branch of internal iliacs

but note two other pedicles also present which bleed furiously

Fig. 15.2. Rich blood supply of the bladder from branches of the internal iliac artery.

Chapter 15/*The Bladder—Structure and Function*

veins. However, from these, there is not only a connection to the inferior vena cava, but also a second 'backstairs' system connecting the bladder and prostate directly with the veins of the innominate bones, the heads of the femora, and the vertebral bodies. Coughing, or the Valsalva manoeuvre, or anything that raises the intra-abdominal pressure, forces blood from the pelvis into these bony plexuses. It is hardly surprising that a favourite place for metastases from carcinoma of the bladder and prostate is the bony pelvis and the upper end of the femur.

Lymphatic drainage

Lymphatics are hard to find in the innermost layers of the bladder: indeed, it would be rather absurd if the bladder, designed to hold urine, were equipped to absorb it. But in the outer layers, especially the deep muscle, there are innumerable lymphatics that drain not only directly to the lymph nodes of the internal iliac and obturator groups, but also, via their own backstairs system, to lymph spaces in the bones of the pelvis and the upper ends of the femora. Here is another system whereby metastases can be formed from primary neoplasms in prostate and bladder.

Innervation of the bladder

The bladder has its own system of ganglia and its own intrinsic nerve network. Superimposed on this system are outside influences.

THE REFLEX ARC OF THE BLADDER

Afferent impulses from the bladder pass up in the parasympathetic nerve filaments of the nervi erigentes, the pelvic parasympathetics, to the S2 and S3 segments of the cord. Some afferent impulses, probably mainly conducting pain impulses, pass up in the sympathetic nerves located in the presacral plexus. Both parasympathetic and sympathetic filaments actually get to and from the bladder along the main arterial supply (Fig. 15.3).

The main afferents that travel in the pelvic parasympathetic filaments, reach the S2 and S3 segments of the cord. The pain afferents from the bladder reach astonishingly high levels in the sympathetic system and to block all pain from the bladder with a spinal anaesthetic it is necessary to go as high as T6.

The reflex arc that is concerned with most of the physiological functions of the bladder is situated in the stump of the spinal cord, in S2 and S3. Remember that this lies just at the level of the junction of the thoracic and lumbar spine—the most vulnerable part of the backbone, the most easily injured in motor or industrial accidents.

Issuing from the reflex arc are three sets of fibres: (a) *Efferent* impulses pass to the detrusor muscle along the pelvic parasympathetic filaments. They cause the detrusor muscle to contract. (b) Other α and β adrenergic fibres supply the

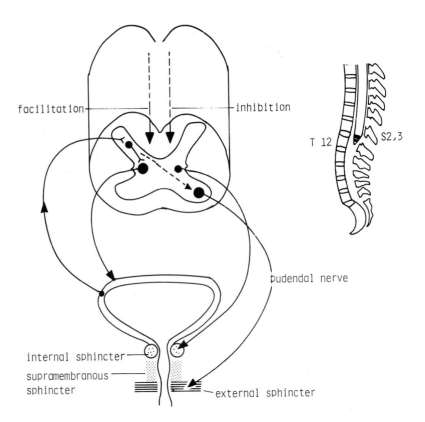

facilitation —————— inhibition

T 12   S2,3

pudendal nerve

internal sphincter —

supramembranous —
sphincter

external sphincter

Fig. 15.3. Innervation of the bladder. The afferent arc from the stretch receptors in the detrusor ascends to the spinal centre in S2 and S3 which lie on the level of the 12th thoracic vertebra. The reflex consists of efferent stimulation to the detrusor muscle, at the same time as inhibition of activity in the external sphincter and the supramembranous and internal sphincters.

supramembranous sphincter and the bladder neck. (c) Somatic efferent myelinated fibres run in the pudendal nerve to supply the striated muscle of the external sphincter.

Micturition (Fig. 15.4)

When the bladder fills, afferent fibres sensitive to stretching, signal to the reflex arc. In the simplest system of all, the reflex arc is completed, and the efferent fibres to the detrusor cause the detrusor to contract, while at the same time efferent impulses to the supramembranous, external and internal sphincter muscles. are inhibited. The internal sphincter at the neck of the bladder relaxes, urine enters the prostatic urethra, the supramembranous ring relaxes, and the external sphincter relaxes. The urine leaves the bladder and when it has all gone, the external sphincter contracts, followed by the supramembranous sphincter which milks back any urine left above the levator shelf. Finally, the internal sphincter contracts again.

   If the time is not convenient, this reflex arc can be interrupted by conscious or unconscious inhibitory impulses from higher up in the central nervous system. Similarly, the reflex can be facilitated by impulses coming down from higher centres, e.g. when under the influence of anxiety or terror.

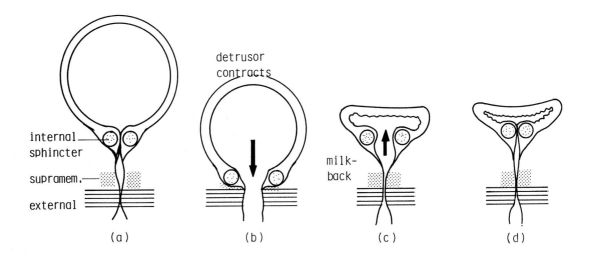

(a)   (b)   (c)   (d)

There are a great many alterations to the pattern of normal micturition that are of concern to the urologist. They can be studied in several ways—the whole system being referred to as *urodynamics* (see page 200).

Fig. 15.4. Sequence of events in micturition. The full bladder (a) is closed off by the internal, supramembranous and external sphincters. As the detrusor contracts, the trigone descends (b) and the sphincters relax. After the bladder is emptied (c), urine above the external sphincter is milked-back into the bladder by the action of the supramembranous sphincter, before the internal sphincter contracts (d).

FURTHER READING

Edwards L. (1976) Incontinence of urine. In J.P. Blandy (ed.), *Urology*, p. 687. Blackwell Scientific Publications, Oxford.

Griffiths D.J. (1980) *Urodynamics.* Adam Hilger, Bristol.

Smith J.C. (1976) The function of the bladder. In J.P. Blandy (ed.), *Urology*, p. 672. Blackwell Scientific Publications, Oxford.

Turner-Warwick R.T. & Whiteside C.G. (eds) (1979) Clinical urodynamics. *Urologic Clinics of North America*, **6**, 1.

Chapter 16
The Bladder —
Congenital
Abnormalities

EMBRYOLOGY

The dome of the bladder and its long tail that connects it to the umbilicus (the urachus) are formed from the primitive hind-gut or cloaca into which drain the Wolffian mesonephric ducts and the ureteric buds. Parallel and lateral to the Wolffian mesonephric ducts run the Müllerian paramesonephric ducts that are going to form the Falloppian tubes of the female. The trigone and the urethra are formed by the tissue contributed by the lower ends of the Wolffian mesonephric ducts, into which are incorporated the ureteric buds (Fig. 4.7, see page 46). The urethra is formed by the inrolling of folds on either side of the midline. There is ample scope for innumerable congenital anomalies to occur. The following are some of the more common or more important ones.

Agenesis

It is exceptionally rare for the cloaca not to be formed at all. Since both ureters are usually obstructed the disorder is usually incompatible with survival.

Duplication

The bladder may be divided by a median septum, sometimes a transverse one, giving an hour-glass appearance.

Patent urachus

The urachus may remain patent allowing urine to escape at the umbilicus. This is usually found in association with obstruction at the neck of the bladder or in the urethra. More commonly the urachal remnant forms small cysts that become secondarily infected. Occasionally the urachus, which is lined with columnar epithelium since it is derived from the hindgut, gives rise to an adenocarcinoma. This typically presents with haematuria and is seen on cystoscopy as a cherry-coloured lesion near the fundus of the bladder. Above the cherry-coloured swelling there is always a much larger lump. It has a very bad prognosis, typically leading to death with the peritoneal cavity full of mucus.

Extrophy

This is usually explained by the formation in early fetal life of an abnormally large cloacal membrane extending up towards the umbilicus, and preventing ingrowth of the tissue that would otherwise go to form the muscle and skin of the abdominal wall (Fig. 16.1). The cloacal membrane normally dissolves in the perineum to open up the anus, vagina, and urethra. In extrophy the solution of the extra-large cloacal membrane leaves the whole triangle of tissue below the umbilicus exposed. The gap varies in extent. It may, at its least severe, form only

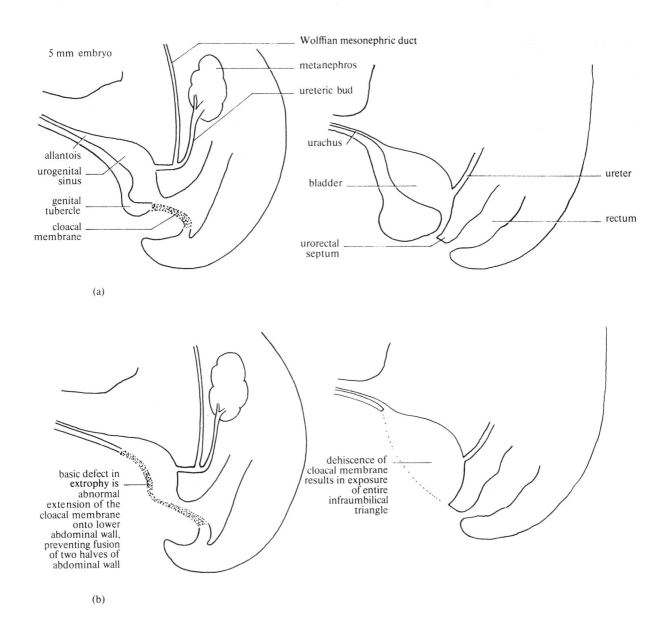

Wolffian mesonephric duct

metanephros

ureteric bud

urachus

allantois

urogenital
sinus

bladder

ureter

genital
tubercle

cloacal
membrane

rectum

urorectal
septum

(a)

basic defect in
extrophy is
abnormal
extension of the
cloacal membrane
onto lower
abdominal wall,
preventing fusion
of two halves of
abdominal wall

dehiscence of
cloacal membrane
results in exposure
of entire
infraumbilical
triangle

(b)

a dorsal cleft in the penis (*epispadias*), or at worst, leave the entire primitive cloaca exposed. Usually the bladder opens like a flat red ulcer on the abdomen, onto which the ureters discharge urine. There is usually associated prolapse of the rectum and undescended testes. The symphysis pubis is usually widely separated (Fig. 16.2).

If nothing is done the exposed urothelium undergoes constant irritation and infection and eventually turns into squamous or glandular epithelium leading to squamous or adenocarcinoma. The sufferers are continually incontinent.

Fig. 16.1. (a) Normal development of the bladder. (b) Extrophy: the error in development.

Chapter 16/*The Bladder—Congenital Abnormalities*

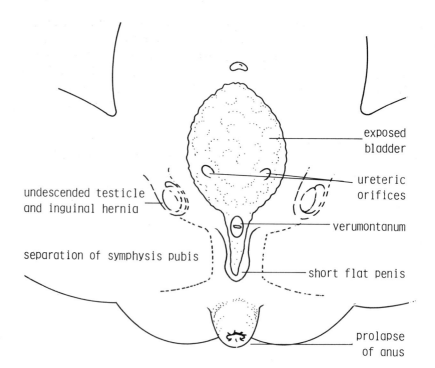

Fig. 16.2. Extrophy of the bladder—the typical combination of deformities.

exposed
bladder

ureteric
orifices

verumontanum

short flat penis

prolapse
of anus

undescended testicle
and inguinal hernia

separation of symphysis pubis

TREATMENT OF EXTROPHY

This is a very uncommon condition and whenever possible it is wise to refer the infant to a specialist paediatric urological centre. In any one country there are hardly likely to be more than one or two experts who have gained enough experience to get the best possible results. It is not a task for the occasional paediatric urologist, and in any event, there is no hurry. The first duty, on diagnosing this distressing-looking condition, is for the doctor to reassure the anxious parents that the child can be made to look normal.

Fig. 16.3. Iliac osteotomy allows the pelvis to be closed together to assist in the closure of an extrophied bladder.

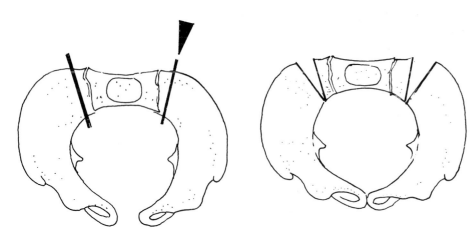

Chapter 16/*The Bladder—Congenital Abnormalities*

When the child is about a year old and is thriving, an operation is done to close the exposed bladder. The bladder mucosa is freed from the surrounding skin, rolled up, and sewn into a ball. To close the abdominal wall over it, it is customary and helpful to divide the iliac bones near the sacroiliac joint: this allows one to close the pelvis like the halves of an oyster (Fig. 16.3). It does not stay closed—but it remains together long enough for the abdominal wall to heal.

At a later stage attempts are made to restore continence to the internal sphincter. This is difficult and unreliable, but it sometimes works. If it fails, then the child needs some form of urinary diversion (see page 306). Sexual function is often good in these children: the girls are capable of having babies and the boys of growing up to be able to penetrate and experience orgasm. Their undescended testicles are however often poorly developed, and many of these children are doomed to be infertile.

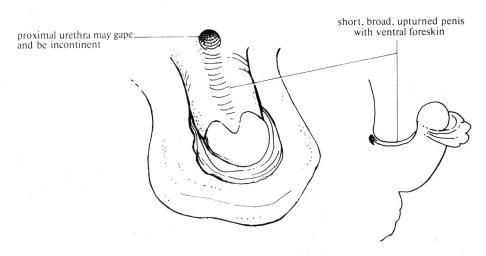

proximal urethra may gape and be incontinent

short, broad, upturned penis with ventral foreskin

Fig. 16.4. Epispadias.

Epispadias

This is a minor version of extrophy (Fig. 16.4). The boy has a urethra opening out on the proximal end of the dorsum of his penis which is flattened, stumpy, and curved upwards. Again, this rare condition requires experience and practice on the part of the surgical team who are looking after the children if one is to hope for the optimum results. Incontinence from defects in the bladder neck is also common. Staged reconstruction of the short bent penis is done first, followed by formation of a new urethral tube, and finally by attempts to restore continence.

FURTHER READING

Jeffs R.D. (1979) Exstrophy. In J.H. Harrison *et al.* (eds), *Campbell's Urology*, Vol. 3, 4th edn, p. 1672. W.B. Saunders Co., Philadelphia.

Johnston J.H. (1976) Congenital anomalies of the bladder and urethra. In J.P. Blandy (ed.), *Urology*, p. 619. Blackwell Scientific Publications, Oxford.

Johnston J.H. (1979) Epispadias. In J.H. Harrison *et al.* (eds), *Campbell's Urology*, Vol. 3, 4th edn, p. 1663. W.B. Saunders Co., Philadephia.

Muecke E.C. (1979) The embryology of the urinary system. In Harrison J.H. *et al.* (eds), *Campbell's Urology*, Vol. 3, 4th edn, p. 1286. W.B. Saunders Co., Philadelphia.

Perlmutter A.D. (1979) Urachal Disorders. In J.H. Harrison *et al.* (eds), *Campbell's Urology*, Vol. 3, 4th edn, p. 1883. W.B. Saunders Co., Philadelphia.

Aetiology

Acute cystitis is so common that in one series it was found that 70% of the healthy wives and mothers accompanying their families to general practitioners surgeries admitted to having experienced its characteristic symptoms. The most common cause is ascending infection from one of the many pathogenic organisms in the bowel, e.g. *Escherichia coli*, *Klebsiella*, *Proteus mirabilis*, *Streptococcus faecalis*. Recurrent infections may be due to reinfection with the same strain of micro-organisms that has continued to multiply within the bowel, or to a different strain.

Not all acute cystitis is caused by such bowel flora: virus infection, e.g. *Herpesvirus hominis*, can give an acute inflammation of the urethra and bladder, so can *Chlamydia* and even *Neisseria gonorrhoeae*.

Bacterial infection often occurs when some other factor has lowered the local resistance to infection: diabetes mellitus must never be forgotten. Often patients with recurrent cystitis will give a history of an upper respiratory infection five to seven days before the onset of the symptoms of cystitis, and many young women find that the minor trauma of sexual intercourse is often succeeded by an acute inflammatory episode.

Chemical cystitis can also occur: the chemicals may be detergents used in beauty preparations put in the bath-water or applied to the vulva. They may be secreted in the urine, e.g. in cyclophosphamide therapy for malignancy or in the treatment with high doses of mandelic acid of urinary infection itself.

Pathology

Whatever the cause of the acute inflammation, its gross macroscopical features are those of inflammation anywhere else in the body. As one would expect, the bladder mucosa is acutely red, swollen and painful. The afferent arc of the reflex of micturition is intensely stimulated, so that the patient has to empty the bladder even when it is hardly half-full. The acute inflammatory exudate makes the urine turbid with exfoliated pus and urothelial cells, and bacterial fermentation of urea may give the urine a typically ammoniacal smell. If the inflammation is very severe, the patients may lose blood.

The cystoscopic appearances of acute cystitis are striking: the mucosa is oedematous, acutely red and inflamed, and bleeds on the slightest touch of the instrument.

A biopsy of the epithelium during acute cystitis reveals that the urothelium is infiltrated with leucocytes, as is the lamina propria.

Clinical features

In many cases the patient has a remarkably sudden onset of the symptoms which may begin with pain in the suprapubic region, intense frequency and pain before and during the expulsion of urine. In a severe attack the unfortunate patient may sit for hours on the toilet with the urge to void every few minutes, made unbearable by the severe pain that accompanies each passage of urine. If the inflammation is confined to the bladder there is seldom a high fever.

Later in many cases of acute cystitis there is pain referred to the loin, followed by fever and often by rigors. It is thought that in such patients oedema around the ureteric orifices has allowed urine to reflux up the ureter, and the loin pain and other evidence of bacteraemia suggest that the inflammation has affected the lining of the collecting system of the kidney.

Investigations

A brief but careful general examination notes other reasons for any lowering of the patient's resistance. There may be considerable discomfort on palpating the suprapubic region, but other signs are usually wanting. The urine is often turbid, and sometimes frankly 'fishy' from its content of bacterial metabolites and ammonia. Microscopy shows many bacteria, many leucocytes and often many red blood cells.

The urine should be cultured at once. If the urine cannot be taken at once to the laboratory, it may be cultured with a dip-slide or put into a refrigerator pending (cold) transport to the laboratory (see page 14).

Treatment

When first seen one can only guess as to the causative organism. If the patient has experienced previous attacks of acute cystitis she will have a good idea of what medicine made her better before, and it is a sound rule to start off with the same antibiotic the second time round, pending the results of laboratory culture and sensitivity studies.

Choose a safe and cheap antimicrobial, e.g. trimethoprim, a simple sulphonamide, or nitrofurantoin. Reserve the more wide-spectrum and expensive substances for severe cases, and use them whenever possible under microbiological control. In the first attack a short course of medication (for three days) works as well as a long course.

It will take 24 hours for the antimicrobial treatment to kill the organisms and another 24 hours for the acute inflammatory changes to resolve. It may help the patient to make her urine alkaline (e.g. giving sodium bicarbonate up to 6 g/24 hours or a similar dose of Potassium citrate). Dilution of the urine may help to weaken its stimulating effect on the inflamed vesical epithelium so it is good sense to encourage her to drink a very large amount of fluid. Some patients find alcohol makes the bladder more uncomfortable, and it is best to stick to watery beverages. In Britain it is traditional to offer the patient 'barley water'. This is an ancient tradition; the fluid resembles infected urine, and so *must* do good according to the immutable Laws of Magic. (At least it does no harm.)

Follow-up investigations

Acute cystitis is so exceedingly common that it is always very necessary that the doctor should keep a sense of balance. In males, acute cystitis hardly ever occurs without some predisposing, and often serious, underlying cause e.g. urinary stasis or a stone. In women, the reverse is true. Hence it is reasonable in a female to treat two or three attacks of acute cystitis before insisting on a full urological investigation. But medicine is an art, and in this, as in so many clinical conditions, your experience and your clinical sixth sense will guide you.

The investigations are going to search for some undrained pocket of urine leading to stasis, some foreign body or calculus that may act as a hiding place for micro-organisms or some other, more sinister mimic of urinary infection e.g. carcinoma of the bladder (see page 302).

Haematuria will always demand an excretion urogram and a cystoscopy (after the acute attack has settled). *Sterile pyuria* will always need to be regarded as tuberculosis or cancer until proved otherwise.

CHRONIC CYSTITIS

Aetiology

Many patients suffer frequently relapsing acute cystitis. The causative organism is usually hiding in the intestine. If the faecal flora have been changed by a long course of a wide-spectrum antibiotic, e.g. in the course of a hospital admission, then the invading organisms are often highly pathogenic and very resistant to antimicrobials. If the patient has been treated only with short courses of simple medicaments, it is likely that the infecting organism will be straightforward *E. coli* and sensitive to second or third courses of simple sulphonamides or trimethoprim.

In other patients the cystitis is not so much relapsing, as persistent. Here the cause may be some specific organism such as *Mycobacterium tuberculosis* or *Schistosoma haematobium*, or one may have to search very diligently for some other reason why the infecting organism cannot be got rid of. In this search, it is helpful sometimes to recall what are the natural defences that the bladder offers against urinary infection.

NATURAL DEFENCES OF THE BLADDER

It has been said that the bladder is like a not-very-well-designed dustbin: to keep it clean it needs to be emptied out regularly. If one tries on purpose to infect the bladder with an inoculum of micro-organisms, and the patient empties it frequently, and has no predisposing abnormality, it is virtually impossible to establish an infection. Given that an ordinary *Escherichia coli* takes 15 minutes to grow and divide into two, it needs no great mathematician to realize that at the end of three hours a little inoculum of a hundred organisms will have become four million (see page 77). But if they are all emptied out, then the survivors have to start again. On the other hand, if the patient holds her urine for six hours, or if, when she voids, she does not expel all the contents of the bladder, then not only will the bladder contain billions of micro-organisms for the best part of the day, but the residual inoculum will be enormous. Frequent and complete emptying of the bladder is the patient's first and most important line of defence.

To ensure this, the patient must drink plenty of fluid. This has an added benefit, for it dilutes the nutrient on which the micro-organisms live, and slows down their rate of division.

When the bladder is emptied, some bacteria can be shown to cling to the urothelial cells even when all the urine has been got rid of. In a healthy individual, these will be killed off by the weak natural bactericidal action of the urothelium. In patients with a damaged urothelium this resistance, this protective effect, is weakened. This may be one reason why diabetics are more susceptible to secondary urinary infection, why a previous virus infection is succeeded by one with *E. coli*, and why carcinoma of the bladder frequently present with urinary infection.

Pathology of chronic cystitis

Just as one would expect, when a patient suffers one attack after another of acute inflammation in the mucosa of the bladder, she will eventually develop local collections of lymphocytes. These are quite obvious on cystoscopy: they look like little yellow pimples, and are most marked on the trigone. The appearance is often called *cystitis follicularis*. Biopsy of one of these pimples reveals a collection of lymphocytes, sometimes large enough and active enough to have a 'germinal follicle' in the middle.

The urothelium may be completely shed during a severe attack of cystitis. If so, then it is quickly replaced by ingrowth from the adjacent normal epithelium. If one or two cells have survived the loss of a patch of urothelium, they can become buried under the regenerating layer, and may then multiply, forming first a little 'nest' (named after *Von Brunn*) and later a little hollow cyst (*cystitis cystica*) (Fig. 17.1). Inside the cyst a kind of mucus collects, and as time goes by and as the cause of the inflammation persists, more and more of these cysts are formed. Eventually the urothelium is transformed into something that closely resembles the lining of the large intestine (adenomatous metaplasia). Unchecked, this may go on in the end to form an adenocarcinoma.

Certain types of persistent infection, such as one sees in association with urethral stricture or bladder calculus, lead to *squamous metaplasia* of the urothelium, and in time this may proceed to *squamous cell carcinoma*.

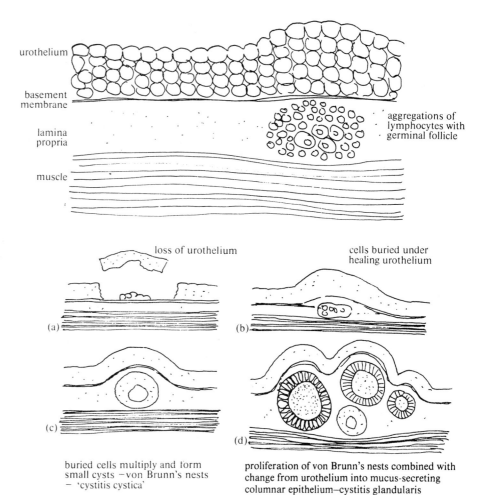

urothelium

basement membrane

lamina propria

muscle

aggregations of lymphocytes with germinal follicle

loss of urothelium

cells buried under healing urothelium

(a)

(b)

(c)

(d)

buried cells multiply and form small cysts − von Brunn's nests − 'cystitis cystica'

proliferation of von Brunn's nests combined with change from urothelium into mucus-secreting columnar epithelium–cystitis glandularis

Fig. 17.1. Changes in chronic cystitis.

Malakoplakia is the term given to a particularly odd kind of chronic inflammatory change: lymphocytes and leucocytes and strange histiocytes containing calcified 'Michaelis—Guttman bodies' clump together to form large, pale, brownish lumps on the surface of the bladder. They may bleed, but their chief importance is that they may be mistaken for a bladder cancer unless biopsies are taken.

Finally, the inflammation may dig deeper into the wall of the bladder. In one variety round cells and fibrous tissue are found in the lamina propria, accompanied by loss of the superficial urothelium. This is seen in a wierd condition named after *Hunner* (the gynaecologist who first noticed it)—*Hunner's ulcer*. The patients—middle aged women—have intense pain when the bladder is half-filled. It is partially relieved by voiding, and so they have intense frequency. Nobody has discovered its cause, and new treatments are published every year. On cystoscopy there are odd 'cracks' in the mucosa which bleed when the bladder is overdistended, but nothing else is ever found wrong.

In another variety, round cells and leucocytes, accompanied by calcification, are found to extend right through the substance of the bladder to the deepest layers of its muscle. This is the rare *alkaline encrusted cystitis* found in association with persistent *Proteus mirabilis* infection. One sees it occasionally in patients who have worn an indwelling catheter for many months, but it is also seen in other unfortunate women for no good reason. It causes very severe pain, dreadful frequency, and on cystoscopy, the entire lining of the bladder is crusted with flakes of mixed magnesium phosphate crystals. The urine smells like smelling salts.

Clinical features

Many patients give a clear-cut history of recurrent acute cystitis. Each attack clears up, only to be succeeded by another, often within a few days of stopping the last course of antibiotics. In these patients you may obtain a distinct history of preceding upper respiratory infection, a relationship to menstrual cycle, or to the mild trauma of love-making. In many others there is no obvious reason for the frequent, tiresome, wearying relapse.

Investigations

In most cases there will be pus in the urine and an easily identifiable organism found on culture. But if no organism can be discovered on routine culture, a more diligent search has to be made. The urine needs to be cultured anaerobically, a time-consuming investigation which is not a routine practice unless specifically asked for, and early morning specimens must be sent for culture on Loewenstein–Jensen media for tuberculosis.

An excretion urogram should be performed in all such patients. You are looking for stagnant urine in a diverticulum of a calix or the bladder, for a foreign body or calculus, and for old scars in the renal parenchyma where organisms may lurk and resist antibiotics. In a male you are above all things seeking evidence of outflow obstruction and residual urine.

Cystoscopy and urethroscopy may give the diagnosis of the cause of the recurrent infection: you may find a stricture in the urethra or a diverticulum along its course. You may find changes of follicular cystitis or malakoplakia in the vesical mucosa, or (more commonly) the rough necrotic surface of a carcinoma on which organisms have settled. Stones may be found in this way when they have been missed in the urogram.

Treatment

At this stage treatment must be determined by your complete investigations. Tuberculosis calls for its own management (see page 88). Cancer requires its own further investigations and therapy (see page 188). Pockets of stagnant, undrained urine contained in diverticula, a hydronephrosis or in the form of residual urine, may demand appropriate surgical treatment, and stones will usually have to be removed. But at the end of your investigation you will be left with a number of people in whom there seems to be no obvious mechanical reason for their persistent infection and their recurrent misery. What should you do for them?

First, advice about the need for a very high fluid throughput has to be reiterated, and this alone often limits the numbers of relapses very drastically. But in addition your patient should be supplied with enough of an appropriate antibiotic to deal with the earliest symptoms of a relapse when it occurs. In practice it is seldom possible for your patient to supply the laboratory with a specimen for culture at the time the symptoms of recurrent cystitis come on. Ideally this should always be done, but it is generally more useful to supply the patient with enough tablets to counter one or two relapses.

If this simple regime does not help, you may reinforce her own natural defences against urinary infection by giving ascorbic acid (to make the urine more acid) and combine this with methenemine mandelate or hippurate day in and day out for months at a stretch. These substances act by releasing formaldehyde in the urine, as well as raising the concentration of undissociated organic acid molecules. One needs to follow the patient carefully for these medications may themselves cause chemical irritation of the bladder.

Finally, if this does not work, your patient may need to take a small dose of a suitable antibiotic every day for several months at a time, or according to some microbiologists, on alternate days. Trimethoprim sulphonamide preparations or nitrofurantoin are most suitable for this purpose.

Having said this, you will even then be stuck with a number of difficult clinical problems.

Interstitial cystitis—Hunner's ulcer

It is no good pretending that anyone knows how Hunner's ulcer arises or how to treat it. At the time of revising this book the fashionable method of treating it is to distend the bladder under deep spinal anaesthesia for two hours. Over-distension of this kind may give prolonged relief of symptoms. If it fails, one may need to remove the greater part of the bladder and replace it with caecum (see page 92).

Alkaline encrusted cystitis

Irrigation of the bladder with buffered Solution G is said to help get rid of the phosphatic encrustations, while intensive antibiotic treatment is administered to kill the underlying *Proteus mirabilis*. The patient is often left at the end of otherwise successful treatment with a small fibrotic bladder.

Tuberculous cystitis (see page 89).

Schistosomiasis

The adult trematode fluke *Schistosoma haematobium*, *mansoni*, and *japonicum*, belong to the order *Digenea*—flatworms with complex life cycles involving at least one stage parasitic in vertebrates and one stage in molluscs. Hardly a vertebrate species is unaffected by similar flukes. In man, there are three principal species of importance: *S. haematobium* and *mansoni* occur throughout Africa, the West Indies and north-east Brazil extending even into southern Portugal and Spain; *S. japonicum* occurs in China and Indo-China.

The adult flukes are about 0.5 cm in length, and live inside human veins, attached to the endothelium by a sucker (Fig. 17.2). The male fluke enfolds the female in a long slit down his belly, hence the name *schisto* (split) *soma* (body). They were first discovered inside the portal vein of Egyptian children dying with portal hypertension, hepatosplenomegaly and ascites, by the great German pathologist Theodor Bilharz, working in Cairo. Hence the disease is often called *Bilharziasis*.

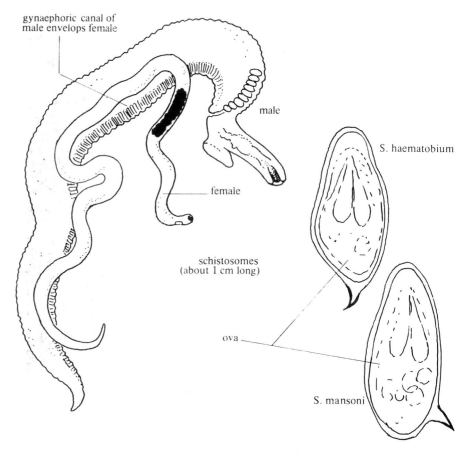

Fig. 17.2. Schistosoma.

Chapter 17/*The Bladder—Inflammation*

The female continually lays eggs. They are provided with sharp spines. The main species have eggs with characteristic terminal (for *haematobium*) or lateral spines (*mansoni*), while the *japonicum* species has a blunted lateral spine.

If the adult pairs of flukes have taken up residence in the veins of the submucosa of the bladder (which is very common) the eggs work their way through the urothelium making tiny holes (and leading to haematuria). The trouble is caused by the foreign-body giant cell and granulomatous reaction set up by the live and dead eggs. This gives rise to 'bilharzial polypi', 'sandy patches' and ulcers in the bladder which can be readily seen and biopsied with the cystoscope. The continual irritation of these living and dead ova leads in time to squamous metaplasia of the urothelium, and eventually to carcinoma. Millions of dead ova, which become calcified, lead to the formation of a line of

Fig. 17.3. Bilharzia life cycle.

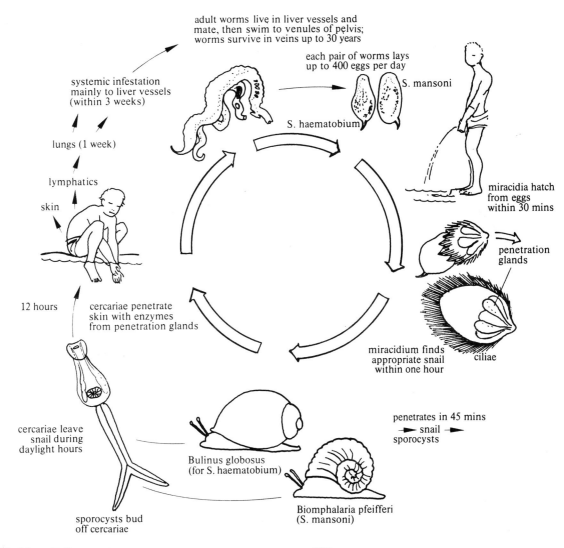

calcification in the muscularis and submucosal tissue of the bladder and ureters. It should be remembered that the flukes are not particularly choosy where they live. The pairs of worms are to be found in almost any vein in the pelvis, so that in heavily infested areas the uterus, fallopian tubes, vagina and vulva and the wall of the rectum are infested as well as the bladder and ureters. The vasa and seminal vesicles are typically outlined in lines of calcification.

If the urine is not voided into a proper sewage system or simple pit latrine (where the concentration of ammonia would quickly kill the ova) then they hatch out (Fig. 17.3). Inside each ovum is a tiny hairy creature, the *miracidium*, which is actively motile, and swims vigorously around until attracted by chemotaxis to a suitable snail. Several species of snail are parasitized by these miracidia which penetrate the skin of the mollusc. They there enlarge to form a 'mother sporocyst', from which 'daughter sporocysts' are formed, and from which in turn little, free-swimming flukes with forked tails, the *cercariae*, emerge. Cercariae find their way from the daughter sporocysts towards the digestive gland of the snail, and thence to the water-exposed surface of the snail from which they are shed, usually at a time when humans are most likely to be visiting the rivers to wash or to bathe. If one watches one of these infested snails cruising on the surface of a glass of water, myriads of cercariae can be seen issuing from its under surface, shimmering like specks of dust in a ray of sunlight.

The unwary human who puts his hand or foot into water containing these cercarieae is bound to be bitten by them within 10 seconds. They can bore through normal cornified skin. Once inside the body, they lose their little forked tails, work their way into the dermal lymphatics, thence into the bloodstream, and are distributed throughout the entire body.

During the stage where they have just penetrated the dermis, the patient may experience a *swimmer's itch*—a mild skin rash. (Identical but fortunately less serious 'swimmer's itch' is encountered by swimmers around the British sea-coast when their skin is similarly penetrated by cercariae—fortunately of non-pathogenic avian species.)

During the stage when the little schistosomes are being spread haematogenously around the body the patient may experience fever, rigors and other evidence of an allergic response. It is as well to remember that this is a widespread dissemination of the little flukes, and that they can fetch up in veins in the spinal cord, brain and skin, not just in those of the pelvic viscera or portal vein. But there is no doubt that they prefer the habitat of the portal vein and pelvic veins. In little children, who spend most of their infancy playing in infested water, repeated reinfection may carry hordes of schistosoma flukes to their portal vein, leading to secondary thrombosis and obstruction with all the usual features of portal venous occlusion. As a late sequel of this, fibrosis and cirrhosis of the liver leads to much morbidity from oesophageal varices and ascites in adult Egyptians.

Finally we return to the copulating couples of worms, firmly attached to the intima of veins in the submucosa of the lining of the bladder, ready to begin the life cycle all over again.

In passing one must notice that schistosomiasis poses one of the major public health hazards in the world. Curiously, governments prefer to spend money on ways of eradicating the snail, or of the adult worm in the patients, rather than upon the much more obvious simple and effective method of introducing latrines and adequate water supplies. Every spadeful of earth dug up from a dried river bed is found to contain hundreds of infected snails, many of which can survive desiccation for many months. It is difficult to prevent villagers from urinating in the local canal, when they have no alternative latrine, or from washing in its polluted water, when there is no other supply. Extensive irrigation schemes such as the Aswan High Dam, only spread the scourge of schistosomiasis. The beautiful lakes that grow upstream of the dams, inviting sailing and swimming and water-skiing, are teeming with deadly cercariae.

TREATMENT

If a poor villager is obliged to return at once to the source of his original infection, treatment of his infestation is of highly questionable value. Nevertheless treatment can be offered using antimony preparations (sodium or potassium antimony tartrate), niridazole (a nitrofuran), lucanthone and hycanthone, and metrifonate. All these drugs are exceedingly toxic and must be used with great care. Efficacy of treatment is assessed by measuring the numbers of eggs shed in the urine.

More pertinent, in most patients, is surgical relief of obstruction of the ureter caused by the fibrosis set up around the live and dead eggs, or the removal of calculi caused by secondary infection upstream of the damaged ureter. The whole range of operations for obstruction and reflux have been employed in the treatment of schistosomiasis. The tissues the surgeons are obliged to work with are stiff, ischaemic, thick and fibrosed. They heal poorly and secondary infection often complicates the operation.

When cancer supervenes it is usually an anaplastic squamous carcinoma. Many cases are inoperable when first seen, for the sufferers from schistosomiasis are so used to haematuria that it is not worth complaining about. Their end is one of dreadful suffering. If operable, total cystectomy is usually performed, but very few, good, long-term follow-ups have been published.

Since this disease is entirely preventable, one cannot help marvelling that so much money is still expended in the search for a vaccine, in ever new medications for the infested patients and in better and more expensive snail-killers, when what is really needed are the most simple of all sanitary measures, the pit-latrine and a stand-pipe for water.

STONE IN THE BLADDER

Vesical calculi are still very common in some parts of the world, e.g. Thailand,

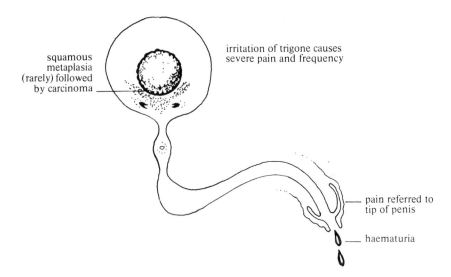

squamous metaplasia (rarely) followed by carcinoma

irritation of trigone causes severe pain and frequency

pain referred to tip of penis

haematuria

Fig. 17.4. Clinical features of vesical calculus.

the Yemen, and Turkey. They are rare in Europe except when seen in association with outflow obstruction from enlargement of the prostate in males. Occasionally they are found on non-absorbable sutures used to suspend a catheter in the bladder or used in pelvic surgery, migrating into the bladder. Sometimes they form on fragments of catheter accidentally left in the bladder.

Vesical calculi rub and irritate the bladder, provoking squamous metaplasia and ultimately, the risk of squamous cancer (Fig. 17.4).

Clinical features

Patients with stone in the bladder typically complain of pain when they are walking rather than lying down at night. The pain is referred to the tip of the penis or vulva, is accompanied by frequency and an intense desire to void. Little boys with this condition tug constantly at their foreskin to try to relieve the pain there.

Investigations

The diagnosis is made in a plain radiograph, but an excretion urogram is usually needed to show the causative outflow obstruction.

Treatment

Most calculi can be crushed and evacuated using a *lithotrite*. Modern versions of this instrument employ high frequency ultrasound to shatter the calculus. In Russia a high energy electric spark is applied through a concentric electrode to the surface of the stone with a similar effect. There are lithotrites that permit the surgeon to watch the crushing of the stone and make sure all the pieces are removed.

In boys, and in men with very large stones, where the risk of injury to the urethra is great, it is usually safer to remove the stone by suprapubic *lithotomy*, the bladder being opened and the stone extracted. A biopsy is usually taken in an adult to make sure there is no squamous carcinoma.

FURTHER READING

Hafner R.J., Stanton S.L. & Guy J. (1977) A psychiatric study of women with urgency and urgency incontinence. *British Journal of Urology*, **49,** 211.

von Lichtenberg F. & Lehman J.S. (1979) Parasitic diseases of the genitourinary system. In Harrison J.H. *et al.* (eds), *Campbell's Urology*, Vol. 1, 4th edn, p. 597. W.B. Saunders Co., Philadelphia.

Marsh F.P. (1976) The frequency-dysuria syndrome. In J.P. Blandy (ed.), *Urology*, p. 734. Blackwell Scientific Publications, Oxford.

Singh M. (1976) Tropical parasitic infections of the urinary tract. In Blandy J.P. (ed.), *Urology*, p. 261. Blackwell Scientific Publications, Oxford.

Smith J.M. & O'Flynn J.D. (1977) Transurethral removal of bladder stone: the place of litholapaxy. *British Journal of Urology*, **49,** 401.

Walsh A. (1979) Interstitial cystitis. In J.H. Harrison *et al.* (eds), *Campbell's Urology*, Vol. 1, 4th edn, p. 693. W.B. Saunders Co., Philadelphia.

Chapter 18
The Bladder—
Neoplasms

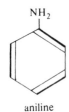

aniline

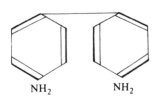

2–naphthylamine

4, 4–diaminodiphenyl (benzidine)

Fig. 18.1. Structural formulae of some carcinogens.

The bladder being lined by urothelium, most of its neoplasms are urothelial (transitional cell carcinomas). But the urothelium may undergo metaplasia into squamous and glandular epithelium, and squamous-cell and adeno-carcinomas are occasionally seen there. Rare neurofibromas, sarcomas, and even phaeo-chromocytomas may be seen that originate in the bladder. Secondary carcinoma, invading the bladder from the colon or the uterus, is occasionally seen. The chief, and unfortunately, all too common neoplasm, arises from the urothelium, and is similar in all respects to the tumours that arise in the renal pelvis, calices and ureters.

AETIOLOGY

In 1894 Rehn noticed that people working in the aniline dye industry were developing an undue proportion of cancer of the bladder. Investigation subsequently showed that it was neither aniline nor the finished dyestuffs that caused the trouble, but a group of nitrophenols (Fig. 18.1) of which the most dangerous were 2-naphthylamine and benzidine. Industries in which these, and similar compounds were used, included chemical works, dyeing, rubber moulding and cable covering, pitch and gasworks, the optical industry (when pitch was used to hold the lenses steady in the grinding and polishing processes), hairdressing, nursing, leather work and, probably, medical practice. In the case of cancer in the upper urothelial tract, as we have observed (see page 73), analgesic abuse and Balkan nephropathy give rise to cancer. Smoking is increasingly indicted as a contributory factor—and year by year the list of hazards grows. In Britain there is a considerable disparity between the numbers of men and women who die every year from cancer of the bladder, and the numbers who are notified as suffering from 'prescribed disease number 39' i.e. industrial cancer. This is almost certainly because it takes some 20 years for exposure to a carcinogen to be followed by bladder cancer, a period during which records are lost, memories have faded, and evidence to pinpoint the danger has been hopelessly diluted. Epidemiologists toiling in this area of research keep, at great trouble, closing stable doors from which the horses have long since bolted.

On a world-wide scale, the chief cause of bladder cancer is schistosomiasis (see page 182), where prolonged irritation from living and dead ova (perhaps exacerbated by tobacco and hashish smoking) gives rise to squamous metaplasia and squamous cancer.

PATHOLOGY

Macroscopic features

Bladder tumours may be single or multiple. On cystoscopic examination they

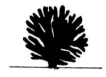
Cauliflower
(papillary)

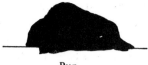
Bun
(solid)

Ulcer

Fig. 18.2. Macroscopic features of bladder cancer.

appear (as do cancers anywhere else in the body) as a cauliflower (papillary), a solid lump, or as an ulcer (Fig. 18.2).

Microscopic features

UROTHELIAL TUMOURS

Papilloma

This name is often used when one ought to be saying carcinoma. Real benign papillomas in the bladder are exceedingly rare—less than 1%. The diagnosis should always be questioned and a second opinion on the section should always be sought. Moreover, the patient ought to be strictly followed up.

Carcinoma

Three Grades of malignancy are recognized, according to internationally agreed criteria, which are no different from those that apply to cancer in other organs: they may be well-differentiated (G1), poorly differentiated (G3), or in between with a 'medium degree' of differentiation (G2).

SQUAMOUS CARCINOMA

Here one must be careful not to include patients with nasty G2 solid tumours which are going a little bit squamous here and there. The real squamous cancer has a thick layer of keratinised 'skin' and epithelial pearls, and carries a dreadful prognosis.

ADENOCARCINOMA

Glandular metaplasia is found in some instances of chronic infection and irritation, e.g. in the exposed bladder of children born with extrophy (see page 172). It is also seen in carcinoma originating in the urachus—a remnant of hindgut—that links the apex of the bladder to the umbilicus. Fortunately both these conditions are exceedingly rare, for the tumour has a miserable outlook.

Spread of bladder cancer

Bladder cancer spreads by direct invasion through the muscle of the wall of the bladder, across the surrounding fat, and into the adjacent organs such as the rectum, prostate and uterus. Curiously it virtually never crosses the barrier of Denonvilliers' fascia, the doubled fold of peritoneum that stands like a fire-resisting door, between rectum and prostate. Hence bladder cancer is never seen fungating into the rectum: it may encircle it or squeeze it, but it never invades it.

Staging of bladder cancer

Like cancers in all other organs of the body, there is now an internationally agreed system of staging that allows surgeons in one centre to compare their results with those obtained in another. This, the TNM (tumour, nodes, metastases) system has a number of detailed rules and regulations which the research worker in the field needs to be familiar with. For the student, it is enough to understand its principles. N (lymph nodes) draining the bladder are almost impossible to depict at present. Current techniques of lymphography are too inaccurate for routine use. The CAT scan is too expensive and not really much more accurate either, and although distant metastases do occur, the M category is of little clinical importance, when the most necessary task is to control the local disease. Hence it is the T category which concerns the surgeon and his treatment plan more than the N or M groups (Fig. 18.3).

If one can discover a bladder cancer before it has begun to invade the bladder muscle, it can usually be cured by quite simple endoscopic means without a cutting operation, and the long term cure rate is excellent. If the

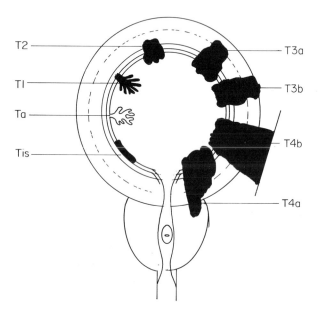

Fig. 18.3. Summary of the T staging system for carcinoma of the bladder.

Chapter 18/*The Bladder—Neoplasms*

bladder cancer is only detected when it has begun to invade the muscle of the bladder, the outlook is much worse. Much more heroic measures need to be employed: the patient needs to undergo cystectomy, with or without radiotherapy, and perhaps several courses of very toxic chemotherapy. The importance of getting the T stage right cannot be overestimated. Because the outlook for the patient with a bladder tumour is so much much worse when it has reached the stage of invading the muscle, it is of crucial importance that the diagnosis should be made if possible at an earlier stage.

SCREENING OF SYMPTOMLESS PATIENTS

Patients may be screened, when they are known to be in hazardous occupations, by looking in their urine for malignant cells by the Papanicolaou test. Urine that has not been kept in the bladder overnight has the best chance of keeping cancer cells undistorted and recognizable. The urine should be fixed at once with 10% formalin or some similar fixative, and then sent to the laboratory where it will be centrifuged, fixed and stained. Unfortunately the diagnosis of cancer depends on recognition of a huge nucleus in the cell and relatively little cytoplasm, and if the cells are originating from a very well-differentiated carcinoma, they will not be distinguishable from normal transitional epithelium unless by chance an entire broken-off papillary frond is included in the smear.

Similarly, if a patient has had some of his urothelium scraped off by a stone, or lost after a severe attack of bacterial cystitis, the lost urothelium will be replaced by mitosis and inward migration of cells from the edge of the defect. If these rapidly dividing and growing cells are lost, they may give rise to a false-positive appearance of 'malignant' cells in the deposit. The Papanicolaou test is of very great value, but it must be used intelligently and its results must be interpreted with caution. The skills necessary to recognize cancer cells are not inexpensive and to provide enough technicians to screen the whole population, let alone prevent them from dying of boredom, would be impossible. Hence 'screening' of urine for malignant cells should only be carried out in high-risk populations, or in patients where cancer is suspected, e.g. in men with symptoms of 'prostatism', in people with haematuria, or in those in suspected occupations. In practice, the most important need is to educate the public to complain of the early symptoms, and for doctors to take note of them.

CLINICAL FEATURES

Haematuria is noticed by 80% of patients with bladder cancer (Fig. 18.4) and this is the cardinal reason why every patient with haematuria must be cystoscoped sooner or later. Almost equally important is the realization that 20% of people with bladder cancer have *not* noticed haematuria: their symptoms are even more deserving of note. How are we to guard against overlooking cancer in these patients?

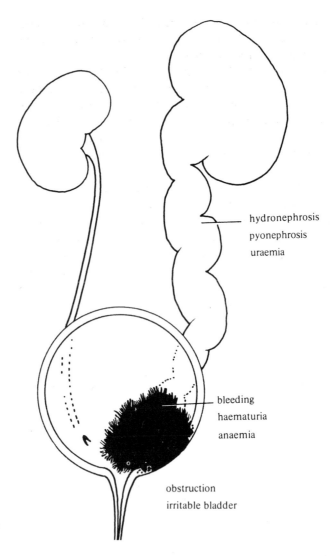

hydronephrosis
pyonephrosis
uraemia

bleeding
haematuria
anaemia

obstruction
irritable bladder

Fig. 18.4. Clinical features of bladder carcinoma.

The bladder cancer irritates the epithelium of the bladder: it makes the surrounding urothelium red and oedematous, and it rubs against the adjacent tissues. Thus the afferent limb of the reflex arc of the micturition reflex is over-stimulated and the patient experiences *frequency*. Many also have discomfort on voiding. They go to their doctor with pain and frequency, and it is exceedingly easy to jump to the conclusion that they have cystitis. Indeed, in some patients, they may very well have infection as well, since the rough necrotic surface of the tumour is a good breeding ground for organisms. However, in the early case, this is not common. How can the alert doctor spot the one patient in a whole group who seem to have identical symptoms of 'cystitis'? The give-away is the absence of micro-organisms from the urine,

Chapter 18/*The Bladder—Neoplasms*

combined with the presence of 'pus' (since cancer cells shed from a tumour under the ordinary microscope used to look at urine look very like pus). *Sterile pyuria = cancer or tuberculosis until proven otherwise.*

In elderly men, (and most bladder cancers occur in elderly men) the symptoms of irritability of the bladder, may well suggest prostatic outflow obstruction (see page 222). How can one avoid this error? The answer is to insist on testing the urine in each prostatic patient for haematuria (e.g. with a stix test, see page 11), to follow this with a Papanicolaou, and in the end, to make sure that before any operation is done on the prostate, the bladder is meticulously inspected with the cystoscope.

Other symptoms may bring the patient with a bladder cancer to the doctor, but they are all late. *Pain*—a boring unremitting pain radiating to the perineum and sacrum, usually signifies extension of cancer outside the bladder. *Anaemia* out of all proportion to the size of the tumour, from long continued loss of blood in haematuria, may reduce the haemoglobin to 3 or 4 g and bring the patient to hospital with angina pectoris. Finally, true urinary *infection*, particularly when it occurs in an elderly man, should be regarded as secondary to outflow obstruction or cancer (or both).

Physical signs

They are usually absent or unhelpful. Occasionally you will feel an indurated mass in the suprapubic region or a hard lump on rectal examination, but these are late features.

INVESTIGATIONS

Engraven on every urologist's heart is the simple equation *Haematuria = IVU + cystoscopy*. Today these are preceded by measurement of the blood creatinine, culture of the urine, and Papanicolaou staining of the urinary sediment for cancer cells.

The excretion urogram may show a filling defect in the bladder (Fig. 18.5) and obstruction to one or other ureter. If the ureter is obstructed it nearly always means that the muscle near to the ureteric orifice has been invaded by tumour and hence the growth is T2 or worse.

Cystoscopy for neoplasms in the bladder

A deep general anaesthetic with full relaxation is needed, for it is essential to feel the muscular wall of the bladder carefully in order to try to assess how far the growth has penetrated. Then the bladder must be carefully inspected so that the size, number and type of tumours can be recorded. A *biopsy* is taken with cup-forceps or resectoscope loop. This biopsy must include a sample of the bladder muscle deep to the tumour so that the pathologist can tell how far the

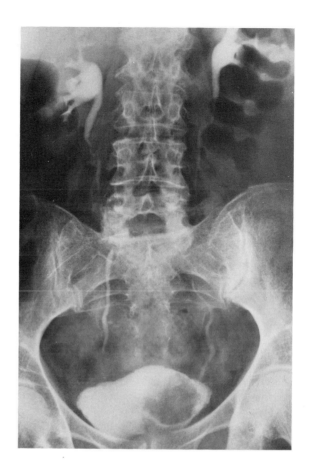

Fig. 18.5. Excretion urogram from a 68 year old man with a three month history of haematuria. Note the large filling defect in the left half of the bladder. The ureter is not obstructed. This was found to be a G2pT1 carcinoma and was treated by transurethral resection.

growth has penetrated (i.e. give its T stage). (When adequate histology is available, the modified staging is referred to as the pT stage.)

TREATMENT

Only after this preliminary examination and biopsy has been done can the surgeon plan treatment properly. It is easiest to consider each stage of tumour in turn.

Tis—flat pre-invasive carcinoma (pTis G3) (Fig. 18.6)

This is a nasty but fortunately very rare entity. It presents as 'cystitis' in middle-aged men, usually without any haematuria. Very anaplastic cells are detected in the urine on Papanicolaou staining. On cystoscopy the bladder looks normal, or just a little inflamed. The diagnosis depends on the alertness of the surgeon doing the cystoscopy and his being prepared to take a biopsy from

Chapter 18/*The Bladder—Neoplasms*

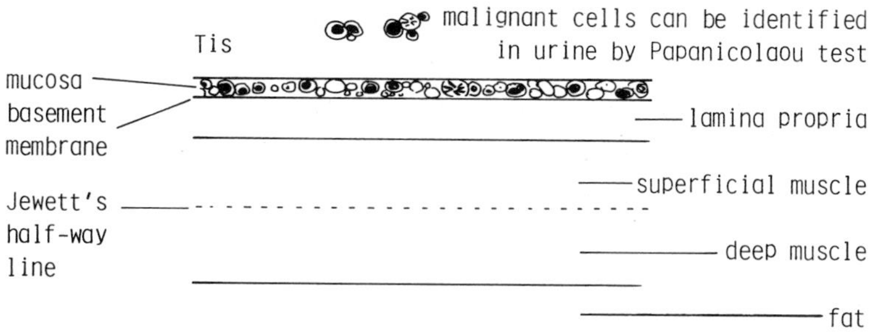

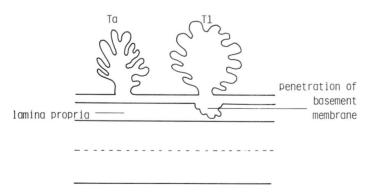

Tis

mucosa

basement
membrane

malignant cells can be identified
in urine by Papanicolaou test

lamina propria

superficial muscle

Jewett's
half-way
line

deep muscle

fat

Fig. 18.6. Tis carcinoma of the bladder—'flat *in situ*' or 'malignant cystitis'.

the mucosa of anyone with unexplained 'cystitis' or sterile pyuria. In days gone by this condition carried a very high mortality because it usually went unrecognized. When detected, surgeons at once proceeded to total cystectomy. Today we have available several chemotherapeutic agents, including systemic cyclophosphamide and intravesical Adriamycin and Mitomycin, all of which seem able to discipline this malignant urothelium and restore it to something approaching normality.

Ta—papillary non-invasive carcinoma

Here one finds pretty, little, pink cabbages, often multiple, growing out from the bladder wall. The distinction between these Ta tumours and the next group T1 rests on the fact that in Ta there is no detectable break-through of the basement membrane. Treatment is the same.

T1—microscopically the tumour does not extend beyond the lamina propria

These look the same as Ta tumours. There may be one or many (Fig. 18.7). The important thing is that muscle underneath the stalk of the tumour is not invaded. Hence it is important that any biopsy or resection-specimen of these tumours must include an adequate portion of the muscle in the stalk or stalks.

Ta   T1

lamina propria

penetration of
basement
membrane

Fig. 18.7. Ta and T1 carcinoma of the bladder. In Ta there is no break-through of the basement membrane into the lamina propria. Unfortunately this is a very rare tumour and T1 is more common.

To this the international system adds, that after complete resection of the tumour no mass should be palpable on bimanual examination.

Treatment of these tumours depends above all on skill and patience on the part of the urological surgeon: skill to enable him to resect large or numerous tumours with the resectoscope, patience to make him continue on and on, hour after hour if necessary, and perhaps on more than one session, until the bladder is entirely clear of the tumours. Bleeding obscures the view and in a bulky tumour it is discouraging and difficult to keep well-orientated. There is a danger, in unskilled hands, of perforating the bladder. But the reward is immense—a clear bladder, and a good prognosis.

ADJUVANT CHEMOTHERAPY FOR TA AND T1 TUMOURS

Every superficial Ta and T1 tumour patient will be kept under regular and repeated endoscopic review. His bladder will be carefully examined under anaesthesia every three months for a year, every six months for two years, and then annually for the rest of his life. Sometimes a whole new crop of little tumours is seen at every cystoscopy. The bladder is clearly the seat of active tumour formation. It is daunting and difficult to deal with endoscopically. Fortunately in such patients we have a whole group of very useful chemical agents that can be instilled into the bladder, *after* destroying all the salient and visible tumours, which will very substantially limit the number and frequency of tumour recurrence. Of these agents the most useful is *Thiotepa* (so long as it is used in a low dose or else there is a risk of absorption and marrow suppression). Others in common use include *Epodyl*, *Mitomycin* and *Adriamycin*.

T2 microscopical invasion of superficial muscle (Fig. 18.8)

If the tumour proves to be G1 and well-differentiated on section, many surgeons are content to remove the tumour and its base with the resectoscope. If the tumour is G2 or G3, less well-differentiated, the writer feels that there is a considerable chance that the neoplasm will have gained access to the lymphatics

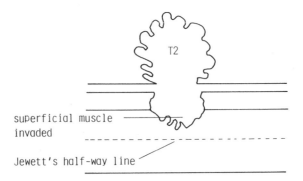

Fig. 18.8. T2 tumour of bladder, where there is invasion of the muscle but not more than half-way through the bladder wall.

Chapter 18/*The Bladder—Neoplasms*

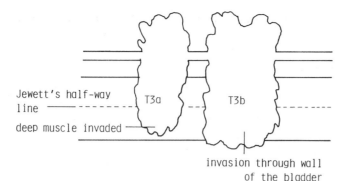

Jewett's half-way line

deep muscle invaded

T3a

T3b

invasion through wall
of the bladder

Fig. 18.9. T3 tumours of the bladder. In T3a the tumour is into the deep muscle; in T3b it has reached the outside of the bladder wall.

of the bladder, and so will have spread beyond the reach of the resectoscope. For this reason resection is supplemented by radiotherapy.

T3 microscopic invasion of deep muscle (Fig. 18.9)

It is here that controversy has been most intense in the last few years. Today it is agreed by all urological surgeons that to remove the bladder without a previous course of radiotherapy is ineffective. Some surgeons give a 'flash' dose of radiation (2000 rads over a five day course) and follow this with a total cystectomy. Better results are obtained with a larger preceding dose of radiotherapy. Current British practice is to attempt to eradicate the tumour with a maximum course of radiation (5500 rads) and see if the tumour resolves or not. If it goes away, one may expect a 70% five-year-cure rate. If the tumour does not go away, then total cystectomy is performed. We hope that in the next few years a more accurate way than the existing method of trial and error to foretell whether tumours will be radiosensitive or not may be forthcoming.

ADJUVANT CHEMOTHERAPY

At the time of writing several clinical trials are in progress to see whether the patient's outlook can be further improved by combining radiation and cystectomy with pre- or postoperative chemotherapy with a number of agents of which today *methotrexate* offers considerable promise.

ALTERNATIVE FORMS OF TREATMENT

The reader must understand that the results of the treatment of bladder cancer are continually improving, and the current methods are under constant review, usually by means of multi-centre clinical trials. To get good results in bladder cancer it is undoubtedly better for the patient to be referred to a specialist centre where the most up-to-date and least invasive methods of treatment are in daily use. Generally abandoned today are the operations of open cystodiathermy and implantation of radioactive gold or radon seeds, and of partial cystectomy supplemented by radiation.

Helmstein's treatment

If a rubber balloon is very tightly blown up inside the bladder until the superficial mucosa is rendered ischaemic, then exophytic tumours on the surface of the bladder urothelium may be killed. When the technique was first announced it was hoped that this process would in some way stimulate the immune defences of the body and control more deeply infiltrating tumours. This has not been the general experience, but the balloon distension technique is useful to get rid of very large bulky tumours, and to control bleeding. It is also employed in a few units for the treatment of Hunner's ulcer (see page 179).

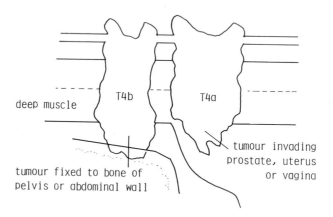

Fig. 18.10. T4 tumours of the bladder. In T4a the growth is invading the prostate uterus or vagina, i.e. in theory it could be removed surgically; in T4b it is invading the bony wall of the pelvis, or at least, is fixed to it on bimanual examination.

Inoperable bladder cancer T4 (Fig. 18.10)

At the end of the day, treatment often fails, and we are left with the elderly patient, racked with pain, voiding blood-stained urine with pain and difficulty every few minutes day and night. Sleeplessness adds to their misery, and the breaking down necrotic tumour inside the bladder is often irremediably infected. Surgery has much to offer, not by way of cure, but by way of relief of suffering. If the urine is *diverted*, either with a ureteroureterostomy (see page 307) or through an ileal conduit, the patient is spared the misery of painful frequency. When pain-relieving medicines fail, then *cordotomy* may bring profound and lasting relief of suffering. Short 'palliative' courses of radiotherapy, if it has not been used before, may stop haemorrhage and bring long lasting relief of frequency. Above all comes the time when the surgeon must be there at the bedside, from time to time, not that he has anything left to offer, but to show that he is still the patient's friend, and that he cares.

Chapter 18/*The Bladder—Neoplasms*

FURTHER READING

Blandy J.P., England H.R., Evans S.J.W., Hope-Stone H.F., Mair G.M.M., Mantell B.S., Oliver R.T.D., Paris A.M.I. & Risdon R.A. (1980) T3 bladder cancer—the case for salvage cystectomy. *British Journal of Urology*, **52,** 506.

Clayson D.B. (1976) Occupational bladder cancer. *Preventive Medicine*, **5,** 228.

Crawford E.D. & Skinner D.G. (1980) Salvage cystectomy after irradiation failure. *Journal of Urology*, **123,** 32.

Fox A.J. & Collier P.T. (1976) A survey of occupational cancer in the rubber and cable-making industries. *British Journal of Industrial Medicine*, **22,** 249.

Kipling M.D. (1976) Occupational considerations in carcinoma of the urogenital tract. *British Journal of Hospital Medicine*, **15,** 465.

Koontz W.W., Prout G.R., Smith W., Frable W.J. & Minnis J.E. (1981) The use of intravesical Thio-tepa in the management of non-invasive carcinoma of the bladder. *Journal of Urology*, **125,** 307.

Wallace D.M. (1976) Carcinoma of the urothelium. In J.P. Blandy (ed.), *Urology*, p. 774. Blackwell Scientific Publications, Oxford.

Skinner D.G. & de Kernion J.B. (eds) (1978) *Genitourinary cancer*. W.B. Saunders Co., Philadelphia.

Chapter 19
The Bladder—Urodynamics and Functional Disturbances of Micturition

NORMAL MICTURITION AND THE INNERVATION OF THE BLADDER

Afferent impulses from the mucosa of the bladder, and perhaps arising from stretch receptors in the muscle, pass up in the pelvic parasympathetic filaments to the S2 and S3 segments of the spinal cord (which lie in the tip of the conus medullaris of the spinal cord, just about opposite the disc between T12 and L1 vertebrae) (Fig. 19.1).

There the afferent impulses synapse in the cord, to stimulate the efferent limb of the reflex arc. Efferent impulses pass back down the parasympathetic filaments to stimulate the detrusor muscle to contract.

But the bladder is provided with a series of sphincters, and to permit the bladder to empty, these must be allowed to relax. Hence an essential ingredient of the reflux action of the spinal centre that controls the bladder in S2 and S3 is *inhibition* of impulses that pass to the internal sphincter, the supramembranous sphincter, and the external striated spincter urethrae, which is part of the levator ani shelf. The motor nerves to the internal and supramembranous sphincter are mainly in the parasympathetic fibres, while those to the external sphincter are carried in the pudendal nerve.

As with any other reflex arc in the nervous system, it is influenced by higher centres, which can either facilitate the reflex or inhibit it. In man these higher influences are represented at every level of the central nervous system, and it is a common observation that from time to time the urge to empty an overdistended bladder may drive all other thoughts from one's consciousness. Equally, when anxious or frightened, one may feel an overwhelming urge to empty a bladder that is barely half-full.

There are very many clinical conditions in which the normal functioning of

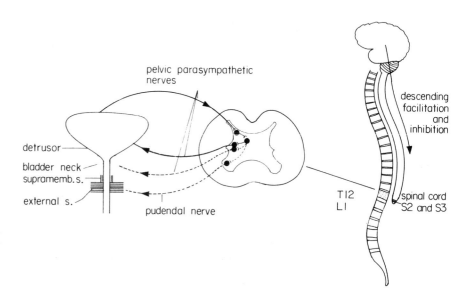

Fig. 19.1. The nervous pathways for micturition are sited in the S2 and S3 segments of the spinal cord, opposite the disc between the T12 and L1 vertebrae. Stimulation—solid lines; inhibition—dotted lines.

the human bladder is altered by disturbances of its innervation. The science of measuring and recording the physiological performance of the bladder is called *urodynamics*. It relies upon certain important methods of measurement.

Cystometry

The oldest of these investigations consisted of the measurement of the pressure inside the bladder as it was filled with water (*static cystometry*) (Fig. 19.2) or as it emptied during ordinary micturition (*voiding cystometry*) (Fig. 19.3). In its most simple forms a catheter attached to a manometer measured the pressure inside the lumen of the bladder, while it was filled at a steady rate from another tube. The pressure inside the bladder however recorded not only the pressure due to the contraction of the detrusor muscle, but also that transmitted from

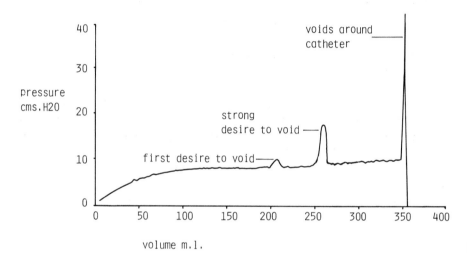

Fig. 19.2. Static cystometrogram.

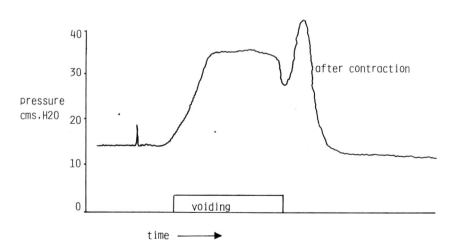

Fig. 19.3. Dynamic or voiding cystometrogram.

Chapter 19/*The Bladder—Urodynamics and Micturition Disturbances*　　201

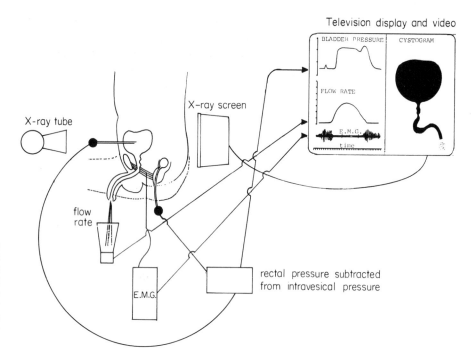

Television display and video

BLADDER PRESSURE CYSTOGRAM

FLOW RATE

E.M.G.
time

X-ray screen

X-ray tube

flow
rate

E.M.G.

rectal pressure subtracted
from intravesical pressure

Fig. 19.4. Diagram of the elements of the videocystourethrogram (VCU). The true intravesical pressure (the measured bladder pressure *minus* intrarectal pressure) is recorded as well as the flow-rate and electromyogram while the radiographic image of the bladder filled with contrast medium is shown on the same television screen and recorded on video-tape.

any other cause of raised intra-abdominal pressure, e.g. coughing or straining. To remove this unwanted component, modern systems have a second manometer, recording from a small balloon inside the rectum (to record intra-abdominal pressure). A simple electronic system subtracts the rectal from the bladder pressure.

More information is obtained from observation of the voiding cystometrogram than from the static record. An even more vivid and useful appreciation of a disturbed bladder at work is obtained from the use of a radio-opaque contrast medium, rather than water, which can be X-rayed and observed fluoroscopically, and recorded along with the corrected voiding cystometrogram on the same television videotape. This expensive equipment is regarded as essential in a modern urodynamic laboratory where it is referred to as 'videocystourethrography' or VCU for short (Fig. 19.4).

Flow-rate

If the detrusor is slack and floppy, or if the urethra is narrowed by stricture, then the jet of urine escaping from the external meatus is a thin one. Much can be gained by the careful doctor who is prepared to spend time watching his patient pass water, but this gives only subjective information, it cannot be recorded, and it is often very difficult to arrange in a busy clinic. Accurate methods of measuring the flow-rate out of the meatus are now available. These 'flowmeters' give a record expressed in volume of urine per unit of time, ml/second. They require a certain minimum volume of urine to be in the bladder (more than 200 ml) for the trace to be repeatable or meaningful. With suitable electronic connections, the flow-rate can be simultaneously recorded on the videocysto-urethrogram trace along with the corrected pressure in the bladder.

Electromyography

In many circumstances it is useful to know what the external sphincter is doing during micturition, and fine needle electrodes can be placed in the external sphincter adjacent to the urethra and be made to record the electromyographic activity of the striated muscle bundles in the vicinity of the needle. Again, the EMG can, if need arises, be recorded on the VCU tape.

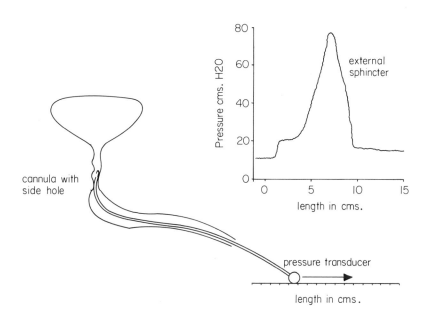

Fig. 19.5. The urethral pressure profile is the plot of the intraurethral pressure against the distance travelled by the cannula down the urethra. Not shown in the diagram is the slow continuous perfusion of the cannula.

Urethral pressure profile (Fig. 19.5).

Where the sphincter squeezes the urethra a fine balloon or cannula with a side-hole, will record an increase in pressure. If the cannula or balloon is slowly withdrawn along the whole length of the urethra it will record the rise and fall of the various components of the sphincter, the internal (or bladder neck), the supramembranous, and the striated external sphincter. This system is usually measured with an XY recorder which automatically notes the distance (from the lumen of the bladder) at which the pressure is being recorded.

COMMON DISORDERS OF MICTURITION

Disorders of the bladder reflex arc

1. AFFERENT OVERSTIMULATION (Fig. 19.6)

Any lesion that makes the lining of the bladder more sensitive, or stimulates it unusually severely, will set off the detrusor reflex contraction before the bladder has become filled to its normal capacity. Common causes of this include bacterial cystitis, a stone, or carcinoma. The clinical symptom that dominates all others is the frequency of micturition accompanied by an intense desire to void, and 'urge incontinence' if the patient cannot reach the toilet in time.

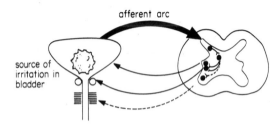

Fig. 19.6. Overstimulation of the afferent side of the reflex arc sets off the detrusor reflex before the bladder is really full.

The patient will show a prematurely early detrusor contraction in the static and voiding cystometrogram. The detrusor pressure will be normal or perhaps a little increased during contractions. The flow-rate is normal, allowing for the fact that the volume voided is often very small. The performance of the external sphincter and the bladder neck is normal.

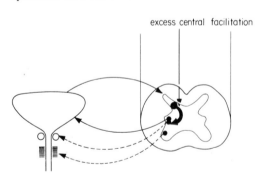

Fig. 19.7. Excessive central facilitation of the reflex arc triggers it to empty before it is really full.

2. EXCESSIVE CENTRAL FACILITATION (Fig. 19.7)

Nobody who has ever had to face an important examination will be ignorant that facilitation from higher centres may sensitize the bladder reflex arc. It is a common and distressing feature of many anxiety states. Clinically it may be very difficult to distinguish this from the first group, in which there is something irritating the bladder, but usually, when the cause is anxiety, the frequency of micturition occurs only in the daytime, and does not disturb the patient's sleep.

Cystometrography will reveal a bladder that empties at a reduced capacity. Under anaesthesia the bladder will be found to be entirely normal, and to hold 3–400 ml without difficulty. The functions of the sphincters are normal and the flow-rate normal too.

3. LACK OF CENTRAL INHIBITION (Fig. 19.8)

Enuresis—bed-wetting

In its most simple form, the higher inhibitory influences that in civilized man stop the bladder from emptying until it is convenient to do so, are acquired as a result of childhood conditioning. In children who sleep very deeply, there may be a failure to inhibit the reflex emptying of the bladder during the night. This is the usual type of bed-wetting, or nocturnal enuresis. It is difficult to know when to begin to investigate or treat this tiresome condition: children develop the sleeping inhibition at different ages, and there are many perfectly normal boys and girls who are not reliably dry at night until they are 8 or 9 years old. In some otherwise normal individuals the reflex is never entirely inhibited—*adult enuresis*. Urinary infection may make things worse by adding an element of afferent stimulation to the reflex arc, but the usual routine investigations show nothing wrong at all. It is doubtful if more than simple testing of the urine for bacteria is needed in most cases. In older children one must always be extremely cautious before embarking on a full series of urodynamic investigations which are always demeaning for the child, at least uncomfortable, and at worst terrifying.

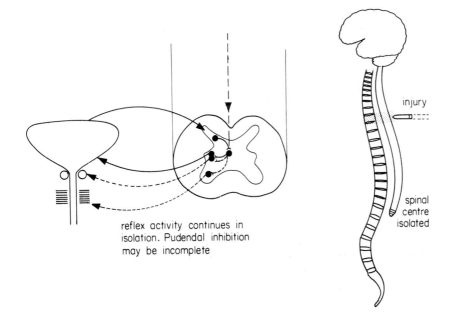

reflex activity continues in isolation. Pudendal inhibition may be incomplete

injury

spinal centre isolated

Fig. 19.8. Lack of central inhibition may occur in sleep (enuresis) or when the higher centres are cut off by some physical injury (paraplegia). In paraplegia, the co-ordinated inhibition of the pudendal and internal sphincter innervation is disturbed.

At the end of the day, treatment nearly always employs three methods. (a) The child is encouraged to pass his or her urine by the clock, learning what it feels like to experience a full bladder, and also to be able to inhibit the detrusor contractions until it is time to go to the toilet. It is obviously impossible to train the cortex to inhibit urination during sleep, but it can be most useful if practised during the day. (b) This is supplemented by medication that lightens the level of sleep, since most of these children sleep very deeply indeed. A wide variety of drugs have been used and one should take care to use the most simple and safe. At the time of writing the author prefers a proprietary capsule containing isopropamide, phenylpropanolamine and diphenylpyraline* but many other alpha-stimulators have been used with good effect. (c) Finally, one may treat the child like a Pavlov dog: he sleeps on two thin sheets, which separate two perforated tinfoil sheets connected to a buzzer and battery, so arranged that when soaked in urine the buzzer goes off. When this system is used, it is essential that the child is fully awakened, and made to urinate. Before long his sleeping inhibitory centre gets the idea that the sensation of a full bladder will be associated with waking up and urinating. It is quite futile to misuse the buzzer alarm: to let it sound, wake up the rest of the family and let the mother change the wet sheets, but allow the child to sleep deeply and obliviously on. Used intelligently this threefold method of treatment works well.

Paraplegia

In high spinal cord injury, the higher inhibitory influences are cut off from the S2 and S3 segments. As a result, the detrusor reflex works automatically when the bladder is more or less full. In practice, this ideal state of affairs is seldom reached in high spinal cord injuries. For reasons at present little understood, the isolated spinal cord centre for the bladder does not react in the same co-ordinated way as the normal one. The chief problem is that the internal and external sphincter muscles are not inhibited in harmony with contraction of the detrusor. The effect of this is to oblige the detrusor to work against resistance at the outlet to the bladder. It becomes hypertrophied, often grossly, and it works inefficiently, so that residual urine accumulates. Urinary infection inevitably occurs in this residual urine. In practice, one is often forced to cut through the sphincters in order to get the bladder emptied and enable infection to be controlled.

Urodynamic evaluation of the paraplegic patient is of great importance and great practical value. The static and voiding cystometrograms will show tremendous 'uninhibited' detrusor contractions when the bladder is half-full. The pressure rises to great heights owing to the increased outflow resistance from the unrelaxed sphincters. Profile measurements show huge pressures at the internal and external sphincter zones, and the videocystogram shows how poorly the contraction of the detrusor is co-ordinated with the relaxation of the sphincters, and often shows reflux up the ureters.

* Eskornade® Smith Kline and French.

Similar though very variable pictures of disturbed bladder function are seen in multiple sclerosis and other lesions involving the long tracts of the spinal cord.

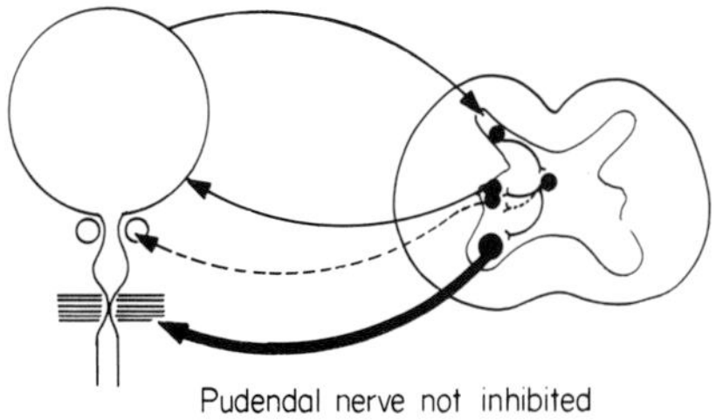

4. EXTERNAL SPHINCTER DYSSYNERGIA (Fig. 19.9)

A rare but extraordinary lack of co-ordination occurs in some children and occasionally adults whose detrusor and whose internal sphincter work harmoniously, but whose external (voluntary) sphincter remains tightly shut while the bladder is trying to empty itself. This can produce the most bizarre clinical picture: huge bladders and often obstructed or refluxing ureters, associated with a poor flow-rate, typically interrupted and 'stuttering'. When studied urodynamically, one finds a large capacity bladder, with a normally performing detrusor, but an external sphincter (measured with the electromyogram) that remains tightly clenched when it ought by rights to be relaxed. It seems very probable that this is an error in behaviour more in the category of bad habit than disease of the nervous system. Patients with this disorder can sometimes be trained to void normally, once they get the knack of relaxing their levator ani at the right time.

Pudendal nerve not inhibited

Fig. 19.9. External sphincter dyssynergia: when the detrusor contracts, the external sphincter does not relax. This is probably caused by some central disorder.

5. DESTRUCTION OF THE SPINA CENTRE S2, S3 (Fig. 19.10)

Unfortunately the bladder centre in the tip of the spinal cord lies just where the patient is most likely to break his or her back—at the junction between the stiff thoracic spine and the mobile lumbar vertebrae. Hyperflexion, or dislocation-

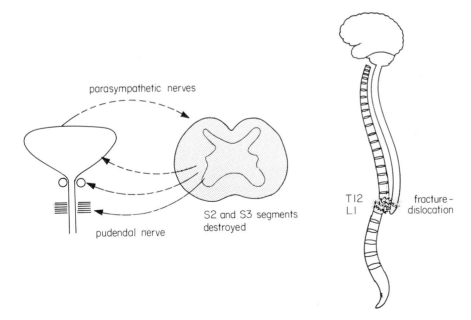

parasympathetic nerves

pudendal nerve

S2 and S3 segments destroyed

T12
L1
fracture-dislocation

Fig. 19.10. If the spinal centre S2 and S3 is destroyed, e.g. by fracture dislocation at the thoraco–lumbar junction, the bladder is entirely denervated. It behaves like an inert rubber bag.

fractures at this level often destroy the tip of the spinal cord completely as well as producing a variable amount of damage to the long nerve roots that surround it in the cauda equina. One useful reflex may be examined to determine whether the spinal centre is intact or not, namely the contraction of the bulbospongiosus muscle that is elicited by tweaking the glans penis (*bulbospongiosus reflex*). If the spinal reflex arc is completely destroyed, then the bladder is left as a denervated bag made of muscle.

Clinically it is difficult, in many cases, to be quite sure of the diagnosis for four to five weeks after the initial injury. The bulbospongiosus reflex may return relatively early and indicate that the spinal centre is intact. Urodynamic studies after this same interval may detect detrusor contractions in response to filling of the bladder, or to irrigating it with ice-cold, sterile water. But when the centre is entirely destroyed, filling the bladder with the static cystometrogram gives a long, flat curve without a flicker of evidence of detrusor contraction.

The electromyogram of the levator ani sheet shows no action potentials. Such a patient may empty the bladder past the flaccid sphincters relatively easily with compression over the lower abdomen, but the utmost vigilance is needed in the follow up to make sure that residual urine (i.e. infection) is not accumulating to bring the hazard of reflux of infection to the kidneys.

6. DESTRUCTION OF THE PELVIC PARASYMPATHETIC NERVES

Very similar paralysis of the bladder follows surgical operations in which the pelvic parasympathetic pathways are cut or removed. These include radical operations for the removal of carcinoma of the uterus or rectum, in which attempts are made to take away the lymph nodes along the internal and external iliac vessels and all the tissue attached to the lateral wall of the pelvis. One may see a very similar disturbance of function after fractures of the pelvis, probably because the fracture line crosses the line of the nerves and tears them across.

Clinically and urodynamically there is the same big, floppy bladder without any detrusor contractions on filling, but here the somatic motor innervation of the levator ani continues to remain intact, and the external sphincter offers an important obstruction to emptying out of urine from the bladder. Hence there is a risk of infection (Fig. 19.11).

In certain neuropathies involving the autonomic nervous system, of which that seen in diabetes mellitus is the most important and most common, there is a failure of function of the pelvic parasympathetics which, in the bladder, may give rise to one of two clinical pictures. In some men the bladder appears to be hypersensitive, to empty when less than completely full, but to empty incompletely. This is in many clinical respects very similar to the changes seen in prostatic outflow obstruction, but the patient's symptoms of frequency and sometimes of urge incontinence are not relieved by removing the obstructing prostatic tissue. The other clinical picture which is seen perhaps more often, is that of a large, overdistended bladder with a big residual urine. Urodynamics will show that the detrusor contractions are weak, the residual urine is large,

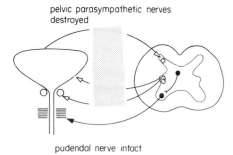

pelvic parasympathetic nerves destroyed

pudendal nerve intact

Fig. 19.11. If only the pelvic parasympathetic nerves are destroyed, e.g. after surgery, the pudendal nerve and external sphincter continue to work; there may be residual urine and infection.

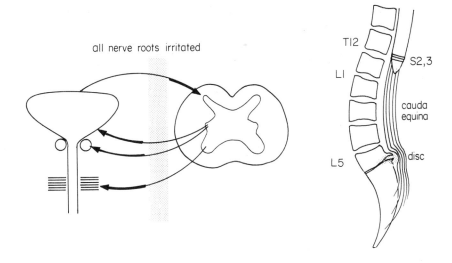

all nerve roots irritated

T12
L1
L5
S2,3
cauda equina
disc

Fig. 19.12. Lesions affecting the cauda equina may irritate the afferent and efferent limbs of the reflex arc. A lumbosacral disc is one such cause of this disorder.

and there is a relative obstruction at the bladder neck. Such patients may be much improved by resecting the prostate, even though the primary problem lies in the detrusor.

7. IRRITATION OF THE SPINAL REFLEX ARC (Fig. 19.12)

One must take care in making this diagnosis, which is obviously going to present clinical and urodynamic features that mimic those caused by failure of central inhibition, or increased sensitivity of the bladder mucosa. One sees rare examples of patients with an apparently irritable bladder, where the cause appears to be a prolapsed intervertebral disk that juts back (usually between the last lumbar and first sacral body) to irritate the most medial fibres of the cauda equina. It is important to bear it in mind, for prompt neurosurgical intervention can prevent irreversible damage to the bladder and bring a complete return of bladder function.

It is possible that some of the clinical symptoms of frequency and urgency seen in pelvic inflammations are related to similar hypersensitivity in the pelvic parasympathetic nerves.

Disorders of bladder function caused by mechanical factors

A. DIURESIS

It may sound absurd to need to point out that if a patient has to pass a large volume of urine, he will experience frequency of micturition. It is not at all uncommon for patients to be referred for the investigation of frequency in whom simple testing of the urine discloses that they have *diabetes mellitus*. Less often seen are those patients with *diabetes insipidus* of pituitary origin, or those with a failure of renal medullary function, caused perhaps by preceding, long-continued, upper tract obstruction, who are unable to concentrate their urine, and must perforce produce large volumes of urine.

Easy to overlook too, are those elderly men, referred for prostatectomy, whose frequency, so troublesome at night, turns out to be caused by that strange aberration of urine concentration, caused by *heart failure*. Oedema fluid, that accumulates during the daytime, is returned to the circulation when the patient lies down, and is presented to the kidneys as a fluid load that needs to be got rid of. The diagnosis in these cases is easily made if the patient is asked to keep a fluid chart. The tell tale signs are that he passes a *large volume* throughout the night.

Curiously enough, a very similar change of renal function is seen in the *renal transplant* patient recovering from his operation. The transplanted kidney seems often to put out the majority of the urine during the night. It may be that this represents some curious alteration in the pattern of secretion of the pituitary anti-diuretic hormone, which is known to be responsive to light and darkness.

Urodynamic investigations are not called for in such patients, but if done, will show no abnormality.

B. BLADDER OUTFLOW OBSTRUCTION

There are many possible causes for an increased resistance downstream of the bladder. Common examples are the enlarged prostate and urethral stricture. Whatever the cause, if there is an increased resistance at the outflow, the pressure inside the bladder has to be increased to get the urine out. To meet this increased demand, the detrusor muscle responds by *hypertrophy*. As with other muscles that undergo hypertrophy in the body, the bladder wall becomes more thick and its texture more coarse (see page 222). At the same time in the early phase of this hypertrophic response, the detrusor becomes—like the highly

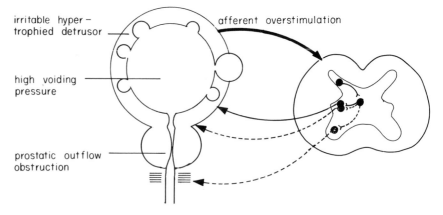

Fig. 19.13. Urodynamic changes in outflow obstruction, e.g. prostate or urethral stricture. The hypertrophied detrusor is also hyper-irritable; its trabeculated and sacculated muscle is abnormally jumpy from afferent overstimulation. There is a high voiding pressure, poor flow, and often abnormal, uninhibited detrusor contractions as the bladder is filled.

irritable hyper − trophied detrusor

afferent overstimulation

high voiding pressure

prostatic outflow obstruction

tuned muscles of the athlete—more jumpy and more quick to respond to distension. Urodynamic studies will show a high pressure in the static and voiding cystometrograms. The flow-rate will, if thoroughly compensated, be normal, but the voiding pressure will be enormous. Pressure profiles may show an exaggerated ridge of high pressure in the region of the offending prostate (Fig. 19.13).

Clinically the patient with these early features of compensatory hypertrophy to outflow obstruction complains of frequency and even of urge incontinence. The symptoms characteristically vary considerably from time to time. At this stage it is very difficult to draw a clear distinction between the bladder that is reacting to increased outflow resistance and the bladder that is irritable from some other cause, and most urological surgeons are very cautious indeed before offering any surgical procedure to patients whose chief complaint is of urinary frequency.

In time the clinical and urodynamic picture of detrusor hypertrophy is succeeded by *detrusor failure*. Like any muscle anywhere in the body asked to continue to work against unfair resistance, the detrusor becomes inefficient. Instead of emptying the bladder completely, it gives up its contraction before the bladder is empty, and there begins to be a residual urine. As the process continues, the wall of the detrusor begins to be chronically stretched, and in amongst the coarsened muscle fibres there appear more and more strands of fibrous tissue. In the end the active, hypertrophied detrusor turns into an inert, atonic bag. There is a huge residual urine. Urodynamic investigations now show hardly any detrusor contractions as the huge bladder is filled on cystometrography. The flow-rate is very poor. Since the detrusor now hardly contracts, it is difficult at this stage to prove that there is increased outflow resistance (Fig. 19.14).

Unfortunately by this stage, even if the cause of the mischief is removed, the

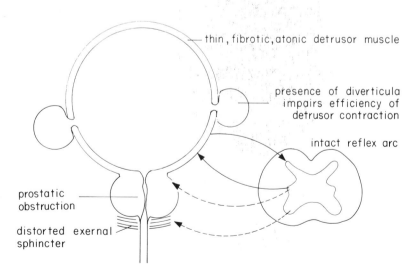

thin, fibrotic, atonic detrusor muscle

presence of diverticula impairs efficiency of detrusor contraction

intact reflex arc

prostatic obstruction

distorted exernal sphincter

Fig. 19.14. Detrusor failure. After continued, unrelieved outflow obstruction the detrusor finally gives up: its wall becomes inert, floppy, and partly replaced by fibrous tissue. There is chronic retention, a very poor flow-rate, and a low voiding pressure.

big, floppy, sacculated detrusor muscle may not contract and the only way the bladder can be got to empty may be by abdominal straining. One may have to 'rest' the detrusor by prolonged drainage with a catheter before it regains something of its former size and (if the patient is fortunate) something of its former ability to contract.

C. OVERDISTENSION

It is claimed that relatively short periods of overdistension of the bladder may give rise to a kind of ineffective detrusor function rather similar to that seen in neglected outflow obstruction, but to prove this entity is extremely difficult, and the writer (at present) is very sceptical that this really happens. Men who are admitted with acute urinary retention, with grossly distended bladders, regain normal micturition afterwards. Before assigning this diagnosis—which is so tempting—one must be very sure that all other causes for a disturbed bladder performance have been excluded.

D. SURGICAL DIVISION OF THE SPHINCTERS

Accidental surgical division of the external and supramembranous sphincters of the bladder may occur during prostatectomy. A similar consequence follows when carcinoma of the prostate has invaded the sphincters, and rendered them stiff and permanently half-open. A very similar thing may follow fracture of the pelvis complicated by tearing-across of the urethra. If the bladder neck (internal sphincter) is also destroyed, then the patient is incontinent of urine (Fig. 19.15).

Urodynamics will show, as a rule, a normal detrusor, possibly made more jumpy and sensitive than normal as a consequence of being kept always in the empty state, and sometimes as a result of being infected. But the detrusor contraction is not excessive. The outflow resistance, when measured, is negligible. The pressure profile shows no peak at any of the sphincters.

Clinically the patient may be dry when lying down in bed, but as soon as he rises, the urine runs away. If the injury to the sphincter is incomplete, he may be able to interrupt the flow of urine by voluntary contraction of the external sphincter. In some patients it seems as if re-education and exercise of this contraction is all that is needed to restore continence. Electrical stimulators may be inserted into the rectum, or applied to the perineum, to help re-educate the external sphincter. But in most patients who cannot raise the external pressure profile and interrupt the urine stream voluntarily, and in whom the external and supramembranous sphincters are quite destroyed, then there is no remedy but to apply some pressure to the urethra as an artificial device to keep the urine inside. A padded clip may be applied to the penis (*Cunningham's clip*), (Fig. 19.16). This is useful, but must be applied with care or it will give rise to a bedsore on the external skin of the penis or the internal lining of the urethra.

A similar principle is utilized in Kaufman's incontinence device: a silicone rubber balloon is fixed so that it compresses the bulbar urethra up against the

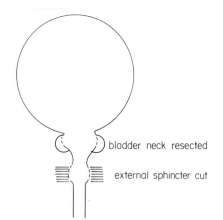

Fig. 19.15. Incontinence from surgical division of both the internal and external sphincters.

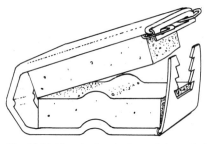

Fig. 19.16. Cunningham's clamp: it is applied across the penis to keep the urethra closed. The pads are made of sponge rubber.

symphysis. The pressure inside the balloon must be adjusted to be exactly enough to keep the urine in at rest—but not too much, or else the patient will develop residual urine. Other devices are even more complex. Rosen has designed a simple inflatable clip that grips the urethra between three silicone-rubber fingers. Scott has an elaborate system, with a cuff (implanted around the membranous urethra) that is inflated by one balloon in one side of the scrotum and deflated by pressure on another in the other side.

E. HERNIATION OF THE BASE OF THE BLADDER THROUGH THE PELVIC FLOOR

After childbirth many women develop a hernia through the levator ani shelf (Fig. 19.17). It descends, carrying the posterior wall of the bladder with it, along the anterior wall of the vagina, to present various degrees of prolapse at the vaginal opening. As a result the internal sphincter comes to lie outside the levator ani. When the abdominal pressure is raised, instead of the pressure being automatically applied to the urethra above the levator sheet, it merely adds to the pressure inside the bladder. Patients complain of being incontinent of urine, at first only when they laugh or cough or strain. Later the urine dribbles away all the time except when they are lying flat in bed. There is usually a certain degree of prolapse of the anterior wall of the vagina and of the cervix of the uterus.

Clinically there is usually a distinction in the history between this 'stress

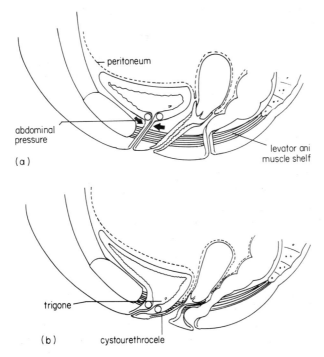

Fig. 19.17. (a) Diagram of the normal perineal floor in a women. When she strains or coughs, the increased intra-abdominal pressure is transmitted to the urethra to compress it and keep the urine in. (b) When there is herniation of the pelvic contents through the levator shelf, the internal sphincter finds itself outside the levator, the intra-abdominal pressure no longer helps keep the urine in and the angle between trigone and urethra is flattened out. The patient is wet at the least exertion. There may be a cystocele.

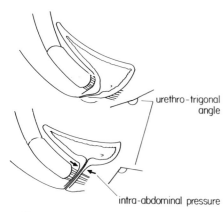

Fig. 19.18. The aim of all operations for 'stress incontinence' is to lift the urethra so that it once more comes within the effect of intra-abdominal pressure to restore the urethro-trigonal angle.

incontinence' and the 'urge incontinence' that is described by women who lose the entire contents of their bladder if they cannot get to the toilet soon enough. But the distinction is not always easy to draw: some women get a complete detrusor contraction when the bladder is stimulated by increasing the intra-abdominal pressure, while in other women, with an obvious mechanical problem, associated irritation or infection in the bladder makes it irritable.

Urodynamic investigation is useful in women with such incontinence, for it will detect primary disturbances of the bladder reflex, and the pressure profile can identify at least some of the faults that accompany prolapse.

There are innumerable remedial operations designed to correct the mechanical disorder of stress incontinence. All share the same aim, to lift up the bladder and trigone, bringing it back into the abdomen above the levator ani (Fig. 19.18), so that when the intra-abdominal pressure is raised, it can once more squeeze the urethra and help to keep the urine in. In addition these 'repair' operations may restore the angle between urethra and trigone which some surgeons think may help keep the woman continent. In the Marshall–Marchetti–Krantz procedure (Fig. 19.19) the urethra is stitched up behind the

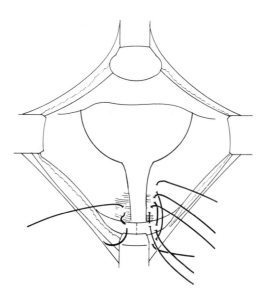

Fig. 19.19. In the Marshall–Marchetti–Krantz operation the urethra is fixed up behind the symphysis in a tunnel made by stitching the vaginal tissues to the back of the symphysis.

symphysis in a sling made of the sturdy tissues of the vagina either side of the urethra. In Millin's 'sling' (and its many imitators) a ribbon made of the rectus abdominis (Fig. 19.20) sheath is drawn under the urethra and lower part of the trigone, and hitched up so as to support them both. Provided that the true reason for the incontinence is the mechanical displacement of the bladder, all these operations work very well. But all too often the patient has, in addition, some of the many other disorders of the bladder reflex which have been referred to above.

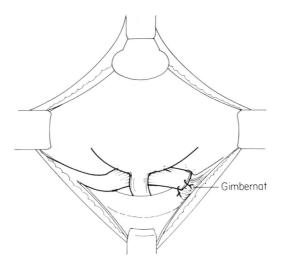

— Gimbernat

Fig. 19.20. In the Millin sling and similar procedures a hammock is made to lift up the trigone and urethra by means of fascia from the rectus sheath or some synthetic material, e.g. mersilene.

PHARMACOLOGICAL TREATMENT FOR DISORDERS OF MICTURITION

Very few medications do any good to common disorders of bladder function. At the risk of oversimplification, think of the control of the unstriped muscle of the bladder detrusor as being cholinergic, and that of the bladder neck internal sphincter, as being alpha-adrenergic (Fig. 19.21).

Hence to get the bladder to empty out, one might use bethanecol to release acetyl-choline in the terminals of the postganglionic fibres in the smooth muscle. Obviously this will not help much if there is unrelieved outflow obstruction.

If the bladder is emptying too frequently, one might expect some assistance by giving atropine to block acetyl-choline receptors, or propantheline which has much the same effect.

If part of the outflow obstruction is due to an overactive internal sphincter, it may help to give an alpha-blocker, such as phenoxybenzamine. In fact it is usually of more importance, to make sure that the patient stops taking alpha-stimulators such as ephedrine.

If the patient has incontinence from want of action, perhaps, of the internal sphincter, one may try the effect of an alpha-stimulator such as ephedrine, imipramine, or phenylproanolamine. Mixtures of the latter with isopropamide and diphenylpyraline seem surprisingly useful in bed-wetting.

Doctors are always under considerable pressure to prescribe 'something' to help to calm the irritable bladder, whatever its cause. One must be particularly careful not to be trapped into prescribing rubbish, especially when the rubbish may have serious side effects.

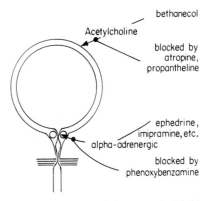

bethanecol

Acetylcholine

blocked by atropine, propantheline

ephedrine, imipramine, etc.
alpha-adrenergic

blocked by phenoxybenzamine

Fig. 19.21. Action of drugs on the bladder. Since the detrusor is under cholinergic control it may be made more active by bethanecol, etc. or inhibited by acetyl-choline blockers, e.g. atropine, propantheline. The internal sphincter is acted upon by alpha-adrenergic stimuli and may be blocked by phenoxybenzamine, stimulated by ephedrine imipramine, etc. Skeletal muscle relaxants are needed to relax the striated external sphincter.

Chapter 19/*The Bladder—Urodynamics and Micturition Disturbances*   215

FURTHER READING

Bradley W.E. & Brantley Scott F. (1979) Physiology of the urinary bladder. In J.H. Harrison *et al.* (eds), *Campbell's Urology*, Vol. 1, p. 87. W.B. Saunders Co., Philadelphia.

Edwards L. (1976) Incontinence of urine. In J.P. Blandy (ed.), *Urology*, p. 687. Blackwell Scientific Publications, Oxford.

Griffiths D.J. (1980) *Urodynamics*. Adam Hilger, Bristol.

Mandelstam D. (ed.) (1980) *Incontinence and its Management*. Croom Helm, London.

Smith J.C. (1976) The function of the bladder. In J.P. Blandy (ed.), *Urology*, p. 672. Blackwell Scientific Publications, Oxford.

SURGICAL ANATOMY (Fig. 20.1)

The normal prostate gland is placed, like a doughnut, around the urethra as it emerges from the male bladder. It lies behind the symphysis pubic to which it is attached by a tough fascia containing large veins. On either side, the pubis and ischium curve around it. Behind the prostate lies the rectum, separated by the 'fire-resisting' layers of Denonvilliers' fascia (made up of two layers of peritoneum fused together). In the groove between the prostate and the bladder posteriorly lie the seminal vesicles, vasa, and the entry of the ureters.

<h1 style="text-align:right">Chapter 20
The
Prostate Gland</h1>

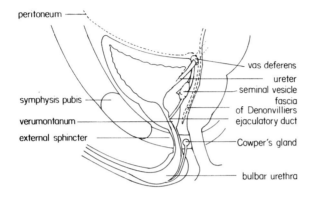

Fig. 20.1. Normal anatomy and surgical relations of the prostate gland.

Structure of the prostate (Fig. 20.2)

The prostate is really, like most secretory glands, a mass of tubes, surrounded by a capsule of muscle. Each tube is supplied with a contractile sleeve of muscle, and the whole is supported by a stroma of connective tissue. Histologically the three elements of the supporting connective tissue, the smooth muscle and the tubules and secretory acini of the glands form a characteristic picture which changes during the different phases of the growth and development of the male. The glandular and muscular elements are hardly detectable in the child, they

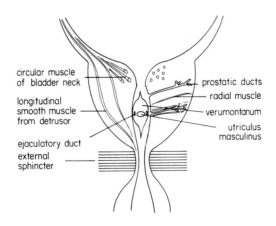

Fig. 20.2. Structure of the prostate in coronal section.

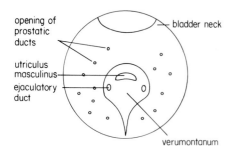

opening of
prostatic
ducts

bladder neck

utriculus
masculinus

ejaculatory
duct

verumontanum

Fig. 20.3. Endoscopic appearance of the prostatic urethra.

hypertrophy with puberty, and then in middle age, they begin to develop the nodules and whorls of benign hypertrophy (see page 210).

The glandular ducts of the prostate run more or less radially out from the prostatic urethra into which they empty. On endoscopy one can easily see their openings in the prostatic urethra (Fig. 20.3). But the chief landmark in the prostatic urethra is the verumontanum which, as its name implies, lies like a mountainous island in the middle of the posterior wall of the prostatic urethra. It is more a volcano than a mountain, because its tip is marked with the crater of the utriculus masculinus—the vestige of the Müllerian ducts that go to form the uterus in a woman. But on either side of the verumontanum are two more important openings, the ejaculatory ducts, which run obliquely down through the back of the prostate.

In the normal, healthy, young man's prostate, there are no true 'lobes' as such. Later on, as the gland is deformed and distorted by the enlargement caused by benign nodular hypertrophy, one can make out distinct bulges and bumps, that are given the names, lateral and middle lobes, but they are only the result of hypertrophy which must take this form owing to the narrow limitations imposed on the prostate by the presence of the symphysis in front and the bladder above.

Below the prostate the thinnest part of the urethra passes downstream through the external sphincter, which is part of the levator ani sheet. The verumontanum always lies just above the external sphincter, even in extreme examples of enlargement of the prostate when the normal anatomy is severely distorted. Urologists make a great fuss of the verumontanum because it is their landmark which stops them cutting away too much tissue, and accidentally making the patient incontinent.

FUNCTION OF THE PROSTATE

Nobody knows what the normal physiological function of the prostate is. Experts reckon that it contributes a tiny fraction (0.5 ml) to the seminal fluid, and that this tiny drop may help the sperms wag their tails. It is thought that the prostate gland contracts thanks to its rich muscular component, during sexual intercourse.

INFLAMMATION

Acute prostatitis

Acute prostatitis may occur out of the blue, often following a systemic type of illness characterized by rigors, fever and muscular pains. Or it may follow the passage of a catheter or cystoscope, or the accidental injection of the prostate with phenol in oil in the attempt to treat haemorrhoids. Clinically the patient is exceedingly uncomfortable, with pain experienced in the perineum, radiating to the thighs and penis. Voiding urine is painful and the stream is thin. There is often frequency of micturition and often a high fever. Rectal palpation reveals an exquisitely tender, swollen gland. The urine may or may not grow pathogenic organisms on culture.

If one can identify the causative organism in the urine then it should be treated by the appropriate antibiotic. *E. coli* or *Streptococcus faecalis* are common pathogens. One difficulty in dealing with acute prostatitis is that few antibiotics really get into the prostatic tissue in adequate dosage. Erythromycin, trimethoprim and cinoxacin have been shown to give rise to high tissue antibiotic levels. It is necessary to continue with the antibiotics for up to six weeks, since the inflamed prostate may take a long time to resolve.

Prostatic abscess (Fig. 20.4)

Acute inflammation in the prostate, as elsewhere in the body, does not always heal with resolution. It may lead on to suppuration. In such cases, which are very rare, a fluctuant abscess forms in the prostate, projecting back towards the rectum as a huge tender mass. Ideally it should be drained per urethram. If it is

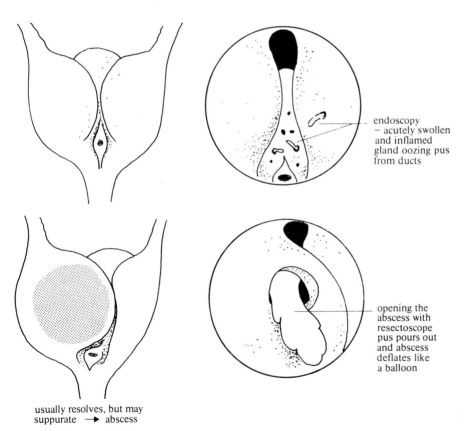

endoscopy – acutely swollen and inflamed gland oozing pus from ducts

opening the abscess with resectoscope pus pours out and abscess deflates like a balloon

usually resolves, but may suppurate ⟶ abscess

Fig. 20.4. Acute inflammation in the prostate.

allowed to point, and work its way through the tough barrier of Denonvilliers' fascia into the rectum there may be a persistent prostatorectal fistula. If detected, a resectoscope is passed and a portion of the roof of the abscess removed with the cutting loop. The pus pours out and the patient is at once relieved.

Chronic prostatitis

As with inflammation elsewhere, healing may proceed by scarring, and the prostate becomes infiltrated with fibrous tissue. In some patients it is very clear that there have been repeated episodes of acute infection, with the clinical features noted above. Some of these men will have, from time to time, a minor exacerbation accompanied by discomfort, fever and pain on voiding. Occasionally organisms may be cultured from the urine or the fluid expressed by firm 'massage' of the prostate. This fluid is found to contain more pus cells than those found in normal men. Sometimes the fluid is shown to grow *Neisseria gonorrhoeae* on careful culture: occasionally *Chlamydia* can be isolated, and in some patients, *Trichomonas* can be recovered from the fluid. In such patients the prostate may be tender to palpation, and the fluid expressed frankly purulent.

For every one of these patients with undeniable evidence of inflammation in the prostate, there are a dozen who complain of discomfort in the perineum, vague symptoms of discomfort on voiding, and even more vague symptoms of sexual inadequacy. In many of these patients the underlying trouble is psychosexual and one must take great care not to make the patient worse by embarking on a course of treatment that can have no justification in terms of pathology or pharmacology. Never fall into the trap of committing the patient to a protracted course of 'prostatic massage' (one of the many fashionable methods of 'therapy' for this condition) without asking yourself candidly whether there is any other chronic inflammation in the body which is better for being deliberately squeezed. Prostatic pain certainly calls for help, for it can be very real and very distressing, but it does not necessarily arise in the prostate. Many of the patients who are most concerned by these symptoms are secretly worried that they may have acquired some loathsome venereal disease: time, explanation, and a consultation with an expert venereologist to provide firm reassurance may bring profound relief.

BENIGN ENLARGEMENT OF THE PROSTATE

Aetiology

Over the age of 40 every man has some degree of benign nodular hyperplasia of the prostate, but only one in ten will have obstruction as a result of it. The size of the enlargement that accompanies nodular hyperplasia is quite unrelated to the degree of obstruction: some of the smallest prostates are accompanied by some of the worst outflow obstruction. Huge glands may be accompanied by no obstruction at all. The type and degree of nodular hyperplasia seems to vary from one race to another: men of Celtic ancestry are thought to have larger and more bulky glands than Anglo-Saxons, and they in turn, larger ones than men of the mediterranean seaboard. But detailed studies of the relationship between genetic factors and the size—let alone the incidence of obstruction—of the prostate have never been performed. No race of mankind is entirely immune from its effects.

Pathology

There are thought to be two zones in the prostate (Fig. 20.5). The inner zone may be a target for oestrogens, since it enlarges for a week or two in the newborn boy, under the supposed influence of maternal oestrogens. The outer zone, is thought to be androgen-influenced. In the normal, young male one can see no histological or anatomical difference between these two zones. The prostate of the 20 year old is composed of acini, interlaced with muscle fibres and supporting stroma.

Often there seems to be pure hypertrophy of the muscular tissue at the neck of the bladder associated with urodynamic evidence of outflow obstruction (see page 210). Sometimes this may be secondary to some other cause, possibly a neurological lesion. It is seen in young men and it may be associated with considerable obstructive changes (Fig. 20.6).

In practice, with the onset of middle age, this change in the bladder neck becomes indistinguishable from the changes caused by nodular hyperplasia (Fig. 20.7). After the age of 40 any man's prostate will show, here and there, little whorls which are composed of hypertrophy of smooth muscle, connective tissue, and duct epithelium. As the years go by the nodules become more numerous and confluent. They take one of two forms. In one, the gland becomes stiff and gristly, though not much enlarged. In the other, large bulky 'adenomas' form, rather like fibroids in the uterus, which displace and compress the remaining healthy prostatic tissue into a more or less thin shell or 'capsule' at the periphery. These more bulky 'adenomas' are the things that grow up through the ring of muscle at the internal sphincter, and because of the rigid confines of the symphysis, must perforce take up the form of the classical three 'lobes' of the prostate. As these bulky adenomas become larger, they push the verumontanum downwards towards the external sphincter.

Pathological effects of outflow obstruction

URODYNAMIC EFFECTS ON THE BLADDER

As we have seen (see page 210) the bladder responds to outflow obstruction, whatever its cause, by increasing the pressure inside it during micturition by

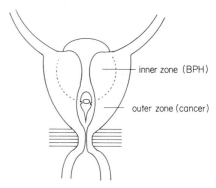

Fig. 20.5. Zones of the prostate.

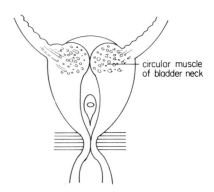

Fig. 20.6. Hypertrophy of the bladder neck, *prostatism sans prostate.*

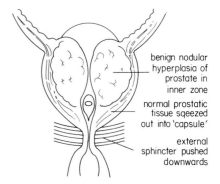

Fig. 20.7. Nodular hyperplasia appears in the inner zone and squeezes the healthy remaining prostatic tissue outwards to form the 'capsule'.

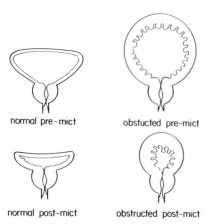

normal pre-mict   obstucted pre-mict

normal post-mict   obstructed post-mict

Fig. 20.8. Radiographic appearances of the normal and the obstructed bladder.

Fig. 20.9.

Fig. 20.10 Progressive failure of the detrusor muscle—at first hypertrophy is weakened by development of saccules and diverticula (left); later on, the muscle becomes slack and atonic (right).

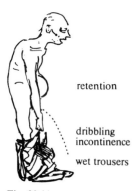

retention

dribbling incontinence

wet trousers

Fig. 20.11.

hypertrophy of the muscle of the detrusor. At first, all that one can detect is thickening of the wall of the bladder, which assumes a spherical shape as the pressure inside it equals or exceeds the ambient pressure inside the abdominal cavity. This hypertrophied detrusor is also a jumpy detrusor. It responds to filling with a smart contraction. At first, this response is enough to keep the bladder emptied out, and the flow-rate may be little if at all affected (Fig. 20.8).

At this stage the patient's symptoms reflect the hypertrophy and irritability of his detrusor. He finds himself obliged to empty his bladder more frequently. He may notice some delay in beginning to pass water, and he may or may not notice that his urinary stream is not as powerful as it used to be (Fig. 20.9).

This is succeeded by a stage—often slow in its course—in which the wall of the bladder gradually loses the battle to keep the viscus empty. At first there is only a small volume of residual urine, but this gradually enlarges (Fig. 20.10).

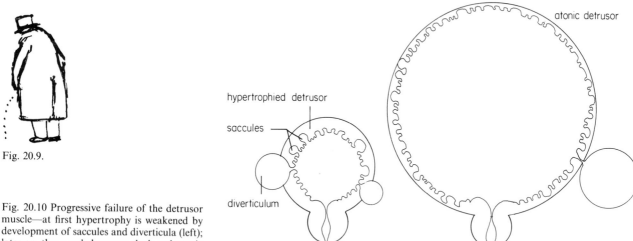

atonic detrusor

hypertrophied detrusor

saccules

diverticulum

At first too, the compensatory hypertrophy of the detrusor is enough to give a reasonable urinary flow. But as time goes by things get worse and worse: the residual urine becomes even larger, until we begin to speak of 'chronic retention'. Eventually the bladder begins to leak a little urine whenever the intra-abdominal pressure is increased. This stage is sometimes called 'chronic retention with overflow' (Fig. 20.11). By now, if one studies the performance of the detrusor, it no longer contracts when stimulated by filling. Along with its atony, we find that its muscle fibres have been replaced by fibrous tissue.

Clinically the march of events is typically for the patient to stop worrying quite so much about his urinary frequency as the bladder gives up the struggle. Instead he may observe that his stream is much worse, and that he has to spend much more time in voiding than he would like to. Incontinence begins to trouble him more and more.

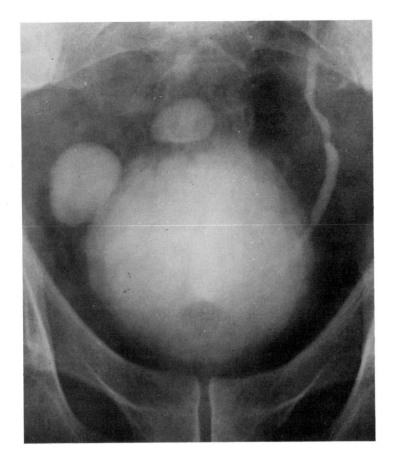

Fig. 20.12. Post-voiding X-ray from an IVU series of a patient with prostatic outflow obstruction showing diverticula.

STRUCTURAL EFFECTS ON THE BLADDER

Because the muscles of the wall of the bladder are arranged, not in neat layers like the muscle of the wall of the gut, but in a fine feltwork, when it undergoes hypertrophy, these change into more and more coarse strands stretched out behind the elastic mucosa. As the pressure rises inside the bladder, the mucosa is pushed out through the ever-growing gaps in between the strands or 'trabeculae' of the bladder. At first these little herniations of mucosa are called saccules, later on they emerge right outside the wall of the bladder to form great balloons called *diverticula* (Fig. 20.12). Once a diverticulum has been formed it never really empties out, and once urinary infection has been inoculated into the system, it remains there. As in other parts of the urothelium, stagnation and infection lead to squamous metaplasia, and carcinoma may arise in a long-continued diverticulum.

EFFECTS ON THE URETERS AND KIDNEYS

Increasing the pressure in the bladder brings about an increase in pressure inside the lumen of the renal pelvis, even before the stage that the ureter has become dilated. But in time this is overtaken by actual nipping of the lower end of the ureter as it traverses the thickened and hypertrophied wall of the bladder (Fig. 20.13). Occasionally the flap-valve at the lower end of the ureter gives way and in addition to an increased pressure inside the bladder, there is free reflux of urine from the bladder to the kidney. On both counts, the kidney suffers. It develops the atrophy of its structure, and the changes in its physiology, that mark obstructive uropathy (see page 73). At first there is impairment mainly of tubular function, with a more and more hypotonic urine and more and more need for a diuresis. This is ultimately succeeded by an impairment of the glomerular filtration rate, and a rising creatinine and urea. Now the deterioration in renal function is reflected in the patients symptoms and signs: thirst,

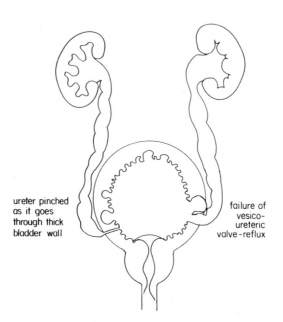

Fig. 20.13. Mechanism of upper tract obstruction in prostatic outflow obstruction: either the ureter is pinched in the thick muscle wall or its valve gives way, allowing reflux.

malaise and confusion are echoed in his general pallor, dehydration and anaemia. To the surgeon the most significant part of this crucial stage in the rake's progress of prostatic obstruction, must be the patient's dehydration, for if a prostatectomy is performed at this stage, with circulating blood volume impaired and anaemia uncorrected, the patient may die needlessly. Time spent in preparing the patient with chronic retention is time well-spent.

Complications

At any stage in this downward course of outflow obstruction two events may suddenly intervene to precipitate admission. Each carries its own special hazards, and multiples the risk of prostatectomy.

If the patient with residual urine develops urinary infection it will not go away until the outflow obstruction has been corrected. Many elderly men first realize that there is something wrong with the prostate only when they are struck down with an acute infection. It may give rise to a high fever and all the features of bacteraemia, it may cause haematuria, or it may present with acute epididymitis. The underlying cause is the volume of residual urine in the bladder. Unfortunately, having once had a urinary infection increases many times the risk of prostatectomy. The condition ought, ideally, to be recognized before this takes place.

ACUTE RETENTION

The overworked detrusor muscle may not always fail slowly: on occasions it fails suddenly. There is often some associated reason: the patient may have become ill for some other cause such as a heart attack or a surgical operation, he may have had to be anaesthetized, or he may have become drunk. In many patients acute retention seems to come on without warning. Traditionally, it is distinguished from chronic retention by the fact that the acutely distended bladder is painful, but in many patients the acute phase is only an exacerbation of a chronic one.

As with infection, it is highly desirable that a patient should be operated on before he develops retention, because otherwise the risks of his hospital admission are much magnified.

Indications for prostatectomy

From the above it is clear that the patient who has developed significant outflow obstruction from his prostate needs the operation before: (a) his bladder wall has become ruined by sacculation and diverticulum formation, and its function changed from a lively contractile viscus into an inert, floppy bag; (b) the ureters have become obstructed or their valves have become blown, and before the kidneys have undergone such atrophy that the level of creatinine has begun to rise; and (c) the patient develops either acute retention or urinary infection.

Early features that take the patient to the doctor include frequency, hesitancy and a poor urine flow. These can of course all be imitated by a number of other conditions. Other bizarre symptoms occur from time to time: patients have been arrested for loitering in public lavatories because they take such a long time to pass their water.

Later, symptoms alter as the condition progresses. Often the very extreme urgency and frequency is lessened as the sensitivity of the detrusor, now getting weary, becomes less marked. The need to pass water disturbs sleep. There is often a tiresome, post-voiding dribble of urine from the urethra.

Later still we move into the realm of overflow incontinence, the distended

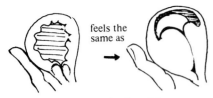

feels the same as

→

Fig. 20.14. Rectal examination of the prostate.

bladder and the wet trousers, accompanied before long by the marks of upper urinary tract obstruction, by uraemia, dehydration, indigestion and confusion.

Physical examination

Since the size of the prostate is unrelated to the severity of outflow obstruction, rectal estimation of the size of the gland is irrelevant. It is of course useful, since it may detect a sinister hardening of the prostate that might betoken carcinoma. One cannot guess very sensibly as to the size of the gland when there is residual urine in the bladder (Fig. 20.14).

Investigations

At the first visit the patient will have the urine examined for malignant cells and sent for microbiological culture. The urine and creatinine will be measured. When prostatic carcinoma is suspected, the serum acid phosphatase is measured too. By way of saving him an unnecessary needle, it is a kindness to the patient to order his haemoglobin and blood group.

Unless the patient is in acute retention, the diagnosis rests mainly on the interpretation of the excretion urogram. Its cardinal features are: (a) the thick-walled, 'high pressure' bladder (Fig. 20.15); (b) the presence of residual urine in the postmicturition film; and (c) the presence or absence of upper urinary tract obstruction. One should take (almost) no notice of the apparent size of the filling defect in the base of the bladder—it is so often so misleading.

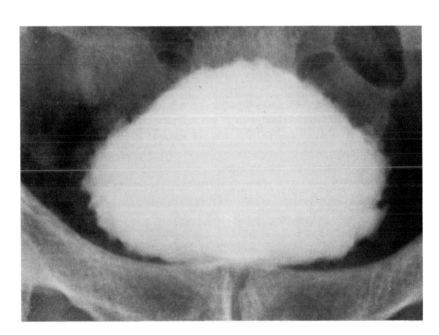

Fig. 20.15. Post-voiding film from an IVU series of a patient with prostatic outflow obstruction, showing the thick bladder wall and the increased trabeculation with a large residual urine.

Chapter 20/*The Prostate Gland*

DIFFERENTIAL DIAGNOSIS

1   *Bladder cancer* may mimic prostatism exactly. Remember that 20% of bladder cancers do *not* have haematuria. There may not be malignant cells in the urine if the tumour is a well-differentiated one. There ought to be filling defects in the bladder pictures if the films are clear and the tumours large: but the only safe test is cystoscopy.

2   *Prostatic cancer.* You may have a hunch that the prostate is malignant from its feel on rectal examination, but you will be wrong half the time. A relatively short history, especially one with early onset of incontinence, should make you alert to the possibility of malignancy. One may of course see metastases in the pelvis and find a raised acid phosphatase.

3   *Stricture.* Urethral stricture giving symptoms without a previous story of urethritis or injury is today very uncommon. You will probably only make the diagnosis when examining the urethra at the time of preliminary urethro-cystoscopy (which is inevitably done before any operation on the prostate).

4   *Neuropathy.* It is among patients whose symptoms arise from non-prostatic causes that one has most difficulty in making a correct diagnosis. They include men with a central prolapse of a low lumbar disc irritating the cauda equina, men with diabetes and diabetic neuropathy, men with diuresis caused by their cardiac condition, men with frequency caused by anxiety, and men who awake in the small hours of the night because they are lonely and depressed, and have nothing better to do than get up, make water, and perhaps have a cup of tea. Depression quite often mimics the nocturnal frequency of the enlarged prostate. There is no simple rule of thumb by which the doctor can distinguish between all these mimics of prostatic enlargement: he must remember that he is still a physician first, and that his skill at listening is what will always distinguish him from the computer.

Treatment

MEDICAL

There is no medical treatment, no pill, hormone or injection that will get rid of prostatic outflow obstruction. The only medication that may help, by buying time, is the alpha-blockade obtained with phenoxybenzamine, which may help by relaxing the smooth muscle element at the neck of the bladder. It should probably be followed by prostatectomy before long.

SURGICAL

1   The elective cold case

When there is residual urine, thickened bladder wall and any of the later, more sinister features such as sacculation and upper tract obstruction, then the patient should be admitted for prostatectomy. Men without these features in the urogram, whose only symptom is frequency, should be treated very conservatively, and not until there is certain urodynamic evidence of outflow obstruction. Even then, a little time spent in observing the natural course of the disease is good practice.

Ideally the patient should be referred to a specialist urological unit where he can be offered transurethral resection (see page 352).

2 Acute retention

Admit the patient. Do not catheterize him and send him home. If you have to transport the patient for a long distance, it is permissible perhaps to empty the bladder before his journey (see page 299). The prostatectomy is performed on the next convenient operating list. Every day that the catheter remains in the bladder increases the chance of the patient acquiring a hospital-transmitted infection. There is no point in performing an emergency prostatectomy, but there is equally no excuse for unnecessary delay.

3 Chronic retention

When the patient arrives with a distended bladder, but without pain, and without a raised creatinine, then his prostatectomy may be done on the next convenient operating list. It is not necessary to drain off the bladder first. But in this decision, there needs to be a little commonsense and judgement, for there is a wide spectrum between normal renal function and the first detectable elevation of creatinine. When in doubt, it does no harm to decompress the bladder.

4 Chronic retention with uraemia

Once one has admitted the patient who has evidence of impaired renal function, the situation is entirely different. The main problem is that he will be dehydrated, his apparently normal haemoglobin level will probably be a falsely high one, which will reveal anaemia when dehydration is corrected. The patient is often on the brink of heart failure and will be improved by digitalization. The deficiency of water salt and haemoglobin all need to be corrected by careful intravenous infusion. Time to allow the renal function to recover is well worthwhile: it may take several days for an obligatory post-obstruction diuresis to settle down.

Do not omit to give some thought and care to the patient's mental condition. He is a sick and frightened old man, more than a little confused by his strange surroundings, often fuddled by drugs and by pain. He often has other equally serious medical and surgical problems. Do not isolate him when he becomes confused: avoid sedation as a substitute for attention. He needs kind voices to talk to, plenty of light, company and stimulation. There is no company

Chapter 20/*The Prostate Gland*

he desires so much as that of his relatives and friends. Waive visiting hours in his case. A little alcohol, in reason, is a great comfort in his time of need, and never did the kidneys any harm, whatever evils it may do to the liver. There is no place at all for emergency prostatectomy in this brittle and hazardous group of patients.

5 Clot retention

Big veins on the surface of the middle lobe may bleed furiously, without warning, bringing the patient to hospital with acute clot retention. This is rare, but it demands emergency clot-evacuation with the resectoscope sheath and Ellik evacuator (see page 321). At this operation scrupulous care is taken to hunt for a carcinoma. *Beware the decoy prostate*—the big adenoma which hides a little cancer on the trigone.

6 Infection

First drain off the urine and keep the bladder empty, then give time for infection to be thoroughly controlled before embarking on surgical removal of the prostate. To rush in to operate courts the risks of bacteraemia.

CARCINOMA OF THE PROSTATE

Aetiology

A very different incidence of carcinoma of the prostate is reported in different countries, perhaps this arises from different criteria used in making the diagnosis. Unlike many other cancers it does not appear to be increasing, nor is it related to any industrial agent or even to smoking. It has nothing to do with benign hyperplasia, though the two conditions occur so often that they inevitably coexist. Genetic factors as in benign hypertrophy, deserve much more study than they have received: cancer is more common in men of blood Group O, and is rare in native Japanese and in emigrants of Japanese ancestry. It is unrelated to social status or fertility.

Incidence

Its incidence depends upon how you define carcinoma of the prostate. Small, latent cancers can be found in 14% of 50-year-olds, and this proportion increases to 80% of 80-year-olds. There is, today, endless and heated argument as to what these figures really mean. Similar small 'latent cancers' are to be found in lungs, adrenals, thyroid, kidney and stomach. Pathologists conjure with the notion of a critical mass needed before cancers can spread. The real and practical problem facing the urologist is that in some 10% of prostates he has to

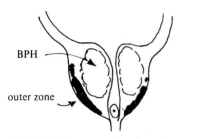

Fig. 20.16. Diagram to show the most common site for carcinoma of the prostate.

resect because the patients cannot void, he finds cancer and wonders what he should do about it.

Site of origin (Fig. 20.16)

We usually seem to see cancers originating in the periphery of the prostate, in the 'capsule' squeezed there by enlargement of the benign nodular tissue in the inner zone. This is not entirely true, and one often finds cancer in the inner part as well. Nevertheless it means that cancer can still occur after so-called prostatectomy since this only removes the obstructing inner fibromyoadenoma.

Pathology

Macroscopically a cancer of the prostate has no well-defined edge and it spreads as a hard, irregular mass around the rectum, into the pubis, but avoiding Denovilliers' fascia. It is very odd how prostatic cancer may squeeze the rectum to the calibre of a pencil, and yet will not invade its wall.

Microscopically one sees a complete spectrum of all the degrees of anaplasia even in the same patient. Classifications based on differing degrees of anaplasia are notably suspect unless strict attention is paid to the amount of the different *grades* that are present in each specimen. Here Gleason's system, based on correlation between more than 3000 specimens and their ultimate prognosis, seems to be really useful: he notes five different 'patterns', and then decides which two are the most important ones, i.e. which make up the bulk of the tumour in each specimen. Each is given a number, 1–5, and by adding the numbers assigned to the primary, to those assigned to the secondary tumour, one ends up with nine different possible tumour 'grades'. Complicated as this system sounds, it correlates very neatly with the survival of the patients. Using Gleason's criteria the original histological appearance of the tumour has important prognostic influence, but ordinary 'grading' based on a single biopsy, without any attempt at quantification, is probably far less useful.

STAGING OF PROSTATIC CANCER (Fig. 20.17)

Tis—pre-invasive carcinoma

It is difficult to be sure what this really means, since in most patients we cannot be sure how far the *in situ* tumour has really got.

T0—no tumour palpable

This is the common variety, where cancer is found unexpectedly on removing a prostatic 'adenoma' that felt normal and benign. It is subdivided into pT0 if, on

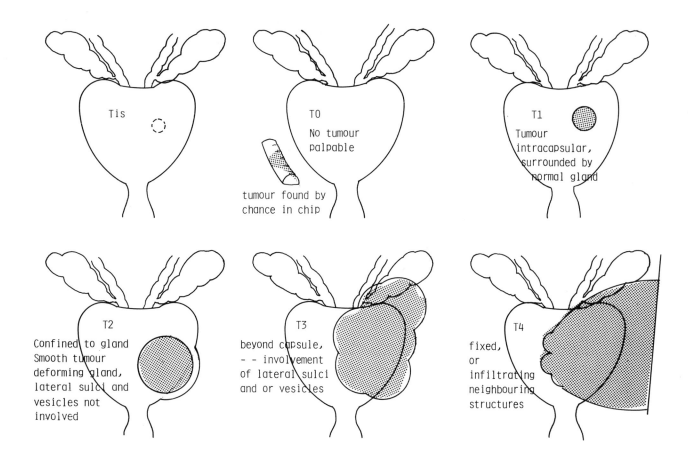

Fig. 20.17. T-staging of carcinoma of the prostate.

subsequent removal of the prostate, the pathologist cannot find any tumour, i.e. it was all removed in the biopsy, and pT1.

T1 and pT1—focal (single or multiple) carcinoma

Clinically the tumour is intracapsular, and as far as the finger in the rectum can determine, it is surrounded by a palpably normal gland.

T2 and pT2—tumour confined to the gland

Smooth nodule deforming contour but lateral sulci and seminal vesicles not involved. Histologically there is diffuse carcinoma with or without extension to the capsule.

T3 and pT3—tumour extending beyond the capsule

With or without involvement of the lateral sulci and/or seminal vesicles.

Chapter 20/*The Prostate Gland*   231

T4 and pT4—tumour fixed or infiltrating neighbouring structures

It must be obvious that this staging system is open to very serious sources of error since so much depends on the palpating finger in the rectum and on the sampling errors inherent in any method of examining histological tissue obtained from the prostate.

The N part of the TNM system is so open to error that most surgeons do not use it. Lymphography is particularly valueless in this context and has been quite given up, and CAT scanning has yet to be shown to be any more accurate.

We are left with the M category, i.e. the hunt for *metastases*. We have three techniques for detecting distant metastases. Each is open to errors of interpretation, but together can be most useful.

Serum markers—serum acid phosphatase

Normal prostatic tissue secretes acid phosphatase, and if there is an excessive bulk of well-differentiated prostatic acini either in the prostate or in metastases, then some of the excess production of acid phosphatase spills over into the blood where it can be measured. More recent refinements in technique enable smaller and smaller amounts of acid phosphatase to be detected with radio-immune assay. The catch is that an undifferentiated tumour, however widely disseminated, may have given up making acid phosphatase, so that a negative value does not rule out widespread prostatic cancer.

Skeletal survey

X-rays of all the bones in the body, the so-called skeletal survey, have been done as a routine in some centres. In most units the radiographs are limited to the pelvic bones and spine, where metastases, thanks to the backstairs veins and lymphatics that connect the bladder and prostate to the pelvis and vertebrae, are most prone to occur (Fig. 20.18).

Radioactive isotope bone scanning

Tc^{99m} MDP is taken up by vascular bony metastases, and proves to be a very sensitive index of metastases. It does not necessarily detect them all however, and a negative bone scan does not exclude cancer. It is a good deal more sensitive than an ordinary radiograph, but if one finds a 'hot spot' in the technetium bone scan it must be checked with a radiograph to ensure that the technetium uptake is not caused by local inflammation from arthritis etc. (see page 27).

Clinical features

Many patients have no symptoms at all other than those of outflow obstruction and the carcinoma is found by accident when the specimen taken at

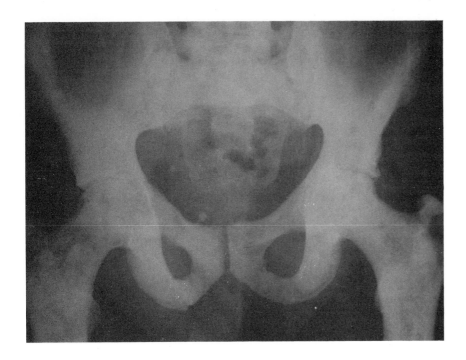

Fig. 20.18. X-ray showing multiple osteoblastic and osteoclastic metastases from carcinoma of the prostate.

prostatectomy is examined histologically (T0, pT1). Others have a progressive tumour that gives an unusually quick onset of the outflow obstruction. Still others only come up with distant metastases. These are usually in bones, and give rise to widespread bone pain that may be mistaken for osteo- or rheumatoid arthritis. Three unexpected manifestations of prostatic carcinoma deserve particular notice, because they are so easily missed.

1. INTESTINAL OBSTRUCTION may be caused by encircling of the rectum by tumour. Spurious diarrhoea and slow large bowel obstruction may be difficult to think of in relation to carcinoma of the prostate in a man who has no urinary symptoms.

2. URETERIC OBSTRUCTION causing insidious uraemia may be due to similar extraprostatic infiltration by the carcinoma. It may resemble closely the type of ureteric obstruction seen in idiopathic retroperitoneal fibrosis (see page 149).

3. HAEMORRHAGES AND SUBCUTANEOUS BRUISING may occur thanks to the secretion of fibrinolysins by prostatic tumour. This may be remedied by aminocaproic acid. Before setting out to resect a prostatic cancer with widespread metastases it is worth having this looked for by the haematological laboratory.

Investigations

In the routine work-up of a known or suspected cancer of the prostate,

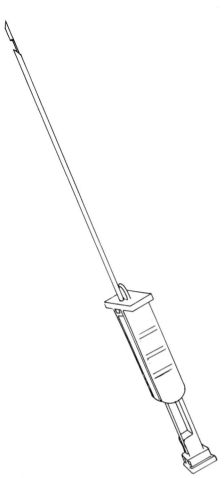

Fig. 20.19. Trucut biopsy needle.

estimations of the acid phosphatase, skeletal survey and where relevant, radiological examination of suspected 'hot spots' are now routine.

In many centres, when a hard nodule is found in the prostate, a biopsy is performed as a routine. This may be with a Trucut biopsy needle (Fig. 20.19) or cells may be aspirated for Papanicolaou examination. It is perhaps marginally easier to get appropriate tissue if the needle is thrust through the rectum into the nodule, but this carries a very serious risk of haematogenous dissemination of infection, and is really difficult to justify. In any event, the thinking doctor must ask why he wants to subject the patient to any risk at all, if he does not really know what to do with the information he has thus obtained. The use of the thin Franzen needle across the rectum seems to be far less likely to give rise to septicaemia, but the same philosophical objections apply with equal force.

Histological verification of the diagnosis is usually obtained by transurethral resection, which offers the patient relief of his outflow obstruction at the same time.

Treatment of prostatic cancer

Nobody knows how to treat cancer of the prostate in any of its stages. We have certain guide-lines, but no certainty.

T1

If a tiny nodule on biopsy proves to be carcinoma, or if by chance some of the chips of prostate after TUR for obstruction show malignancy, we have no sound evidence at present that any form of treatment offers the patient a better chance of survival than doing nothing. Hence in many centres controlled clinical trials are now in process to try to discover what of the following ought to be done: (a) nothing (i.e. wait and follow the patient until he does develop symptoms); (b) irradiate the prostate using either teletherapy with linear accelerator, or implantation of radioactive iodine (this form of treatment is often accompanied by a node dissection of some or all of the pelvic lymph nodes in order the better to stage the tumour); or (c) offer the patient some form of hormone treatment.

T2

Again, the choice lies between doing nothing, radiotherapy, or hormone treatment.

T3

Here the cancer has spread outside the capsule of the prostate and probably into the pelvic lymph nodes. The choice lies between doing nothing, pelvic radiotherapy using a big field, or hormone treatment.

234   Chapter 20/*The Prostate Gland*

Local surgery can do no good except in so far as it relieves symptoms. We do not know for certain that hormone therapy will prolong life. If there are symptoms from distant metastases, we know that localized metastases can be very responsive to local irradiation, and widespread metastases may melt away with hormone treatment. However, there is little evidence that this will offer any useful prolongation of life, and hormone therapy may have an unacceptable toll of side effects.

It will be noted that in no section is there mention of *radical prostatectomy*. This is a British idiosyncracy. In other countries T0 and T1 at least, and some examples of T2 stages are treated by radical excision of the prostate, an operation that carries a considerable risk of incontinence, and an appreciable risk of prostatorectal fistula. All patients are rendered impotent. The justification for the British view rests firmly on the statistics that show no benefit from radical surgery. It must however be admitted that radical surgery is still strongly defended by a dwindling band of zealots.

HORMONE THERAPY

It was noted empirically that removal of both testes (*orchidectomy*) sometimes resulted in the disappearance of multiple metastases of prostatic cancer. Later on, Huggins discovered that the synthetic oestrogen-like substance, *stilboestrol*, would have a similar effect on prostatic metastases. Since then numerous natural and synthetic oestrogens have been used with identical results. Similarly, trichloroanisene (TACE), which blocks the action of stilboestrol on receptors in the prostate, has been shown to give benefit.

Not all prostatic cancers respond to hormone therapy, and it is not at all clear whether any hormones prolong life, even if they certainly relieve pain and may get bony lesions to heal completely. The dose of stilboestrol that is required is very small—1 mg three times a day. Higher doses do not have a better therapeutic effect, and court complications from cardiovascular side effects.

Unfortunately, if a patient has once responded to stilboestrol and later on relapses, he usually will not respond a second time to orchidectomy. But he may still show a subjective improvement to destruction of his pituitary either by surgical removal (transethmoid *hypophysectomy*) or ablation with radioactive Yttrium rods. Adrenalectomy was formerly used for this purpose and had occasionally very good results but they were so unpredictable and the operation had such a morbidity that it has been given up.

No chemotherapeutic agent has yet been shown to benefit a prostatic cancer, though many have been tried. Linking nitrogen mustard to stilboestrol may possibly give some advantage over high doses of stilboestrol alone, but the question has still to be put to the rigid tests of controlled clinical trials. The difficulty in carcinoma of the prostate is that it only causes death in 0.2% of elderly men, and yet most of them can be shown to have it in the prostate on serial section and many of these will have small metastases in the bones. Hence it is always necessary to be quite sure that treatment, however attractive in theory, is likely to do more good than leaving nature to take its course.

FURTHER READING

Ansell I.D. (1976) Histopathology of the prostate. In D.I. Williams & G.D. Chisholm (eds), *Scientific Foundations of Urology*, p. 331. Heinemann, London.

Blacklock N.J. & Bouskill K. (1977) The zonal anatomy of the prostate in Man and in the Rhesus Monkey (*Macaca mulata*). *Urological Research*, **5**, 163.

Blandy J.P. (1976) Benign enlargement of the prostate gland. In J.P. Blandy (ed.), *Urology*, p. 859 Blackwell Scientific Publications, Oxford.

Blandy J.P. (1978) *Transurethral Resection*, 2nd edn. Pitman Medical Publishing Co., Tunbridge Wells.

Oates J.K. (1976) Prostatitis. In J.P. Blandy (ed.), *Urology*, p. 914. Blackwell Scientific Publications, Oxford.

Catalona W.J. & Scott W.W. (1979) Carcinoma of the prostate. In *Campbell's Urology*, Vol. 2, 4th edn, p. 1085. W.B. Saunders Co., Philadelphia.

Gee W.F. & Cole J.R. (1980) Symptomatic Stage C carcinoma of prostate. *Urology*, **15**, 335.

Schmidt J.D. (1980) Chemotherapy of hormone resistant stage D prostatic cancer. *Journal of Urology*, **123**, 797.

Scott W.W., Menon M. & Walsh P.C. (1980) Hormonal therapy of prostatic cancer. *Cancer*, **45**, 1929.

Walsh P.C. & Jewett H.J. (1980) Radical surgery for prostatic cancer. *Cancer*, **45**, 1906.

Yagoda A. (1980) Chemotherapy of metastatic bladder cancer. *Cancer* **45**, 1879.

ANATOMY OF THE MALE URETHRA (Fig. 21.1)

The urethra is a tube made of epithelium that varies from being transitional urothelium near the bladder, skin near the external meatus, and a modified columnar epithelium in the middle. Into the urethra enter the mouths of many 'paraurethral' glands whose ducts lead down into the spongy tissue of the corpus spongiosum which encloses the tube. The corpus spongiosum is an integral part of the glans penis and is firmly joined to the two other erectile structures, the corpora cavernosa that make up the penis (see page 258).

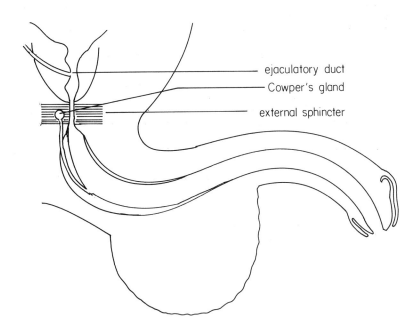

ejaculatory duct
Cowper's gland
external sphincter

Fig. 21.1. Diagram of the anatomy of the normal male urethra.

The narrowest part of the normal adult urethral is just inside the external meatus; the weakest part is where it pierces the perineal membrane and is surrounded by the external sphincter. This is the 'membranous urethra' and it is at this point that it is so easily torn across when the pelvis is fractured.

Above the perineal membrane the urethra passes into the prostate as the prostatic urethra (see page 243). Two large paraurethral ducts have long courses, and end up in distinct glands lying in the external sphincter itself: these are Cowper's glands, important only because they sometimes become infected.

The urethra is easily seen through the urethroscope, and is seen to be pitted with the openings of the paraurethral glands. Its lining is marked with helical 'riflings'—the rings of Moorman. These are not strictures: they are quite normal, but in an erection they become much more pronounced.

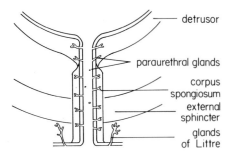

Fig. 21.2. Diagram of the anatomy of the female urethra.

detrusor

paraurethral glands

corpus spongiosum

external sphincter

glands of Littre

ANATOMY OF THE FEMALE URETHRA (Fig. 21.2)

The female urethra is a similar but shorter tube. Where it leaves the bladder it is fringed by a thick roll of internal sphincter often thrown into little folds and oedematous frills. The tube is lined by squamous epithelium exactly like that of the vagina, for a varying distance from the external meatus. In about one in three women the squamous lining is seen to extend right onto the trigone where it is easily recognized as a thin, whitish film of so-called vaginal metaplasia: this is in fact normal, and does not need treatment (Fig. 21.3).

The female urethra is surrounded by erectile, spongy tissue which continues down to the glans of the clitoris. The whole tube is provided with mucus-secreting glands which may on occasion become infected.

Fig. 21.3. Variations in the junction between the squamous (vaginal) epithelium and the transitional (urothelium) of the bladder.

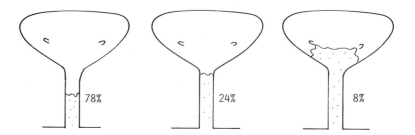

The muscular arrangement of the female urethra has been the subject of considerable study. There are at least two elements: an inner sleeve made mainly of smooth muscle, continuous with the detrusor fibres of the bladder, surrounded by an outer sleeve of striated muscle derived from the levator ani (Fig. 21.4).

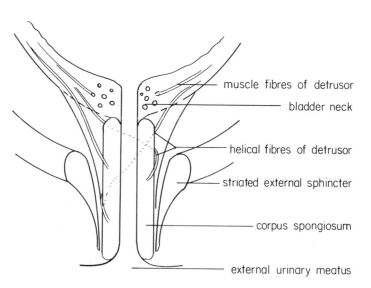

Fig. 21.4. Muscle structure of the female urethra.

muscle fibres of detrusor

bladder neck

helical fibres of detrusor

striated external sphincter

corpus spongiosum

external urinary meatus

238   Chapter 21/*The Urethra*

CONGENITAL LESIONS OF THE URETHRA

Hypospadias (see page 260)

This is essentially a failure of development of the genital folds that leads to atresia of the distal part of the urethra and an external meatus that opens too far proximally.

Epispadias (see page 171)

The result of a congenital error in the growth of the cloacal membrane, of which the most serious manifestation is complete extrophy of the bladder.

Congenital diverticula

In the male these appear to be an attempt at the formation of a double-barrelled urethra (Fig. 21.5). There is more than one slit connecting the two barrels. When the child passes water, the lower of the two urethrae fills out with urine, the slit is closed like a valve, and the urine then dribbles away. If seen in childhood one may simply enlarge the slit to get rid of the valve-like effect, throwing the two channels into one, or one may need to reconstruct the urethra. Both channels are surrounded by corpus spongiosum.

In females diverticula are also seen: they may arise from abscesses in the paraurethral glands, but some of them in a very striking symmetrical form, like two saddle bags on either side of the urethra (Fig. 21.6). They extend as long, thin processes right up through the sphincter layers towards the pelvis, and it seems probable that they represent abortive forms of ectopic ureterocele

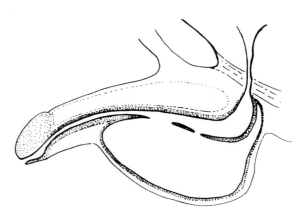

Fig. 21.5. Anterior diverticulum of the male urethra ('anterior urethral valve').

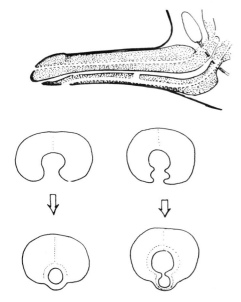

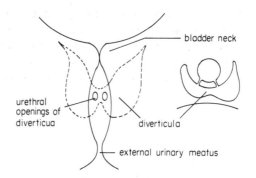

Fig. 21.6. Urethral diverticula in the female—saddle-bag type.

formation (see page 48). They sometimes, as with other pockets of stagnant urine, give rise to repeated infections, stones, and occasionally, to cancer.

Congenital posterior urethral valves (Fig. 21.7)

These occur in boys. There is a pair of sail-shaped valves adjacent to the

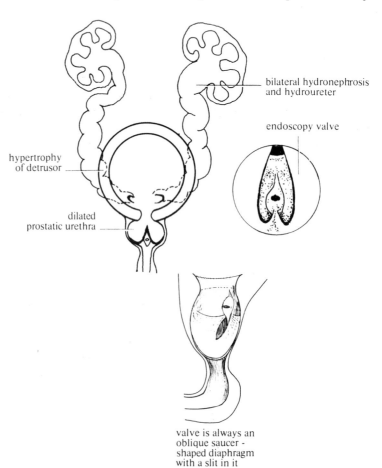

Fig. 21.7. Congenital posterior urethral valves in the male.

Chapter 21/*The Urethra*

verumontanum which look like the valves in a vein. Urine cannot get past them without difficulty. Little boys with this condition characteristically 'dirty when they wet', because they must strain so hard. Often they are born with severe obstructive changes in the bladder ureters and kidneys. Voiding cystography shows a characteristic picture and the treatment is to resect the valves with a miniature children's resectoscope.

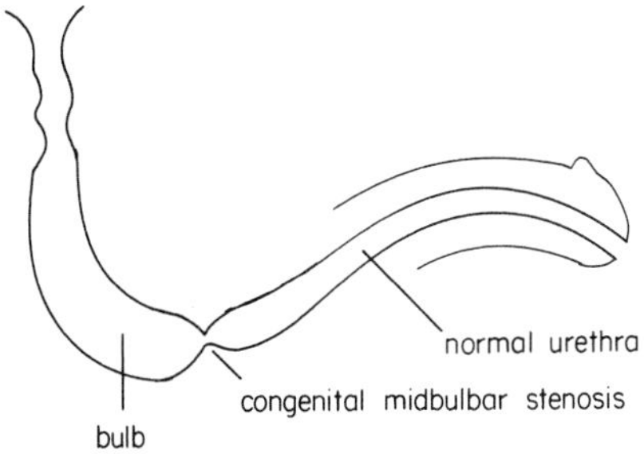

Congenital mid-bulbar stenosis (Fig. 21.8)

This is a different entity to the above. It seems to represent an exaggeration of Moorman's rings, that normally form the 'rifling' of the bulbar urethra. A tight ring, containing hypertrophied muscle, is found in the middle of the bulbar urethra. There is often obstructive uropathy upstream of the stenosis. It is difficult in some cases to be sure that this is not an acquired stricture from perineal injury. It is treated just like any other stricture in this position.

TRAUMA TO THE URETHRA

Perineal urethral injury in the male

Fall-stride injury of the urethra has been known from time immemorial (Fig. 21.9). In the days of sail, ship's crew used to fall from the rigging astride a spar: in the days of coal, Johnny head-in-air would fall astride a manhole cover in the street: today it is seen in motorcycle injuries, traffic accidents and sport. A blunt force squashes the perineal urethra hard up against the firm under surface of the

Fig. 21.8. Mid-bulbar stenosis of the urethra: a very similar stricture is caused by perineal trauma.

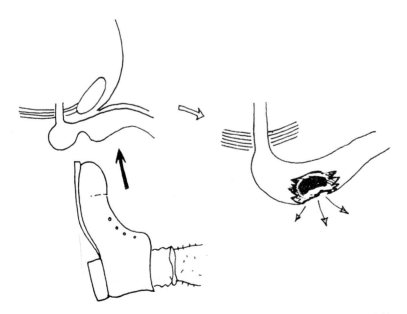

Fig. 21.9. 'Kick-in-the-crutch' injury.

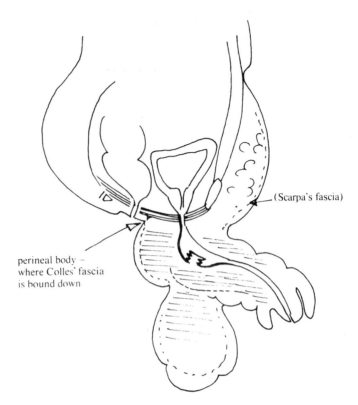

(Scarpa's fascia)

perineal body –
where Colles' fascia
is bound down

Fig. 21.10. Closed injury of the bulbar urethra.

pubic symphysis and tears it. In severe forms of the injury the pelvis is fractured as well. Fortunately the testicles slip to either side and escape injury, and the corpora cavernosa at this site are far enough apart to escape injury as well. The hole in the torn urethra is a ragged one, and blood escapes into the fascial compartment enclosed by Scarpa's fascia, forming a huge haematoma (Fig. 21.10).

The chief danger here is that urine may escape into this haematoma, and if the urine is concentrated, or worse if it is infected, it may give rise to necrosis of the surrounding tissue. In the past neglected extravasation of urine used to be followed by sloughing of the skin of the scrotum, perineum and lower abdomen as the urine sought out the barriers of Scarpa's and Colles's fascia. Today this sight is still occasionally seen when medical aid is not available.

MANAGEMENT

The patient gives a history of the typical injury, and then usually notices blood coming from the external urethral meatus. Sometimes he only has discomfort on attempting to pass urine, when he is seized with severe pain in the perineum from the extravasated fluid. At this stage one may attempt to pass a *soft* narrow rubber catheter. It may go easily into the bladder and drain off clear urine.

Chapter 21/*The Urethra*

More often it cannot get past the laceration because the tissues are so oedematous and bruised. If there is already a large haematoma and suspicion of extravasation of urine, then it ought to be drained through a perineal incision. If the catheter cannot be got through the injury, a suprapubic cystostomy is performed. No attempt is made to effect a primary repair: the tissues are so lacerated and ragged that no neat repair can be attempted.

After 10–14 days when all the perineal haematoma has settled down, the urethra is examined with a urethroscope. Often one cannot see any trace of the original injury: sometimes there is a stricture, and this can be dealt with by internal urethrotomy, dilatation or (rarely) by a one-stage patch urethroplasty (see page 358).

Fractured pelvis with rupture of the membranous urethra

This is a most important type of injury, and one that is becoming increasingly common thanks to the growing number of motor traffic accidents. Essentially the basic problem is a fracture with displacement of part of the pelvic ring. It may be useful to consider it in three degrees of severity.

1. MINIMAL DISPLACEMENT INJURY (Fig. 21.11)

Compressed violently from front to back, the pelvic ring is broken either in two places in front, so as to give a mobile middle segment, or in one place in front and another at the back—just to the side of the sacroiliac joint is the usual place—to allow the entire innominate bone to slide back and upwards.

As the displaced part is forced backwards, because it is firmly bound to the prostate, it carries the prostate back with it. The bulbar urethra however is equally firmly attached to the corpora cavernosa, and these in turn to the ischial rami, so that they hold the urethra firmly, and it has to part at its most weak point—the membranous urethra.

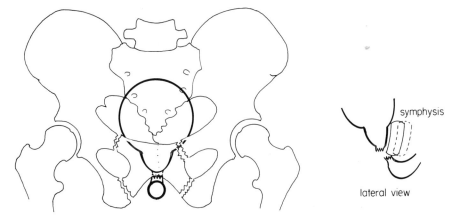

lateral view

Fig. 21.11. Fracture of the pelvis with minimal displacement of the prostatic from the bulbar urethra in AP view (left); but note that it is significantly dislocated posteriorly in the lateral view (right).

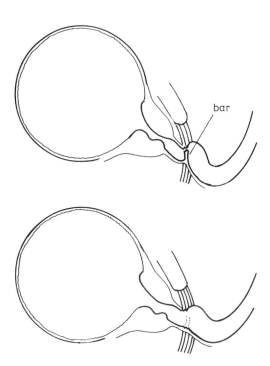

Fig. 21.12. If there is minimal displacement, a thin septum divides the proximal from the distal bulbar urethra which can be divided endoscopically.

When this happens there is a tearing of the bulbar corpus spongiosum and often very severe local bleeding. Blood escapes, often profusely, from the external urinary meatus. The patient is usually unable to pass water, and develops acute urinary retention. Associated with the fracture of the pelvis there is nearly always gross soft-tissue damage and considerable loss of blood into the pelvis from laceration of tributaries of the internal iliac veins.

But if the patient is fortunate, the initial displacement of the broken parts of the pelvic girdle is restored, or almost completely restored, and so the dislocated prostate is brought back nearly to its original alignment with the bulbar urethra.

Characteristically, there is usually some residual posterior displacement, and the lumen of the prostatic urethra fetches up a little behind, and often to one or other side of, the lumen of the bulbar urethra. At worst, an oblique septum of scar tissue separates the two cavities. When all the haematoma and oedema have settled down, and the patient is in a fit state to be examined, one can slit this septum and restore continuity between the prostatic and bulbar urethra (Fig. 21.12). If there is a stricture (and there is not always a stricture at all, but only a kink) then it is a short one, needing perhaps internal urethrotomy and dilatation from time to time, and at worse, an easy one-stage urethroplasty (see page 358).

2. GROSS DISPLACEMENT WITH RUPTURED URETHRA (Fig. 21.13)

Here there is far more dislocation of the parts of the pelvic girdle. Often there is

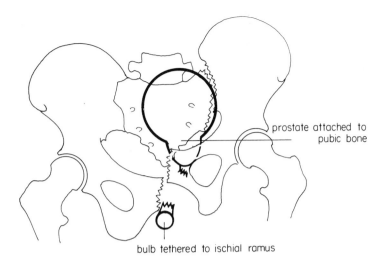

prostate attached to
pubic bone

bulb tethered to ischial ramus

Fig. 21.13. Gross displacement of the fractured pelvis holds the prostate away from the bulb, leaving a long gap that has to be bridged.

a fracture of the acetabulum and more than one additional fracture of the femur. Such patients are always shocked, many have multiple injuries of the head and thorax in addition to their injured pelvis, and all need massive transfusion of blood to correct the blood that is shed into the tissues of the pelvis.

When the patient has recovered from his more important injuries, one often finds that the pelvis is in a grossly displaced position, one innominate bone riding several centimetres up from the other. In consequence the gap between the ends of the torn prostatic and bulbar urethrae is long, and filled with haematoma.

If this gap is not reduced, and the ends are not brought together, one is faced with a difficult task to fill the gap with a suitable tube. When possible (and it is not always possible) one aims to try to shorten the gap by mobilizing the prostate from its firm attachment to the bone of the pelvis, to bring it down to the upper torn end of the bulbar urethra, so as to make the subsequent and inevitable stricture relatively short and so relatively easy to deal with.

3. GROSS DISPLACEMENT, MULTIPLE INJURIES, COMBINED INJURY OF THE RECTUM (Fig. 21.14)

In the third category the soft tissue damage is even more severe. Often the cause is massive crushing combined with rolling, as when one of my patients was run over by a tank-transporter. Skin and muscles are torn down from the pelvic bones which are crused and broken in several places. The front of the rectum is split across, and the tear in the urethra often runs right up, splitting the prostate, and extending up into the bladder. Tremendous loss of blood is combined with many other internal injuries to liver, spleen and bowel.

Chapter 21/*The Urethra*   245

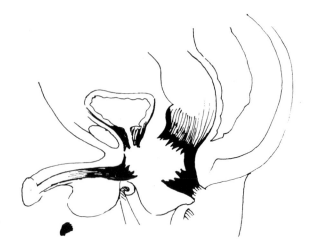

Fig. 21.14. Massive crush injury with rectal damage.

Management of fractured pelvis with ruptured urethra

DIAGNOSIS

Always suspect that there might be an injury to the urethra when there is a severe pelvic fracture, blood is seen at the external urinary meatus, and the patient has not passed urine. In many instances, the rupture of the urethra is the least dangerous of the patient's problems, and the first task of the accident surgeon must be to resuscitate the patient and deal with internal haemorrhage, sucking wounds of the chest, haemopneumothorax, etc. In such a case with multiple injuries, to monitor the response of the patient to transfusion may require measurement of his urine output. Even if this is not needed, sooner or later a catheter should be passed, and here the greatest care, and the most experienced surgeon available, should be brought to the patient as soon as possible.

Given an experienced urologist, using a *soft* narrow catheter, with strict aseptic precautions, no harm can possibly come from a gentle attempt to pass the catheter into the bladder. If the laceration of the wall of the urethra is incomplete, or if there is no injury to the urethra at all, then the catheter slips in and clear urine escapes. The catheter can be left in as long as is necessary to monitor the patient's response to resuscitation, or until he is sufficiently well to be allowed to use the bottle in bed.

If there is the slightest difficulty in passing the catheter, then no attempt should be made to force it into the bladder. In particular, the use of the rigid introducer should be banned, and never should the surgeon resort to stiff coudé catheters. The decision should be made at once to introduce a suprapubic tube. Since these patients often have very considerable bruising of the lower abdomen it may be safer to make a formal suprapubic cystostomy, but in many centres a blind suprapubic tube is introduced.

Chapter 21/*The Urethra*

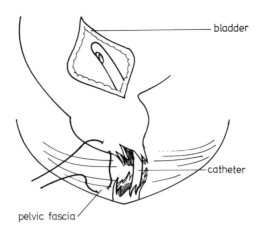

Fig. 21.15. When the patient has recovered from the initial injury and shock the prostate has to be separated by sharp dissection from the pubis and approximated to the urethra over a suitable splint.

REDUCING THE DISPLACED RUPTURED ENDS OF THE URETHRA (Fig. 21.15)

If the patient is perfectly well, and has obviously not lost much blood, and if the severity of the fracture is not great, then it is my firm opinion that the sooner one attempts to get the displaced ends of the urethra more or less together, the better. Through a midline or Pfannenstiel incision the blood is aspirated from around the displaced prostate, which is always found lying stuck firmly to the side wall of the pelvis, and separated from the torn membranous urethra, often to one side. To get the lower end of the prostatic urethra to come down to the bulbar urethra without any tension, it is first necessary to divide the puboprostatic ligaments attaching it to the pelvis. When this is done the ends can be approximated without tension. A few catgut sutures will hold the prostatic capsule down to the pelvic fascia. A narrow splinting catheter is left to bridge the gap.

In older textbooks elaborate instructions were given for methods whereby a foley catheter was to be 'railroaded' into the bladder, and then by traction on the balloon of the foley, the displacement of the prostate was to be overcome. This is quite wrong. Traction on the foley is to be strictly avoided since it must lead to pressure necrosis of the internal sphincter. In any event, since the displacement of the prostate is caused by the difficulty in reducing the displacement of the bony pelvis, one is attempting to do with traction on the foley catheter, what all the blocks and tackles of the orthopaedic team have been unsuccessful in achieving.

Alas, few of these men come in with such a simple and easy fracture. The majority have multiple injuries, have lost much blood, and are quite unfit for any surgical intervention when they arrive in hospital. For them, an introduction of a suprapubic tube as atraumatic as possible is all that you can offer in the first instance. However, after a week or so, when the patient has stopped bleeding into his pelvis, and when his other more important injuries have started to get better, one makes as early an attempt as possible to go in and reduce the displacement of the prostate, remembering that it is the ligamentous attachment of the prostate and bladder to the side wall of the pelvis that is holding the two ends of the torn urethra apart.

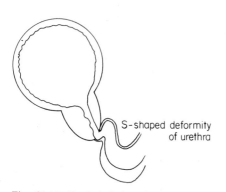

Fig. 21.16. Typical S-shaped bend in the urethra that results from a minimal displacement injury. The lumen may not be narrowed at all.

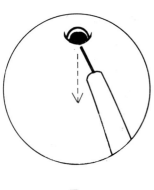

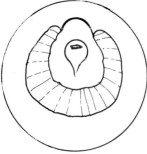

Fig. 21.17. Dividing the septum between the upper and lower urethra with an electrode.

WHEN THERE IS A RECTAL INJURY

One important consideration must be borne in mind when faced with these appalling injuries, the risk of gas gangrene. To start with, every effort is concentrated upon resuscitation. But as soon as possible, the patient must have the faeces diverted away from the massive laceration of the perineum and thighs, or there will be clostridial infection. As early as possible, a defunctioning colostomy must be made, and the lower bowel irrigated thoroughly to get rid of spore laden faeces.

After this, urinary diversion is needed, in order to get the perineal injuries to heal. Since the damage to the urethra extends up through the sphincters, through the prostate, and often into the bladder, a suprapubic diversion is seldom enough to keep the wound dry, and one may have to resort to a temporary ileal conduit to get the urine away from the healing tissues. From then on, the reconstruction of the anal canal and the lacerated urethra calls for the utmost skill and ingenuity, since each case presents a unique problem.

The aftermath of ruptured urethra

IF THE ENDS HAVE BEEN BROUGHT TOGETHER

Here one finds a typical S shaped deformity (Fig. 21.16). There may be no actual narrowing of the lumen of the urethra, and hence no need for any surgery at all. The patient should be followed up by regular endoscopic examination, since late scarring can make the lumen narrow.

In other cases the lumen is narrowed, but there is a way through, and all that is necessary is to slit open the septum which separates the prostatic from the bulbar urethra. This may be done with a knife (the Storz–Sachse urethrotome) or a diathermy electrode (Fig. 21.17). In still other instances, the lumen has been allowed to block right off. This makes incision of the septum much more difficult, but not impossible, so long as the gap is short. If the divided septum closes up again and again, then an easy one-stage urethroplasty is performed (Fig. 21.18) by sewing in a patch of scrotal skin, on its own 'mesentery' of dartos muscle (see page 358). This is only possible when the gap is short, and hence every effort must be made to bring the ends together.

IF THE ENDS ARE FAR APART

This poses the most difficult of all problems in urethral surgery. One must bridge the gap, which is often several centimetres in length. In one method, part or the whole of the symphysis pubis is taken away, leaving a defect in the bony ring. This allows the distal urethra to be brought up through the gap and sewn on to the lower end of the prostate (Fig. 21.19). In another method a long tube is formed from the skin of the scrotum and brought up to the prostatic urethra (Fig. 21.20) and kept there until it has healed on. At a second operation the defect in the scrotum is fashioned into a new urethra (see page 358). None of these operations are easy. All of them involve division of the external sphincter, and if in the initial treatment of the patient, traction has been applied to the trigone and has ruined the internal sphincter, the patient will be left incontinent of urine.

POTENCY AFTER URETHRAL INJURY

Approximately half the patients with severe pelvic fractures and urethral injuries will be unable to obtain an erection or ejaculate afterwards. The cause of this is ill-understood. In some men the pelvic parasympathetic fibres responsible for governing the erectile mechanism are probably torn by the fracture line (and impotence may occur after severe pelvic fractures without urethral injury). In others the terminal branches of the internal iliac artery that supply the spongy erectile tissue of the penis are blocked off (see page 258).

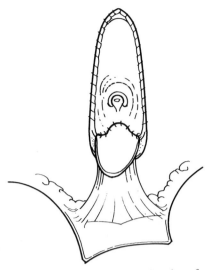

Fig. 21.18. One-stage patch urethroplasty for short, 'easy' strictures where there is little displacement of the upper and lower parts of the urethra.

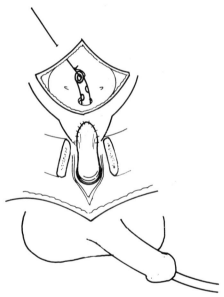

Fig. 21.19. Difficult transpubic urethroplasty where there is a long gap separating the prostatic upper urethra from the bulbar lower urethra.

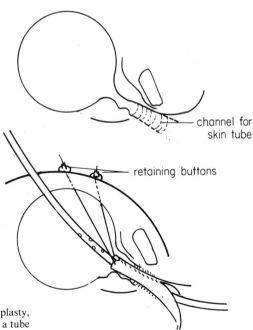

— channel for skin tube

— retaining buttons

Fig. 21.20. Even more difficult urethroplasty, where a scrotal skin flap is formed into a tube and drawn into the prostatic urethra.

Chapter 21/*The Urethra*   249

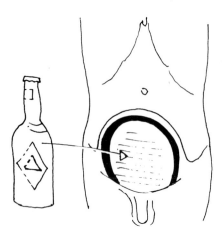
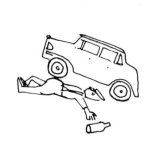
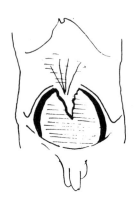
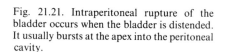

Fig. 21.21. Intraperitoneal rupture of the bladder occurs when the bladder is distended. It usually bursts at the apex into the peritoneal cavity.

TRAUMA TO THE BLADDER

Intraperitoneal rupture of the bladder

1. EXTERNAL INJURY

Typically the patient is drunk, has a distended bladder and is run over (Fig. 21.21). The bladder bursts into the peritoneal cavity. Enormous amounts of (fortunately) dilute, and therefore unirritating, urine escapes into the peritoneum. If recognized promptly the outlook is good. There may be other good reasons for performing laparotomy, e.g. the suspicion of internal haemorrhage or a bloody aspirate on 4-quadrant paracentesis, and the tear in the bladder may only be found on inspection of the abdominal contents. It is easily repaired, and a catheter left indwelling.

2. SILENT PERFORATION OF THE BLADDER

This is an odd condition, worth bearing in mind. Elderly people without a story of injury but often with previous treatment in the bladder for carcinoma by biopsy or diathermy, may be admitted with vague abdominal pain. The clinical features of urine in the peritoneum are notoriously misleading, unless the urine is infected or very concentrated. It is not very irritating when it is dilute. There may be vague discomfort, and perhaps an absence of bowel sounds. In many cases one can only make the diagnosis by a cystogram, and this may require the introduction of large volumes of contrast medium. Seldom do these patients need any treatment other than an indwelling catheter, for so long as the urine is uninfected, the peritoneum will absorb it, and the hole in the bladder will heal on its own.

3. SURGICAL PERFORATION OF THE BLADDER

It is very easy to make a hole in the bladder even when using the greatest care, in

250   Chapter 21/*The Urethra*

the course of transurethral resection of a tumour on the vault. It is recognized by the failure of the irrigating fluid to remain in the bladder, by the 'black hole' appearance of the site of resection, and (rarely, but very obviously) by recognizing loops of intestine down the resectoscope. In some gynaecological procedures, when it has been difficult to separate the uterus from the bladder, a hole is made. In both these instances, the bladder only needs to be sewn up and provided with catheter drainage and all will be well. The important thing is to recognize the damage and mend it at once.

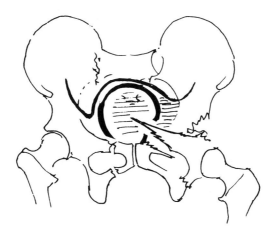

Fig. 21.22. Extraperitoneal rupture of the bladder.

Extraperitoneal rupture of the bladder (Fig. 21.22)

If the wall of the bladder has been damaged outside the peritoneum, blood and urine will collect outside it. It may occur together with damage to the urethra, or damage to other viscera, in multiple injuries. The cause of the laceration is usually a sharp spike of bone. There will always be good reason to perform laparotomy, and the nature and extent of the laceration is readily seen. The pieces of bone are replaced or removed and the wall of the bladder is closed in the usual way, with plenty of free drainage.

Similar extraperitoneal perforations of the bladder occur very commonly when resecting tumours on the trigone and base of the bladder. Unless they are very large, and large volumes of irrigating fluid are escaping, they can be safely disregarded. The holes in the bladder quickly heal with adequate catheter drainage, and there is no need to open the pelvis unless there is a local collection of fluid.

THE INDICATION FOR CYSTOGRAPHY AND URETHROGRAPHY IN TRAUMA

In some centres patients with urethral injury or suspected bladder injury are investigated, as a routine, with the introduction of contrast media into the urethra and bladder. In the writer's opinion this is very seldom necessary, since the urethro- or cystographic findings will not affect the surgeon's actions. There are certain important exceptions to this rule.

In multiple injuries, when there is loss of blood from the external meatus, and genuine doubt as to the possibility of associated injury to the kidneys as well as the lower urinary tract, then an *emergency intravenous urogram* should be performed. It may be very useful later that night to know that the patient has two kidneys.

When you suspect a *silent perforation* of the bladder a cystogram can be useful, and may save the patient from a laparotomy, since if you find a small hole in the bladder with this investigation only catheter drainage is needed.

But in the investigation of the patient with a fractured pelvis the simple decision is whether or not a catheter will slip *easily* into the bladder and let clear urine out. If not, then the patient needs a suprapubic cystostomy, or very exceptionally, is fit for exploration. Cystourethrography produces elegant but confusing pictures, but may introduce infection, and does not help the patient.

INFLAMMATION OF THE URETHRA AND URETHRAL STRICTURE

Aetiology

Stricture of the urethra is as old as surgery: Socrates joked about it; Celsus described operations for it; the Pharoahs took catheters with them to the after life because of it. It has many causes, most of them due to the effects of inflammation in the urethra, although as we have seen, healing of traumatic injury is also followed by a stricture.

In children urethritis of unknown cause may give haematuria, form tiny granulomatous polypi and be succeeded by a stricture usually in the bulbar urethra. In adults urethritis is often caused by *Neisseria gonorrhoeae*, but *Chlamydia* and other agents responsible for non-specific urethritis may lead to a stricture. The reason seems to be either that the raw inflamed lining of the urethra sticks together (Fig. 21.23) or fibrosis following inflammation in the paraurethral glands produces a narrowing of the wall of the urethra.

OTHER CAUSES OF STRICTURE

For completeness one may list the causes of stricture:

1 Congenital (this usually includes the double-barrelled urethra and the congenital mid-bulbar stricture).

2 Traumatic. We have referred to the aftermath of ruptured urethra in the perineum and membranous urethra. Far more numerous are the strictures

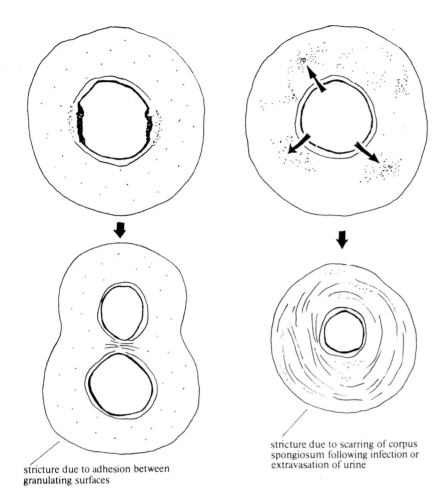

stricture due to scarring of corpus spongiosum following infection or extravasation of urine

stricture due to adhesion between granulating surfaces

Fig. 21.23. Diagram of urethral strictures.

which follow bedsores in the urethra caused by indwelling catheters that press on the internal lining of the urethra at the penoscrotal junction (where the urethra lies at an angle), at the external meatus (where it is naturally most narrow), or just where it is gripped by the external sphincter. The prevention of these strictures is difficult but relies on the use of a very narrow and very soft catheter for as short a time as possible.

3 Inflammatory (these include gonorrhoea and chlamydia).

4 Neoplasms. Carcinoma occurs in the urethra, usually secondary to long standing stricture, with stasis of urine upstream of the stricture leading to squamous metaplasia of the urothelium. It is fortunately rare in Britain.

5 Balanitis xerotica obliterans. This obscure skin disease, known in other sites as *lichen schlerosus et atrophicus* causes a white stiff change in the skin around the external meatus and prepuce. It may also occur in the skin that has been let into the urethra at the operation of urethroplasty, though fortunately this is very uncommon.

Clinical features of urethral stricture

A poor stream is accompanied by a poor flow-rate and the development of the same set of symptoms caused by detrusor hypertrophy that were noted in the context of the prostate (see page 22). Urine is trapped in the urethra upstream of the stricture and dribbles away after the patient thinks he has finished his micturition. Often the patient observes a spraying or a bifurcated urinary stream.

Complications of urethral stricture (Fig. 21.24)

Retention of urine may occur with a stricture, particularly when in addition to the stricture, there has been an acute infection.

Urinary infection is common, due to the residual urine upstream of the stricture.

Obstructed ejaculation may cause pain in coitus and result in such a poor ejaculate that the patient is infertile.

Chordee results from shortening of the inflamed and fibrosed corpus spongiosum, and may be so marked as to prevent intercourse.

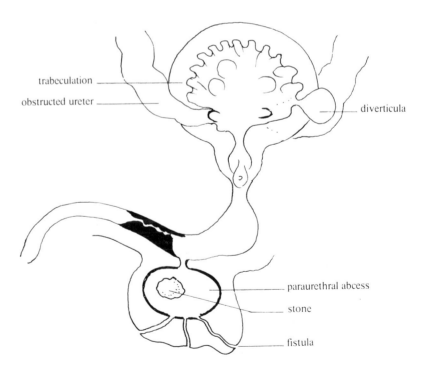

Fig. 21.24. Complications of a urethral stricture.

Chapter 21/*The Urethra*

Calculi form in the dilated urethra upstream of the stricture, or in paraurethral abscesses.

Paraurethral abscess may result in bursting of the pus into the soft tissues of the scrotum. Since the abscess is always upstream of the stricture, the urine finds its way into the soft tissues, leading to *extravasation*, resulting in *necrosis* of the overlying skin and thence to multiple *fistulae*. The end result is a chronically infected, indurated, puckered mass of fistulae, some leaking urine, and others leaking pus. This is called the watering-can perineum.

Squamous cell carcinoma may complicate any long-standing urethral stricture. It seems to occur in the squamous metaplasia of the urethra upstream of the stricture. In my experience successful relief of obstruction, e.g. by urethroplasty, does not necessarily prevent this complication which takes many years to develop. The moral is that in any man with a long-standing history of urethral stricture, one should suspect cancer.

Investigation of urethral stricture

1. FLOW-RATES provide documentation of the stricture, but unfortunately, since flow is proportional to the square of the radius of the urethra, it only needs a very small reduction in the lumen to change a good into a very poor flow-rate.

2. URETHROGRAPHY. Water-soluble or jelly contrast media are used to outline the stricture.

3. URETHROSCOPY AND ENDOSCOPIC PHOTOGRAPHY of the urethra give the best assessment of its nature, extent and severity, and if photographed, the best and most objective record.

Management of urethral strictures

There is an old urological adage 'once a stricture always a stricture'. Even today, when our armamentarium has proliferated greatly, the truth of this dictum is unchallenged. When you read of any new method for treating urethral strictures, always say to yourself, 'and how long is the follow-up?'

BOUGINAGE

Bujiyah is the name of the Algerian town and its adjacent bay, noted in mediaeval times for its honey and its beeswax. For generations beeswax candles were used to dilate strictures. The French named their wax tapers after Bujiyah (*bougie*) and the English named their urethral dilators after the French. Others refer to urethral dilators as 'sounds', from the metal instrument used to detect bladder calculi by clicking against them before the days of X-rays. Today the words *bougie* and *sound* are interchangable (Fig. 21.25).

Using instruments of gradually increasing diameter, the surgeon gently

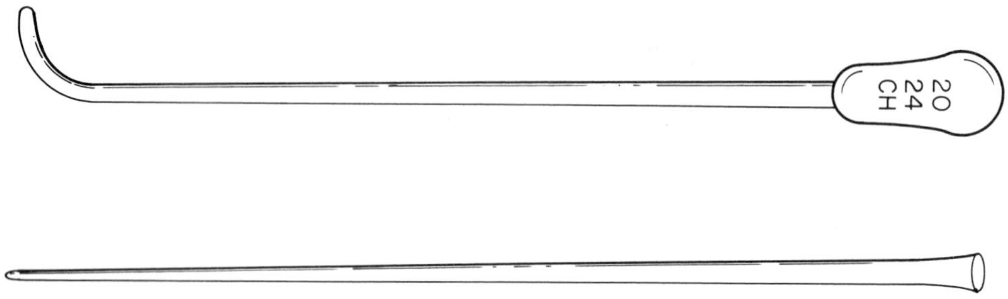

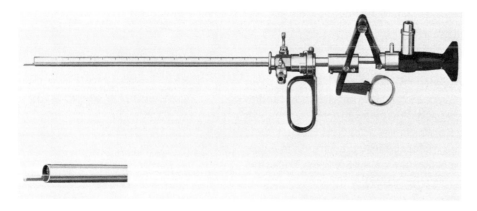

Fig. 21.25. Urethral bougie and urethral sound.

stretches the stricture, hoping to stretch the fibrous tissue of the corpus spongiosum without tearing the mucosa. Urethral bouginage remains the mainstay of the management of a urethral stricture. But it is not perfect: it often gives rise to bacteraemia, it may tear the urethra and cause bleeding, and if the urethra is forcibly overstretched the resulting scar may be tighter than ever.

Bouginage is performed at gradually lengthening intervals until eventually the patient only has to undergo dilatation once a year.

INTERNAL URETHROTOMY

Unfortunately it is not always possible to introduce bougies of the right size, because the scar tissue is too tough. To start the patient off, one may slit the stricture right open. This is done with a variety of instruments, many of them of very ancient pattern. The most useful one (the Storz–Sachse internal optical urethrotome) allows the surgeon to see exactly where and how deep he is cutting (Fig. 21.26). After urethrotomy a catheter remains in the urethra for a few days to prevent extravasation of urine that might make the inflammatory reaction worse.

URETHROPLASTY

Fig. 21.26. Storz–Sachse internal optical urethrotome. (Courtesy Karl Storz.)

Sometimes strictures return so tightly, and cause so much pain and misery when

Chapter 21/*The Urethra*

they are dilated, that some alternative means of dealing with the stricture is sought. There are several methods now available. One may slit open the urethra and insert a patch of skin. The skin may be a free split-skin (Wolff) graft, often taken from the hairless skin of the prepuce, or it may be full thickness skin on a pedicle provided by the dartos muscle (see page 358). The inlay of scrotal skin may be performed in one or two stages. If the stricture is very short, one can excise it and join the ends of the urethra together, but this may result in shortening of the urethra and a bent erection (chordee).

Many are the claims made for modern versions of urethroplasty; none can be guaranteed to be without late complications which include hairs growing in the lumen that form stones, late stenosis of the urethra at either end of the skin patch, balanitis xerotica leading to shrinking of the patch and so on. Urethroplasty is useful, but not perfect. 'Once a stricture always a stricture'.

FURTHER READING

Attwater H.L. (1943) The history of urethral stricture. *British Journal of Urology*, **15**, 39.
Blandy J.P. (1975) Injuries of the urethra in the male. *Injury*, **7**, 77.
Blandy J.P. (1980) Urethral stricture. *Postgraduate Medical Journal*, **56**, 383.
Johnson F.P. (1920) The later development of the urethra in the male. *Journal of Urology*, **4**, 447.
Matouschek E. (1978) Internal urethrotomy of urethral stricture under vision—a 5 year report. *Urological Research*, **6**, 147.
Singh M. & Blandy J.P. (1976) The pathology of urethral stricture. *Journal of Urology*, **115**, 673.
Turner-Warwick R.T. (1977) A personal view of the management of traumatic posterior urethral stricture. *Urologic Clinics of North America*, **4**, 111.

Chapter 22
The Penis

SURGICAL ANATOMY (Fig. 22.1)

The penis is made up of three distensible spongy sacs, the twin corpora cavernosa and the corpus spongiosum that ends in the glans penis. Distension of the sacs within the strong and rigid Buck's fascia results in a firm erection. The spongy spaces of the two corpora cavernosa intercommunicate, but those of the corpus spongiosum are virtually distinct. Each of the corpora cavernosa has a large artery running down its centre. The corpus spongiosum has two smaller arteries. Two more run on the dorsum of the penis on either side of its deep dorsal vein, all within the fascia of Buck, while outside the fascia lies the superficial dorsal vein of the penis.

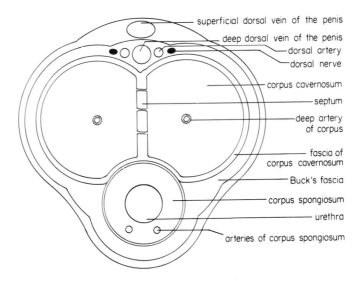

superficial dorsal vein of the penis
deep dorsal vein of the penis
dorsal artery
dorsal nerve
corpus cavernosum
septum
deep artery of corpus
fascia of corpus cavernosum
Buck's fascia
corpus spongiosum
urethra
arteries of corpus spongiosum

Fig. 22.1. Diagrammatic transverse section through the penis.

The physiology of erection

At rest, blood is shunted away from branches of the penile veins, bypassing the corpora (Fig. 22.2). During erection, these arteriovenous shunts are closed off, and the blood fills the erectile spongy tissue (Fig. 22.3). Two distinct elements are at work in this process: first, the AV shunts appear to be under the control of the pelvic parasympathetics, so that lesions of the autonomic nervous system may prevent adequate erection; secondly, filling the corpora requires an intact arterial blood supply and undamaged AV shunts.

Ejaculation is an even more complex process (Fig. 22.4). First, the seminal vesicles secrete fluid and 'pump up'—a process that has been recorded after filling them with contrast medium. In the second phase of ejaculation sperms stored in the vasa deferentia and possibly in the lower part of the epididymis are squirted out through the ejaculatory ducts, to be followed by the third phase in which the seminal vesicles contract and push before them the sperm-rich fluid derived from the vasa. The mechanism of ejaculation requires an intact bladder neck, which must contract to stop sperm refluxing back into the bladder. This

Chapter 22/*The Penis*

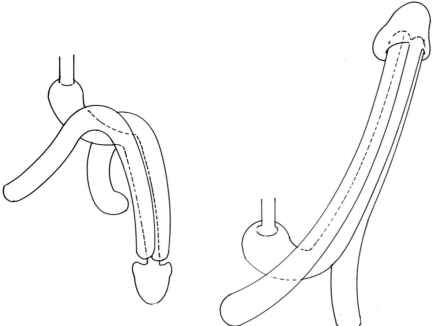

Fig. 22.2. Flaccid penis.

Fig. 23.3. Erect penis.

phase 1

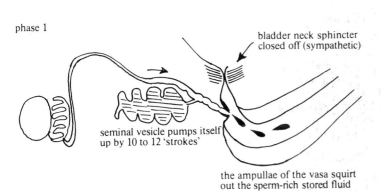

bladder neck sphincter
closed off (sympathetic)

seminal vesicle pumps itself
up by 10 to 12 'strokes'

the ampullae of the vasa squirt
out the sperm-rich stored fluid

ejaculated semen

trace from prostate ? 0·5 ml

4 ml from seminal vesicles
containing bicarbonate
and fructose

0·5 ml containing the inspissated
sperm from the ampulla of the vas
deferens

phase 2

sphincter still
shut off

seminal vesicles suddenly empty and wash
sperm-rich ampullary fluid ahead down the
urethra (held open by corpus spongiosum)
and perhaps squeezed out by bulbospongiosus
muscle

Fig. 22.4. Mechanism of ejaculation.

part of ejaculation at least is clearly shown to be under the alpha adrenergic influence of the sympathetic system. If the last two lumbar sympathetic ganglia are removed then there is retrograde ejaculation. It is also probable that the contraction of the seminal vesicles is also mediated by alpha adrenergic fibres.

CONGENITAL LESIONS OF THE PENIS

Hypospadias (Fig. 22.5)

Failure of fusion of the embryonic genital folds in the midline leads to more or less incomplete formation of the distal part of the urethra. This takes several forms. One sometimes sees adults with chordee (shortening of the urethra) and narrowing of the distal urethra, with a normally placed external meatus. But in most cases not only is the distal part of the urethra shorter and narrower than normal, but the opening is placed further towards the perineum than it ought to be. Hypospadias therefore comprises a spectrum of changes.

In its most common and least important form, the external urinary meatus opens just a little behind the normal site. This is called glandular hypospadias. It

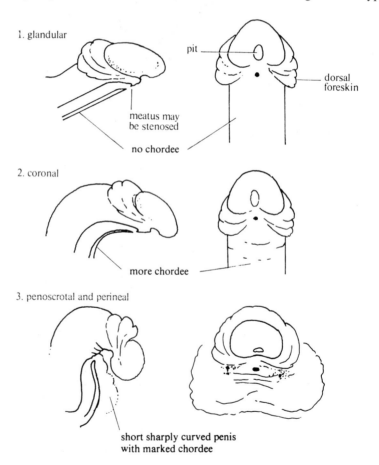

Fig. 22.5. Hypospadias.

Chapter 22/*The Penis*

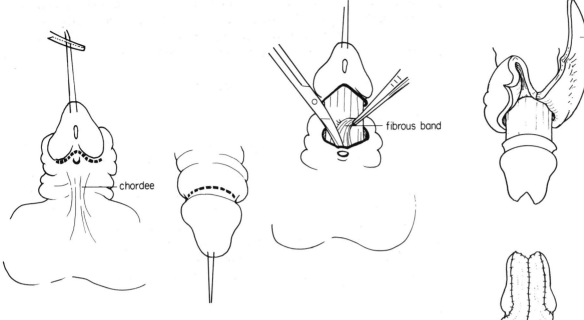

causes no disability. If it is not associated with chordee it gives rise to no trouble in lovemaking or procreation, and it should not be meddled with. Associated with the proximal placement of the meatus is cleavage of the prepuce so that it forms a kind of frill on the dorsum.

In coronal hypospadias this proximal situation of the meatus is accompanied by shortening of the distal urethra resulting in chordee. In penoscrotal and perineal hypospadias, the most severe forms, the penis is extremely short, flat and stumpy, and the testicles are often undescended as well. In such patients one must consider the diagnosis of intersex.

MANAGEMENT

The most mild forms of hypospadias do not need treatment at all. The real indications for surgical interference are when there is gross chordee and when the meatus opens far back on the underside of the penis. In such patients the operation has usually to be done in two stages: (a) the fibrous cord that represents the poorly developed distal urethra is dissected out, to allow the rest of the penis to be straightened out, and at the same time allow the external meatus to drop down (Fig. 22.6); (b) a new urethra is formed by inrolling a tube of skin (Fig. 22.7).

It is usual to perform the first stage of the operation when the little boy is about two years old, the second stage about four so that the entire procedure is completed before he starts school. Very mild cases of glandular hypospadias can be made to look more normal with a one-stage operation.

There is a late aftermath of successful hypospadias operations. Sometimes

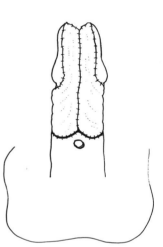

Fig. 22.6. Stages in first-stage hypospadias repair.

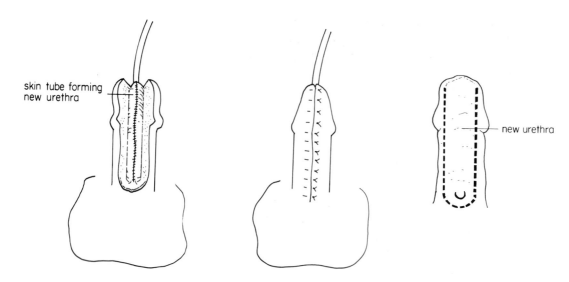

Fig. 22.7. Stages in second-stage hypospadias repair.

the new skin tube that forms the urethra does not keep pace with the growth of the urethra and may give rise to late stricture or chordee requiring late revision in adult life.

Phimosis

True phimosis, i.e. narrowing of the opening of the foreskin is quite rare. The natural separation of the two layers of skin that form the foreskin is usually not complete until the boy is about two years old. After this age one should be able to retract the prepuce in order to clean the glans. Ritual circumcision is a most interesting anthropological remnant of an initiation rite which, with the passage of the ages, has been transposed further and further back in childhood until it is done on the 8th day in the Jewish rite. The prepuce serves quite a useful function in infancy, protecting the glans penis from the scarring that sometimes follows ammoniacal dermatitis (napkin rash).

There is no doubt that neonatal circumcision protects men from developing carcinoma of the penis in adult life. The drawback is that wholesale circumcision of all males to prevent the annual rare occurrence of carcinoma would probably have a greater morbidity and mortality than leaving them alone, so long as it is possible for people to have access to soap and water. In Europe carcinoma of the penis is very rare, and virtually limited to old men with prolonged phimosis with a poor standard of personal hygiene. This observation does not apply to other cultures where water supplies are limited and soap and water hard to come by. There circumcision may prevent large numbers of penile cancers.

TRAUMA

The foreskin is often caught accidentally in zip-fasteners, and less often in industrial and other accidents. Dreadful lesions have been reported when men have inserted their penis into vacuum cleaners. Self-injected paraffin and silicone materials have been the cause of other granulomas in the penis and scrotum. The corpus cavernosum may be ruptured during intercourse. It is usually recommended that the tear be repaired promptly though cases are recorded of obvious ruptures that have healed spontaneously.

INFLAMMATION

Inflammation of the glans penis is called *balanitis*, of the space under the prepuce, *posthitis*. They usually occur together. Acute balanitis is seen in patients with allergic dermatitis, from herpes genitalis, and from non-specific secondary infection in men with diabetes mellitus.

Specific lesions on the glans include the classical Hunterian chancre of primary *syphilis*, the soft painful exuberant chancre of *Haemophilus ducreyi* infection, infected scabies, lymphogranuloma venereum and granuloma inguinale—all lesions that need to be distinguished from syphilis, and that call for expert treatment by a specialized venereologist. Diagnosis by dark field examination may not be too difficult, but tracing contacts and making sure of the efficacy of a course of treatment requires great skill. The penalty for ineffective amateur treatment is disastrous.

Recurrent non-specific balanitis is usually an indication for circumcision. Allowing the glans to become dry and cornified improves its ability to resist infection.

Balanitis xerotica obliterans is an unusual skin condition causing a whitish, sometimes irritating change in the skin around the foreskin and glans penis. Its cause is unknown. It leads to thickening and shrinking of the skin, so that the meatus may be stenosed. The same process seen elsewhere in the skin is called *lichen sclerosus et atrophicus* and occurs on the vulva and elbows. Steroid ointments may arrest its progress, but as a rule the narrow meatus requires a meatoplasty (see page 357).

Peyronie's disease (Fig. 22.8)

Named after the founder of the French equivalent of the Royal Society who described it in 1743, there is a hard white plaque of fibrous tissue in Buck's fascia, and sometimes in the septum between the corpora cavernosa. It may be associated with nodules in the ear lobes, Dupuytren's contracture of the palmar and plantar fasciae, and idiopathic retroperitoneal fibrosis. Innumerable forms of treatment have been used. Whenever any of them are compared with controls, no benefit has occurred. There is a natural but slow tendency for the plaques to resolve spontaneously, but this does not always occur. For many patients the deformity caused by the nodule preventing filling of the corpus cavernosum on the affected side, and the pain that sometimes occurs when the

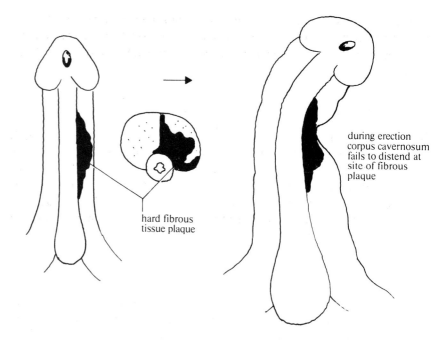

Fig. 22.8. Peyronies disease.

penis is erect, requires more active treatment. Sometimes it is worth dissecting away a particularly dense plaque of fibrous tissue and replacing it with a dermis graft. In other patients Nesbit's operation straightens the penis—tucks are taken out of the fascia on the other, normal side, until the penis is seen to be straight.

CARCINOMA OF THE PENIS

In the West cancer of the penis is a disease almost entirely confined to elderly men with poor hygiene who cannot or do not pull back the foreskin to wash underneath. In Africa it is much more common and occurs in a younger age group unless they have been circumcised. It is very likely that cancer in the penis is initiated or promoted by other local lesions, particularly herpes genitalis and soft chancre.

A precancerous condition occurs in which there is a red moist sore on the glans, which may resemble non-specific balanitis. Biopsy shows *in situ* carcinoma of the skin, and unless treated vigorously (with 5-fluoruracil cream or local irradiation) it will certainly be followed by undoubted invasive cancer. This is called *Erythroplasia of Queyrat* (after the Parisian dermatologist who described it many years after it had been well recognized by Brodie).

Benign warts (caused by a transmissible virus) occur on the penis called *Condylomata acuminata*. They are not premalignant and respond to treatment with podophyllin.

Huge, giant, warty tumours that mostly look benign were described by Buschke and Loewenstein. If treated early and vigorously they may be cured by local surgical excision but in many of the cases reported they have ended up as true invasive cancers.

Pathology of carcinoma of the penis

These are squamous cell carcinomas and metastasize to the inguinal lymph nodes. It is said that the first node to be involved is the sentinel node of Cabana just where the saphenous vein dives down to enter the femoral vein. Two histological types are recognized—those with a 'cord' pattern of growth and those with a 'solid' pattern, and in each of these types three Grades of malignancy are usually noted. Grade 1 tumours with the 'solid' pattern do well; Grade 2 and 3 tumours with the 'cord' pattern do badly.

Clinical features

The elderly, unwashed, uncircumcised man comes up with a discharge issuing from his prepuce, under which one can usually feel a lump. Sometimes on drawing back the foreskin, when this is possible, one can see an ulcer, sometimes a cauliflower growth and sometimes an erosive loss of part or all of the glans penis. The inguinal lymph nodes are always enlarged, though not always with metastasis, more often due to inflammatory change. The first investigation consists of a biopsy which should usually be combined with circumcision in order to allow antiseptic irrigations to help clear up the local infection.

Management

For practical purposes there are two main Stages: those for whom local amputation or the application of an Iridium mould is feasible, and those where the tumour has so invaded the perineal and scrotal skin that no partial amputation will suffice and no Iridium radioactive mould can be devised that will cover the growth.

Stage 1 where the tumour is confined to the prepuce and glans penis, and Stage 2 where the tumour has just begun to infiltrate the shaft of the penis are best treated (after preliminary circumcision and antibiotic treatment) with the application of radioactive Iridium[192] in a specially made mould that fits the penis. Using this technique one may expect 80–100% cures. If there is a local recurrence, it is still possible to perform an amputation.

But when the patient has left the condition so late that no mould can be fitted, then a radical removal of the penis should be performed.

The *inguinal lymph nodes* are treated by delayed intervention. The primary growth, which is always infected, is dealt with first, and the glands are observed. If they are still enlarged, needle aspiration and cytological confirmation of their malignant infiltration is obtained, and then they are treated by radiotherapy. In former times radical node dissection was performed in the groins. It carried a very severe morbidity, and as a rule only cured those patients in whom the nodes were negative. Today node dissection is deferred until the patient has completed a course of radiotherapy to the inguinal regions, and when lymphography has excluded invasion of lymph nodes higher up in the iliac and para-aortic groups.

Bleomycin was found to be very effective for carcinoma of the penis of the type encountered in Japan, but in Britain has given most discouraging results.

IMPOTENCE

When a patient complains of impotence it is necessary to listen patiently in order to discover exactly what has gone wrong. One may distinguish five different syndromes.

A. DISAPPOINTMENT

Some men have exaggerated ideas of what their 'normal' performance ought to be. They forget that in this as in all physical attributes, a man's performance diminishes with age. They may seek some wonder-working pill or injection from their doctor. He has none to offer. Do not be bullied into prescribing androgens or so-called stimulants and aphrodisiacs.

B. EJACULATION NORMAL, BUT COITUS UNSATISFACTORY

This needs delicate enquiry. If your patient ejaculates in his dreams and can masturbate, then there is nothing wrong with the physiological mechanism. You may learn that the difficulty is related to one sexual partner, but not to another. Unless you have had special training and experience in sexual counselling, refer the patient to someone who has.

C. ERECTION NORMAL, EJACULATION UNSATISFACTORY

1 *Trigger set too delicately—premature ejaculation.* Ejaculation may occur before the patient has penetrated, well before his partner has achieved climax. This is a natural phenomenon as may be verified by simple observation of apes in the zoo. The patient needs sympathetic reassurance. Let the couple have a rest and try again a little later. Often all that is needed is some information about the techniques of civilized lovemaking. There is no pill that will replace informed understanding of the matter.

2 *Ejaculation inhibited.* Feelings of guilt, anxiety, or fear of discovery (as every novelist knows) may inhibit the progress of lovemaking. When this occurs

repeatedly, it may blight an otherwise loving and happy relationship. Patient explanation by a skilled counsellor will nearly always bring the problems into the open.

3   *Retrograde ejaculation.* If the last two lumbar sympathetic ganglia have been removed surgically, or if the patient is born with a defect of the bladder neck that renders it unable to close during orgasm, then the ejaculated semen may pass back into the bladder. It may be collected from there and used for artificial insemination. However, it is well worth trying the effect of large doses of alpha-stimulating drugs which may be enough to close the internal sphincter and allow the semen to issue down the urethra.

4   *No ejaculation.* A small number of men do not ejaculate at all. In some there is an obvious cause, e.g. diabetic autonomic neuropathy, or medication with ganglion-blocking drugs. In others the cause remains obscure.

D. NO ERECTION

Two main types of cause need to be looked for. First, are all those lesions that might result in a fault in the *parasympathetic innervation* of the penis: trauma or surgery to the pelvis, autonomic neuropathy of various kinds, particularly that seen so tragically often in young diabetic men. Second, where there is a block in the *blood supply* of the penis. There may be generalized arteriosclerosis, and obstruction of the arteries in the corpora cavernosa is only one aspect of a generalized disease. There may be a block at the bifurcation of the aorta giving rise to the well-recognized syndrome of Leriche. Or the blockage may be from previous priapism that has been followed by damage to the AV anastomoses upon which erection depends.

E. NO DESIRE

Two common conditions fall into this category. (a) *Overwork*—the so-called 'Barrister's impotence' (though barristers are not the only sufferers). The syndrome is easily recognized: hard-working and ambitious middle aged man, workaholic, brings his work home, has no time for anything else, collapses exhausted to bed, uninterested in his wife; result—frustration, recriminations, alcohol and divorce. (b) *Depression.* Watch out for the truly depressed patient whose impotence is only one of many features of the disease. Fortunately it responds to appropriate psychiatric treatment.

Investigation

The careful taking of the history is far the most important investigation, and it will rule out any need to pursue investigations any further in the majority of your patients. Routine examination will detect diabetes and severe arteriopathy. You will be left with a small number of patients presenting a clinical difficulty. To distinguish the 'psychogenic' from the small vessel obstructive type of impotence one may attach a strain gauge to the penis and register its expansion and contraction during sleep. Erections are a feature of 'deep REM' sleep (where rapid eye movements are recorded and a typical electroencephalograph is found). If during sleep there is no erection when REM sleep occurs then one must assume an organic lesion of the parasympathetic nerves or the blood vessels going to the penis.

Careful angiography may reveal a blockage in the terminal branches of the internal iliac artery that supply the bulb and the corpora cavernosa. Plethysmography may reveal an absence of arterial pulsations in the superficial arteries of the penis but do not necessarily detect what is happening in the deep vessels of the corpora cavernosa. Doppler studies similarly give useful information about the superficial arteries but not necessarily about the deep ones.

Treatment of organic erectile impotence

If one can be reasonably satisfied that the impotence is of organic origin (i.e. cannot be put right by a psychiatrist), then the patient may wish to have his penis made stiff by some artificial implanted gadget. They come in several forms. There are permanently stiff silicone rubber splints (the Small–Carrion prostheses) (Fig. 22.9) that are forced into the corpora cavernosa to keep them semi-erect. This is enough to allow the husband to penetrate his wife, and may restore his self confidence. There is another model (Jonas prosthesis) which is provided with a bendable silver wire core so that the penis can be bent and unbent at will. There is a blow-up device in which inflatable cylinders in the

Fig. 22.9. Insertion of the Small–Carrion prosthesis.

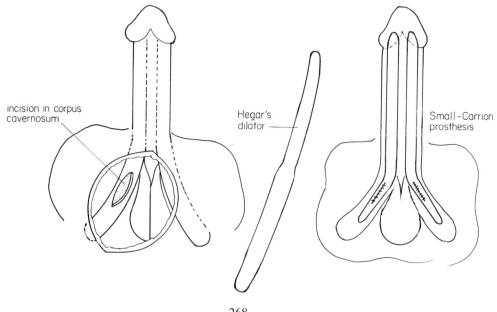

incision in corpus cavernosum

Hegar's dilator

Small-Carrion prosthesis

Chapter 22/*The Penis*

corpora cavernosa can be filled and emptied by appropriate manipulation of small silicone-rubber fluid-filled balloons housed in the scrotum (Scott prosthesis). All of these prostheses are exceedingly expensive, and as with all implanted foreign bodies anywhere in the body, they are apt to become infected and work their way out. Unless the patient is highly motivated and carefully selected it is easy to see that complications may lead to bitterness and recrimination.

Nevertheless there remain a small number of patients for whom these devices offer a new lease of life, and the achievement of the pioneers who have devised them must not be belittled.

PRIAPISM

When the erection will not go down and the corpora cavernosa remain stiff, but the glans and corpus spongiosum become flaccid, the condition is known as priapism. It is painful and very distressing. It is seen more often in males with sickle cell disease and leukaemia, sometimes in men taking ganglion-blockers for hypertension, and sometimes in patients on dialysis. Its pathology is not clear. The blood inside the distended corpora cavernos is thick, like strawberry jam, but it never clots. Anticoagulants, hypotension, ganglion blockers, spinal

Fig. 22.10. Corpus–corpus anastomosis for priapism.

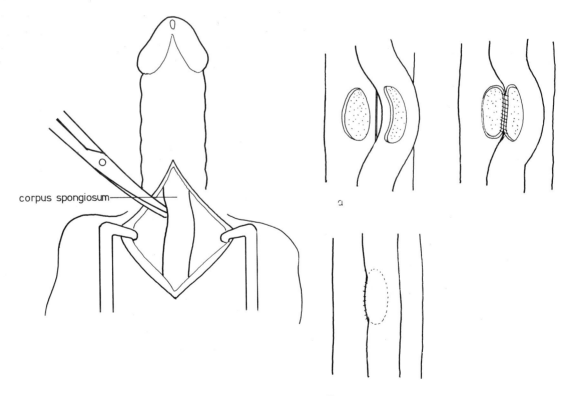

corpus spongiosum

anaesthesia, irrigation with heparin, none of these do any good. The only effective remedy is to make a window somehow between the distended cavernous system and the flaccid spongiosum.

There are several methods of doing this. Waterhouse thrusts a fine knife through the glans penis into the protrusion of the underlying corpora cavernosa. Winter does the same thing, using a Trucut needle. These are easy to do, but do not always work. The next most easy procedure is to remove a small window from the fascia over the corpus spongiosum and corpus cavernosum on one side and anastomose the two to each other (Fig. 22.10). Blood in the distended system leaves via the flaccid one. Even this does not always work. Finally one may take the saphenous vein and anastomose it to the side of the corpus cavernosum, and if this fails on one side, it may work on the other.

Some men who have suffered priapism are left with a permanently flaccid penis. Others recover normal function. It was formerly taught that there was a time limit after which surgical intervention could not be successful. This does not seem to be the case, but there is little doubt that the sooner something is done the better the result in the long run.

FURTHER READING

Blandy J.P. (1976) Penis and scrotum. In J.P. Blandy (ed.), *Urology*, p. 1049. Blackwell Scientific Publications, Oxford.

Blandy J.P. (1976) Male fertility and impotence. In D.I. Williams & G.D. Chisholm (eds), *Scientific Foundations of Urology*, p. 187. Heinemann, London.

Casey W.C. (1980) Penile blood pressure—a clarification. *Urology*, **15**, 47.

Cohen M.S., Sharpe W., Warner R.S. & Zorgniotti A. (1980) Morphology of corporal cavernosa arterial bed in impotence. *Urology*, **16**, 382.

Megafu U. (1979) Cancer of the genital tract among the Ibo women in Nigeria. *Cancer*, **44**, 1875.

Merrin C.E. (1980) Cancer of the penis. *Cancer*, **45**, 1973.

Mira J.G. (1980) Is it worthwhile to treat Peyronie's disease? *Urology*, **16**, 1.

Newman H.F. & Tchertkoff V. (1980) Penile vascular cushions and erection. *Investigative Urology*, **18**, 43.

Salaverria J.C., Hope-Stone H.F., Paris A.M.I., Molland E.A. & Blandy J.P. (1979) Conservative treatment of carcinoma of the penis. *British Journal of Urology*, **51**, 32.

Schmauz R., Findlay M., Lalwak A., Katsumbira N. & Buxton E. (1977) Variation in the appearance of giant condyloma in an Ugandan series of cases of carcinoma of the penis. *Cancer*, **40**, 1686.

Spark R.F., White R.A. & Connolly P.B. (1980) Impotence is not always psychogenic. Newer insights into hypothalamic-pituitary-gondal dysfunction. *Journal of the American Medical Association*, **243**, 750.

SURGICAL ANATOMY

By tradition testis and epididymis are together included in the term 'testicle'. They lie in the scrotum, the testis in front of the epididymis, both slung from the external inguinal ring by the spermatic cord. Around the testis there is a thin space containing a trace of fluid—the cavity of the tunica vaginalis. The testicular artery is a branch of the aorta at the level of the renal arteries which curves round lateral to the inferior epigastric vessels to pass from the retroperitoneal tissue into the groin and along the inguinal canal. There is a rich venous drainage from the testicle, the pampiniform plexus draining upwards to fuse into the spermatic veins that enter the left renal vein and the vena cava directly on the right side.

The testis is composed of sets of tubules containing the sperm forming cells. The tubules drain into the rete testis, and thence along the vasa efferentia into the epididymis. The epididymis is a long, coiled tube lined with ciliated epithelium that issues into the vas deferens (Fig. 23.1).

The vas deferens runs behind the spermatic cord, curls around the inferior epigastric vessels, crossing the ureter, and dives down through the prostate to emerge beside the utriculus masculinus at the side of the verumontanum in the prostatic urethra. Before it enters the crack between the bladder and prostate, it gives off a diverticulum, the seminal vesicle (Fig. 23.2).

Histology of the testis (Fig. 23.3)

Each testicular tubule has a thin basement membrane within which one finds two types of cell—the germinal cells and the Sertoli cells. The germinal cells give rise to generation after generation of spermatocytes, and finally form the spermatozoa. The Sertoli cells stand around in between them, and probably play an important part in the final preparation of the spermatozoa for their long journey to the ejaculatory duct.

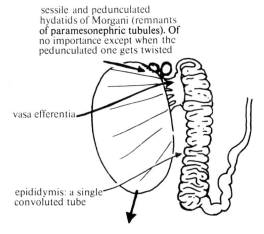

sessile and pedunculated hydatids of Morgani (remnants of paramesonephric tubules). Of no importance except when the pedunculated one gets twisted

vasa efferentia

epididymis: a single convoluted tube

Fig. 23.1. Surgical anatomy of the testis.

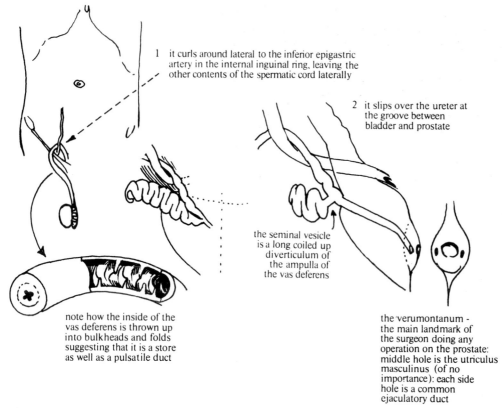

1 it curls around lateral to the inferior epigastric artery in the internal inguinal ring, leaving the other contents of the spermatic cord laterally

2 it slips over the ureter at the groove between bladder and prostate

the seminal vesicle is a long coiled up diverticulum of the ampulla of the vas deferens

note how the inside of the vas deferens is thrown up into bulkheads and folds suggesting that it is a store as well as a pulsatile duct

the verumontanum - the main landmark of the surgeon doing any operation on the prostate: middle hole is the utriculus masculinus (of no importance): each side hole is a common ejaculatory duct

Fig. 23.2. Anatomy of the vas deferens.

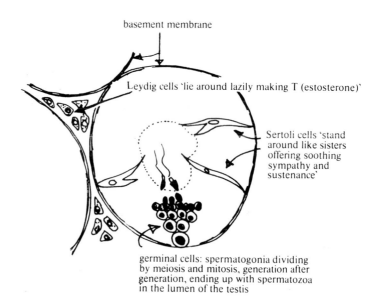

basement membrane

Leydig cells 'lie around lazily making T (estosterone)'

Sertoli cells 'stand around like sisters offering soothing sympathy and sustenance'

germinal cells: spermatogonia dividing by meiosis and mitosis, generation after generation, ending up with spermatozoa in the lumen of the testis

Fig. 23.3. Histology of the testis.

Chapter 23/*The Testicle and Seminal Tract*

The germinal cells have an incredible history. They start off in the primordial yolk sac, make their way to the genital ridge by their own amoeboid movements, burrow into the epithelium of the coelom and finally fetch up forming the core of what are destined to be the seminiferous tubules.

The histology of the testis alters at different stages in its development. In the fetus one can discern primitive germ cells and precursor Sertoli cells. Packed in between the tubules are Leydig cells whose office seems to be to secrete testosterone. They play a most important part in the fetus in differentiation of the male external genitalia, the prostatic bud and the seminal vesicles, and at the time of birth they are quite numerous.

Shortly after the baby is born the Leydig cells vanish, only to reappear again just before puberty. With puberty also the long-dormant germ cells begin to divide and form spermatocytes.

Histology of the epididymis

The epididymis is lined by pseudostratified columnar epithelium from which microvilli protrude into the lumen (stereocilia) whose function is not known.

Structure of the vas deferens

The vas has a huge muscular wall in proportion to its tiny and folded lumen. In animals it is capable of undergoing considerable peristaltic activity. As the vas nears the seminal vesicle its wall is thrown into convolutions which increase its storage capacity.

Structure of the seminal vesicles

Each seminal vesicle is a diverticulum of the vas that arises just before the vas joins the ejaculatory duct. Each one holds from 2 to 5 ml of fluid, and each is made up of a long duct, with branches, coiled and twisted into a compact mass. It is lined with columnar mucosa. The vesicles secrete fructose to a concentration three times that of the glucose in the blood, perhaps because this suits the spermatozoa which have an anaerobic metabolism. It also coats sperms with some substance that gives them an apple-green fluorescence (though nobody knows what this signifies). If the seminal vesicles are diseased then the semen volume is reduced.

CONGENITAL ANOMALIES OF THE TESTICLE

Normal descent of the testicle

The testis originates in the genital ridge, adjacent to the mesonephros, and takes over the mesonephric Wolffian duct to serve as its genital duct, the vas deferens.

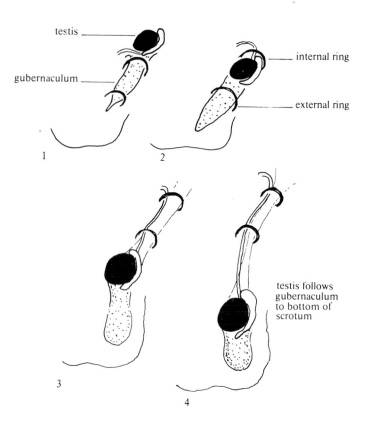

testis

gubernaculum

internal ring

external ring

1

2

testis follows
gubernaculum
to bottom of
scrotum

3

4

Fig. 23.4. Descent of the testicle.

In man the testis migrates into the scrotum. In other mammals it migrates towards the scrotum, but not always so far: in elephants they stop near the kidneys: in whales they remain near the bladder: in hedgehogs just inside the abdominal wall: in pigs they pop in and out of the inguinal canal. In man (like the sheep) they lie at the bottom of a pendulous scrotum.

The testis is preceded in its journey by a lump of jelly, the 'gubernaculum'. It probably oozes through the tissues swelling and expanding to make way for the testis to come after (Fig. 23.4).

If the gubernaculum goes astray, the testis follows the wrong path; hence sometimes testicles are found in ectopic positions. *Ectopic testicles* may be found in the thigh, at the base of the penis, or the perineum. Sometimes they wander up into the fat of the abdominal wall.

If the migration of the testis is on its normal course, but is arrested, then the testicle is held up somewhere between the abdominal situation appropriate to an elephant or a whale, and the proper position in the bottom of the scrotum (Fig. 23.5).

Hence undescended testicles are classified as: (a) ectopic; and (b) incompletely descended ((i) abdominal and (ii) inguinal).

The *inguinal testicles* are further subdivided according to their range of

Chapter 23/*The Testicle and Seminal Tract*

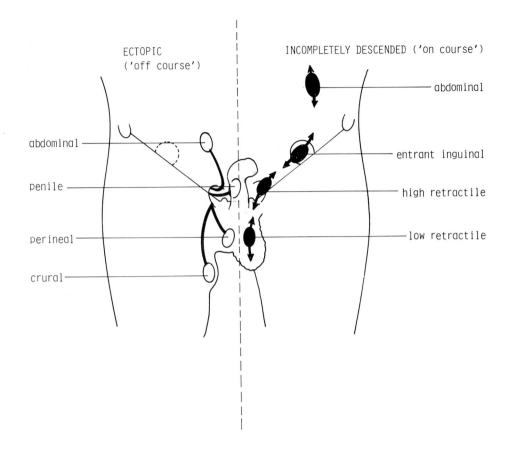

ECTOPIC ('off course')

INCOMPLETELY DESCENDED ('on course')

abdominal

penile

perineal

crural

abdominal

entrant inguinal

high retractile

low retractile

Fig. 23.5. The maldescended testis may either be off course or on course, i.e., ectopic (left) or incompletely descended (right). All types other than the 'low retractile' need orchidopexy.

movement. All normal testicles move up and down according to the contractions of the cremaster muscle which lifts them up out of harms way when threatened by cold or injury (or the cold bony fingers of the doctor). If the normal range of movement includes the bottom of the scrotum, then one can be confident that they will settle there once puberty has come. Such testicles are called 'low retractile' and they are quite normal.

Others can be brought out of the inguinal canal towards the top of the scrotum, but can never be coaxed into the bottom of the scrotal sac. These are 'high retractile', and when puberty comes they usually seem to be a little smaller and lie a little higher than is normal.

Complications of testicular maldescent

1. TORSION OF THE TESTICLE

The undescended testis arrested in its normal course of development nearly always carries with it a voluminous tunica vaginalis within which it can twist round (see page 278).

Chapter 23/*The Testicle and Seminal Tract*

275

2. INFERTILITY

Perhaps because of its high position, perhaps because it is warmer than it would ideally like to be, the undescended testis tends to produce a poor supply of sperms. At the age of three, when the normal testis in the scrotum is beginning to wake up and its tubules are enlarging and the spermatogonia are beginning to divide and multiply, none of these changes can be found in the undescended testis. Instead the tubules remain thin, the basement membrane becomes thicker, and Leydig cells, when they reappear, do so in excessive numbers. Opinions differ as to the age at which definite irreversible changes can be recognized in the undescended testis. Electron microscopy suggests that damage has been done by the age of three, light microscopy shows changes by the age of six.

3. MALIGNANCY

One in ten malignant tumours of the testicle occur in association with maldescent on the same or the other side. Most of these have been found in testicles brought down after puberty or not brought down at all. Although orchidopexy does not entirely protect the testicle from the risk of malignancy, it seems to lessen it.

With this risk, it is really essential that the testis be put in a position where it can be felt if it goes wrong. For this reason testicles in the abdomen, or lying in the inguinal canal where they cannot be felt, must be exposed and either brought down or removed.

Management of the undescended testicle

A. ECTOPIC TESTICLES

These should be fixed in the right place as soon as possible. Ideally the operation should be done by the age of three, and preferably by six.

B. INCOMPLETELY DESCENDED

All but the low retractile (ultimately normal) testicles need to be operated on. Perhaps they should all be brought down before the age of three, but in practice this is not without risk. The vas deferens and the testicular artery are very delicate at this age, and it may perhaps be better to wait until the child is approaching his sixth birthday.

HORMONES FOR UNDESCENDED TESTICLES

By giving pituitary gonadotrophin, puberty can be brought on prematurely, and so the distinction between low and high retractile testicles can be made with certainty. But this distinction can usually be made anyway by gentle palpation in warm surroundings, and gonadotrophins cannot force down gonads that will not eventually descend of their own accord. Moreover, this speeding up of the onset of puberty may be achieved at the price of premature fusion of epiphyses and stunting of growth.

Orchidopexy (see page 360).

The operation to bring down the testicle aims to detach its blood vessels from the back of the peritoneum, to which they are bound by a series of fibrous bands. Dividing these 'adhesions' allows the spermatic vessels more room, and the testicle can often be brought easily into the scrotum without tension. The operation is usually easy and successful when the testicles are ectopic, or high retractile, but the higher up in the inguinal canal towards the internal ring, the more difficult it becomes. It may be necessary to bring the gonad down in two stages, first as far as the external ring, and a year or two later, at a second operation, one hopes to find that the testicular vessels have elongated enough to allow the testicle to be placed in the scrotum. If the testicle cannot be brought down, it should probably be removed, but when both testicles are in this high situation, the parents will usually prefer to accept the slight risk of malignancy rather than the certainty of having their boy rendered eunuchoid.

When a testis cannot be found at attempted orchidopexy, laparotomy is performed at a convenient later date, and if the testicle can be found, it is removed. Recent developments in venography suggest that the patient may be excused this operation if he can be shown to lack a testicular vein on the offending side.

Torsion of the testis

One may have a voluminous tunica vaginalis in a fully descended testicle, and this arrangement may allow the testis and epididymis to rotate on a kind of mesentery or stalk, with the result that first the venous drainage, and later on the arterial supply, are obstructed (Fig. 23.6). Typically these patients have recurrent 'warning' attacks of severe pain coming on and suddenly being relieved. Torsion may occur at any age from infancy to old age. It is most common around puberty. It is worth keeping in mind that epididymitis is exceedingly rare in children (though it can occur), and that mumps orchitis is never seen before puberty. So when a boy comes up with a swollen and 'inflamed' testicle, torsion should be the first diagnosis, and a diagnosis that requires urgent surgical treatment. If seen for the first time, try to untwist the testicle: try to rotate it first one way, then the other. If you are successful you will feel a distinct 'click' and the patient will experience sudden relief.

The clinical signs of torsion of the testicle are indistinguishable from infarction from other causes, from acute epididymoorchitis (unless only the

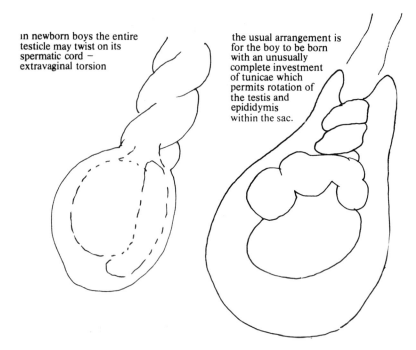

in newborn boys the entire testicle may twist on its spermatic cord — extravaginal torsion

the usual arrangement is for the boy to be born with an unusually complete investment of tunicae which permits rotation of the testis and epididymis within the sac.

Fig. 23.6. Torsion of the testis.

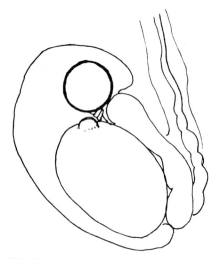

Fig. 23.7. Torsion of the appendix testis.

epididymis is enlarged and tender) and from rare examples of the 'inflammatory' type of tumour.

TORSION OF THE APPENDIX TESTIS (Fig. 23.7)

The signs of torsion of the testicle can be mimicked by torsion of the hydatid of Morgagni—the little pedunculated remnant of the Müllerian duct that sits on the top of the epididymis. Usually one sees a distinct bluish, pea-sized, tender swelling through the skin of the scrotum, but from time to time there is such a tremendous inflammatory reaction to the infarcted hydatid that it is necessary to explore it in case it is torsion of the entire testicle.

Varicocele

The veins issuing from the testis and epididymis are exceedingly tortuous and complicated, and it is widely believed that they serve as a heat exchanger mechanism that keeps the testicle cool, and that this has some useful part to play in spermatogenesis (Fig. 23.8). Claims are made (see page 292) that ligature of the varicocele improves spermatogenesis and the chance of successfully siring a family. These problems are discussed later: on its own account, a varicocele may, very uncommonly, be so uncomfortable as to require supporting with a jock-strap, and rarely, justifies ligation. It is a normal but transient phenomenon in many healthy adolescents.

Chapter 23/*The Testicle and Seminal Tract*

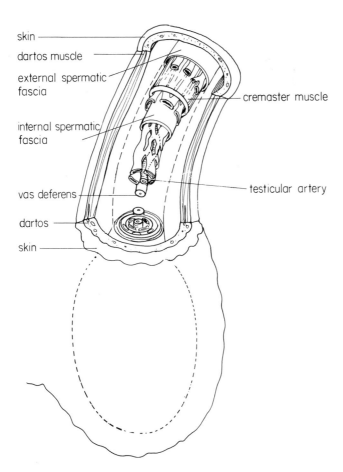

skin
dartos muscle
external spermatic fascia
cremaster muscle
internal spermatic fascia
vas deferens
testicular artery
dartos
skin

Fig. 23.8. Veins of the pampiniform plexus all contribute to the formation of a varicocele: they may enlarge between all the anatomical layers of the spermatic cord.

Hydrocele

The testicle has a series of lymphatic capillaries between its tubules which drain into the lymphatics of the spermatic cord. If these lymphatics are obstructed anywhere along their course, lymph may accumulate in the space between the layers of the tunica vaginalis (Fig. 23.9).

When a cause can be found for the hydrocele, it is called *secondary*. These include hydroceles secondary to injury to the testicle, to tumour, to heart failure, to obstruction of the retroperitoneal lymphatics by fibrosis or cancer, or as a result of surgical removal of para-aortic lymph nodes. When there is no cause, it is called *primary*. Primary hydrocele is very common. It is seen in many middle-aged and younger men for no good reason. Congenital hydroceles, seen in infants (Fig. 23.10), communicate along the patient processus vaginalis with the peritoneum, and, when there is a hernia, should be treated by ligature and division of the processus, for fear of strangulation at this age. The remainder can safely be watched, in the knowledge that most of them go away before the age of 18 months. After this age they should probably be operated on.

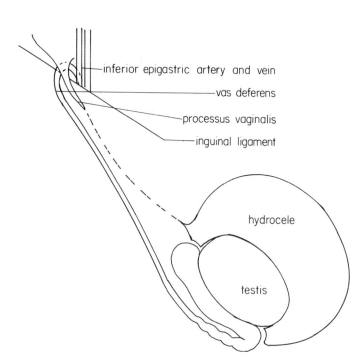

inferior epigastric artery and vein

vas deferens

processus vaginalis

inguinal ligament

hydrocele

testis

Fig. 23.9. Structure and anatomical relations of a hydrocele.

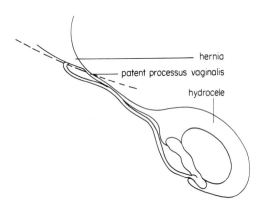

hernia

patent processus vaginalis

hydrocele

Fig. 23.10. Hydrocele in an infant—the processus vaginalis is patent so that it alters in size. A hernia is often associated.

Hydroceles may be emptied regularly with an intracath (Fig. 23.11) (trocar and cannula). The fluid inside them is amber coloured and rich in protein. It fills up again, and needs to be emptied again when it inconveniences the patient. Larger hydroceles, and hydroceles that are painful to aspirate, or in which aspiration is followed by bleeding or infection, should be operated on.

Operations for hydrocele (see page 364) consist of draining and bunching up the surplus sac with a series of sutures, or removing the sac. Either operation often leaves the patient with a large haematoma in the scrotum that will take several weeks to go down, and the patient must be warned that the result does

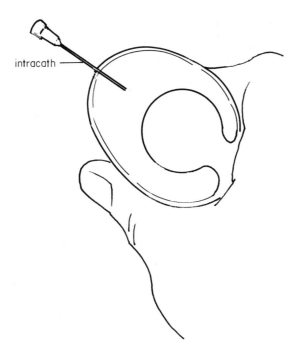

Fig. 23.11. Tapping a hydrocele using an 'intracath'.

not take place at once. In former days surgeons used to inject various potions into the hydrocele to make the walls adhere.

One particular form of hydrocele needs to be noticed. It occurs when adult *Wuchereria bancrofti* worms take up residence in the pampiniform plexus, and give rise to fibrosis and secondary inflammation. This is very common in some tropical countries and may give rise to elephantiasis of the scrotum, and tremendous hydroceles. The fluid inside the hydrocele is rich in fatty globules. Aspiration of such a hydrocele is quickly followed by recurrence.

Cysts of the epididymis and spermatocele (Fig. 23.12)

Most males over the age of 40 can be felt to have tiny cysts in the sulcus between epididymis and testis. These are thought to be diverticula of the collecting tubules of the vasa efferentia testis. In many men they enlarge, forming multiple translucent cysts, like a bunch of grapes, that lie behind the testis, and make the epididymis thin and stretched out. They contain clear watery fluid, sometimes cloudy with dead sperms inside. Occasionally they contain fluid that is thick with sperms and these cysts are sometimes called spermatoceles.

Clinically they present as multiple translucent fluctuant cysts behind the body of the testis. Nothing should be done about them unless they are so big that they give the patient difficulty in putting his trousers on. If any operation is done, it should be the removal of the cysts. Since this may interrupt the vasa efferentia from which they originate, it must not be done unless the patient is

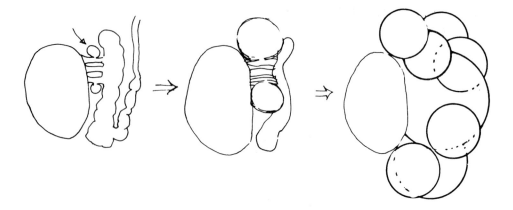

Fig. 23.12. Cysts of the epididymus.

sure he wants no more children. They should not be aspirated: the procedure is painful, it is incomplete because there are so many of the cysts, and they always come back very quickly.

TRAUMA TO THE TESTICLE

The testis is easily injured at sport or at work and the lesion is usually a split in the visceral layer of the tunica vaginalis, through which blood and testicular tubules spill like cotton wool. A large painful hydrocele containing blood (*haematocele*) forms. If left alone it will gradually subside, but the danger is that before it subsides it squeezes the testicle flat within the firm tunica vaginalis, resulting in permanent atrophy and loss of spermatogenic function (Fig. 23.13). To save the testis from this fate it should be explored as soon as possible, the blood-clot removed, and the tear in the visceral layer of the tunica vaginalis sewn up. It is worth remembering at the back of one's mind that some of these

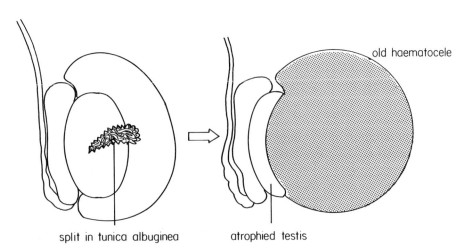

Fig. 23.13. Closed injury splits the tunica albuginea (left) giving rise to (right) a haematocele which, if untreated, will result in atrophy of the testis by pressure of the blood inside the tunica.

split in tunica albuginea   atrophied testis

injuries and haematoceles turn out to be tumours of the testicle—an additional reason for not treating them 'conservatively'.

INFLAMMATORY DISEASES OF THE TESTICLE

Acute orchitis

Most acute infections in the testis are of virus origin—e.g. mumps (never before puberty), Coxsackie and more rarely other viruses. Fortunately mumps orchitis is usually unilateral, but it may occur on both sides, and it may give rise to bilateral atrophy of the testis.

When a man is seen with an acutely swollen testicle and is suspected of having mumps, the diagnosis may be in doubt, since it is clinically so similar to torsion. It is best to explore the testicle. However it is a common complication in adult mumps occurring in 16–20% of cases. Many surgeons have advised incision of the swollen tunicae in order to decompress the testicle in mumps: others have given steroids with the same object, but it does not always prevent atrophy.

Acute epididymitis

In former times acute bacterial infection of the epididymis occurred so often after prostatectomy as a sequel to sepsis in the urethra, that it was routine practice to divide the vas deferens on each side before enucleating the prostate. Today its incidence is so low that this precautionary operation has been given up. It usually occurs out of the blue. In most males in whom it is seen, no identifiable organism can be found in the urine, and only 4% (at most) can be attributed to gonorrhoea. Only a quarter have an identifiable organism. However in this small group is a very important if tiny number whose acute epididymitis is the first clinical sign of genitourinary tuberculosis. Hence it is routine practice in every case with an 'acute' epididymoorchitis to rule out tuberculosis with three early morning cultures on Loewenstein–Jensen media.

In some of these patients there is a convincing history of a heavy physical strain a day or two before the onset of the epididymitis and it seems possible that urine has been injected backwards along the vas, has been extravasated into the epididymis, and has set up an acute inflammation there.

Chronic epididymoorchitis (Fig. 23.14)

Tuberculosis characteristically lodges in the head of the epididymis. It is thought to gain access there by haematogenous spread, rather than along the lumen of the vas from active tuberculosis in the bladder or prostate (although that may, of course, occur too).

When it is seen in the epididymis, the vas is usually beaded and shortened, and the epididymis is nodular and hard, thanks to a series of caseating abscesses

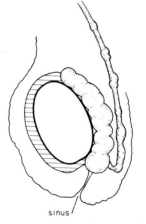

sinus

Fig. 23.14. Genital tuberculosis.

that form along it. The testis is often invaded late in the course of the disease. It is very difficult to be certain of the diagnosis in the early stages of this disease unless acid fast tuberculous bacilli can be recovered from the urine, or unless there are obvious radiological features of the disease in the kidneys and ureters.

Gumma was reported in the testicle in the last century with great frequency and the textbooks of those days were full of directions by which one could distinguish on clinical grounds between gumma and cancer. The writer has never seen gumma of the testis and would get the diagnosis wrong if he were to encounter the condition. When a doctor sees a firm lump in the testis it ought to be regarded as cancer until proved otherwise, with the possible exception of patients of African genetic origin in whom testicular tumours are virtually unknown.

Extravasation of sperm may give rise to a very chronic indurated *sperm granuloma* in the epididymis, rarely in the testis. It is seen today, from time to time, in men who have undergone vasectomy.

Granulomatous orchitis gives rise to a hard lump in the testis in a man who has had repeated attacks of urinary infection. Its cause is not clear: in this it resembles some of the more sinister granulomas seen in the kidney. It gives rise to a painful persistent swelling, fever, and generalized illness. The writer has tried to save the testis in such a patient, with intensive antibiotics and local surgery without success. If sure of the diagnosis, one may try giving the patient steroids.

TUMOURS OF THE TESTICLE

Aetiology

The cause of testicular tumour is not known. Some 500 new cases occur every year in Britain, or about 20 cases per million of the male population. It is very rare in Africans. There are two main groups—seminomas and the rest. Seminomas tend to appear in older men (above the age of 30) while the other, more malignant tumours, occur in post-pubertal boys and young men.

Pathology (Fig. 23.15)

Tumours may arise from any of the cellular elements in the testicle. Most of the testicular growths arise from the germinal cells, Leydig cells or Sertoli cells, and of these the germinal cell tumours are far the most important. When the spermatogonia become malignant they form sheets of uniform cells—*seminoma*. A small group of these resemble spermatocytes, and are worth noticing, because they carry a particularly good prognosis. The other germinal cell tumours are loosely called *teratomas* or 'non-seminomas'. These cover a broad spectrum. At one extreme they are very well-differentiated, looking like benign teratomas elsewhere, with mature tissues such as skin, bone, cartilage and so on, and well formed little organs—'organoid development'—here and

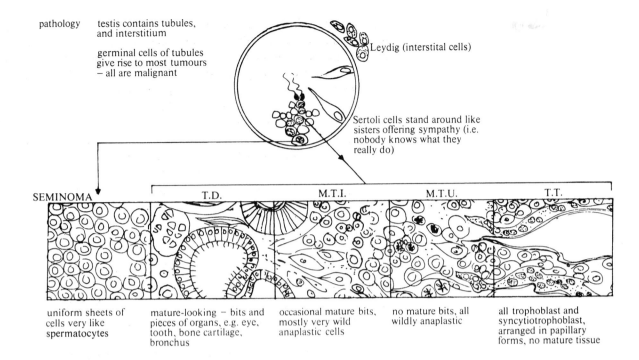

pathology | testis contains tubules, and interstitium

germinal cells of tubules give rise to most tumours – all are malignant

Leydig (interstital cells)

Sertoli cells stand around like sisters offering sympathy (i.e. nobody knows what they really do)

SEMINOMA   T.D.   M.T.I.   M.T.U.   T.T.

uniform sheets of cells very like spermatocytes

mature-looking – bits and pieces of organs, e.g. eye, tooth, bone cartilage, bronchus

occasional mature bits, mostly very wild anaplastic cells

no mature bits, all wildly anaplastic

all trophoblast and syncytiotrophoblast, arranged in papillary forms, no mature tissue

Fig. 23.15. Tumours of the testis.

there. One finds little joints and occasionally a miniature eye or a finger. This kind of non-seminoma is seen in children when it is reliably benign. In adults the danger is that somewhere in amongst all the good-looking bits of *Teratoma Differentiated* lurk more sinister malignant undifferentiated tissue.

At the other extreme the group of non-seminomas include the most wildly anaplastic and invasive cancers seen in pathology where sheets of undifferentiated cells rampage all over the slide. In this wild tissue occur bits of tissue with trophoblast and cytotrophoblast giving the label *chorioncarcinoma* to the growth. This also is rare and account for another 1 or 2% of the whole group.

In between lie the controversial tumours. In one system of classification an attempt is made to quantify the amount of each kind of tissue that can be recognized in any one specimen. In another system a label is assigned according to the most well-differentiated tissue that is present. At present, in Britain, we recognize two groups—a 'good teratoma' (*Malignant Teratoma Intermediate*) which behaves reasonably well after treatment; and a 'bad teratoma' (*Malignant Teratoma Undifferentiated*) which behaves dreadfully. The 'good' MTI is comparable to the American term *teratocarcinoma*, and the 'bad' MTI with *embryonal carcinoma*.

Non-germinal cell tumours of the testicle

Benign and malignant tumours may arise from the other cells present in the testis. Sertoli cells may give rise to gynaeocomastia. Leydig cells, secreting testosterone, may result in precocious virilization. Both are very rare. Rare tumours may also be found that originate in the epididymis, and the coverings of the cord. None of them can safely be regarded as benign until they have been removed.

Spread of testicular tumours

Testicular cancer spreads into the epididymis and tunicae, but seldom outside the tunica into the scrotum unless it has been stupidly meddled with by incision or biopsy, or by performing the orchidectomy via a scrotal incision. Then it transgresses the barrier of the parietal tunica vaginalis, gets into the tissues of the scrotum, and gains entry to the lymph nodes that drain the scrotum in the groin.

Otherwise testicular tumours spread upwards along the course of the testicular lymphatics, which return along the course of the testicular artery, to its origin from the aorta near the renal arteries (Fig. 23.16).

If the epididymis has been invaded then some tumour cells may pass along the lymphatics of the vas deferens to the internal iliac group of nodes.

Blood borne spread occurs early in the most malignant choriocarcinomas and some of the worst kind of anaplastic embryonal cell cancers. Metastases crop up anywhere, but particularly favour the lungs, where enormous cannon-ball metastases are common.

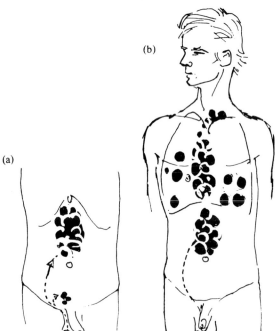

(b)

(a)

Fig. 23.16. Spread of testicular tumours: (a) from the testis via the lymphatics in the para-aortic nodes; (b) from the para-aortic nodes to the mediastinal nodes, thence to the thoracic duct and into the bloodstream.

note inguinal lymph nodes not involved unless previous surgery done in groin, e.g. hernia or orchidectomy

Chapter 23/*The Testicle and Seminal Tract*

Tumour markers

The non-seminomas produce two 'tumour markers'. These are enzymes manufactured by specific groups of cells in these varieties of teratoma. Cells derived, it is thought, from the most primitive gonadal cells that make the embryonic journey from the yolk sac to the gonadal ridge, generate a material called α-*fetoprotein* (AFP). Cells having other features of trophoblast generate a material called β-*chorionic gonadotrophin*. Both of these enzymes can be detected by radio-immunoassay techniques in minute quantities. If they are detected in the plasma it means that the patient has cells making these materials somewhere in the body, usually in metastases. By their means one can chart the rise and fall of the amount of tumour in the body as it responds to radiotherapy, to surgery or to chemotherapy. One is given warning that tumour has returned long before it can be picked up by other methods of investigation.

The cells that manufacture AFP and HCG can be detected in histological sections using modern immunoperoxidase techniques. It is this new technology, perhaps more than any other, which has caused a revision of the pathological classification of these cancers.

Clinical staging of testis tumours

Unfortunately the internationally agreed TNM system has virtually no relevance in the practical management of testis tumours but most centres dealing with large numbers of these rather rare growths make use of the following staging (Fig. 23.17):

Stage 1 Where by using all the means at one's disposal one can find no evidence that the growth has spread beyond the testicle i.e. markers are negative,

Fig. 23.17. Staging of testicular tumours.

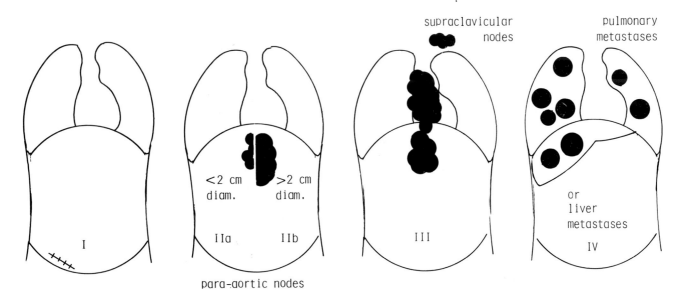

supraclavicular nodes

pulmonary metastases

<2 cm diam.   >2 cm diam.

IIa   IIb

III

or liver metastases

IV

I

para-aortic nodes

X-rays of chest and lymphogram are normal, and when performed, the CAT scan is normal too.

Stage 2 (a) There are lymph node metastases in the para-aortic nodes but they are less than 2 cm in diameter;

(b) there are nodes larger than 2 cm in diameter as measured with CAT scan or lymphography.

Stage 3 There are nodes in the mediastinum of supraclavicular groups, but none in the lung fields or any other haematogenous sites.

Stage 4 Haematogenous metastases in lungs, liver, bone, etc.

Obviously the distinction between these different stages has to be made on the basis of lymphography and CAT scanning, and the more sensitive these methods, the more metastases will be detected.

Clinical features of testicular tumours

LUMP

About 80% of patients with a testicular tumour notice a swelling in the testis: sometimes it is painful, usually not. In many instances the patient is quite certain there is a swelling there, when it is well-nigh impossible for the doctor to feel it. The rule in such cases is to trust the patient—he is usually right (Fig. 23.18).

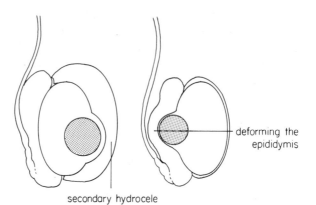

deforming the epididymis

secondary hydrocele

Fig. 23.18. Small lumps in the testis may be misleading if they are smothered by a secondary hydrocele (left) or so near the epididymis that they resemble epididymitis (right).

PAIN AND INFLAMMATION

Pain is not usual in a testicular tumour, but it can occur, and can be associated with overt signs of redness oedema and swelling, that exactly imitate acute epididymitis or torsion of the testicle. It is often very difficult indeed to be certain where the swelling originates, in testis or in epididymis, and the tenderness and 'inflammatory' reaction may be most confusing. Some 10% of most large series record this wrong diagnosis, and account alas for many weeks of pointless treatment with antibiotics.

Chapter 23/*The Testicle and Seminal Tract*

TRAUMA

Some 10–15% of patients will give a story of having injured the testicle in the recent past, and it is only natural that they attribute their swelling to the injury. In many instances it does seem that an injury accelerates the rate of growth of the tumour. For this reason one must be exceedingly suspicious of any lump in the testicle following trauma: an additional reason, if any were needed, to make it a rule to explore every haematocele (see page 282).

METASTASES

Distant metastases in liver or lungs are a rather common method of presentation of the rapidly growing tumours.

HORMONAL EFFECTS

Non-seminomas that secrete human chorionic gonadotrophin may make the patient's breasts enlarge and become painful. Adolescent mastitis is of course a common symptom in otherwise perfectly healthy young men. Nevertheless when such a youngster is seen it should always be the rule for his testicles to be examined.

MALDESCENT

An important group are the tumours associated with testicular maldescent (see page 275). Every testis that is found to be so high in the abdomen or inguinal canal that it cannot be brought down must always be looked at very carefully for histological evidence of tumour. It is not at all unusual to find a small tumour in what otherwise seems a normal if small testis.

CARCINOMA-*IN SITU* IN THE TESTIS

Careful examination of testicular biopsies performed for men with infertility has revealed a surprisingly high incidence of carcinoma *in situ*—seminoma cells inside the tubules without any evidence of breakthrough of the basement membrane. At present these pose a difficult clinical decision, because it is not yet certain how many of these *in situ* patients will proceed to develop an invasive growth.

Management of the patient with a testicular tumour

The first step is to remove the testicle. This is performed through an inguinal incision, first clamping the spermatic cord at the internal ring to make sure the tumour cells in the spermatic veins do not escape into the circulation. The testicle is then delivered, inspected, and removed.

After this a set of investigations to stage the tumour are performed.

Nowadays these will include lymphography, CAT scanning of abdomen and lungs (where available) and serial measurements of AFP and HCG.

Seminomas are treated with radiotherapy to the para-aortic nodes in all stages, with chemotherapy for men with Stage 4 (multiple metastases). Seminomas are very radiosensitive, and if diagnosed before they have escaped from the testicle, are followed by 100% cure.

Non-seminomas form a wide spectrum. At one extreme it seems that no amount of chemotherapy nor the most diligent radiation can cure choriocarcinoma of the testis in the male. At the other extreme, in the equally rare well differentiated teratoma (T.D.), that looks like a dermoid cyst, and has not even the most minute area of undifferentiated tissue, it is possible that the condition is entirely benign—and certainly behaves benignly when seen in little boys.

For the in-between teratomas, there is as much difference of opinion as to the best way of treating them as there is difference of opinion as to how to classify them histologically. Excellent results are reported with *radiotherapy* directed to the para-aortic nodes when the metastases are small (Stage 2a), but not when they are large. Excellent results are reported from *radical removal of the retroperitoneal lymph nodes* when the lymph nodes are small, and only invaded below the diaphragm. One advantage of operating to remove the nodes is that one obtains accurate evidence as to the stage of the tumour, can give a more accurate prognosis, and decide with better judgement whether or not to give chemotherapy. The disadvantage of this operation is that it is often followed by failure of ejaculation owing to the removal of the lowest lumbar sympathetic nodes or their efferent nerves.

When metastases are large or widely disseminated, prolonged and dramatic cures have been achieved with *chemotherapy*, using Einhorn's regime involving cis-Platinum, Vinblastine and Bleomycin. Today, thanks to the very rapid improvement that is seen in detection of metastases, the technique of radiotherapy, and the efficacy of chemotherapy, the outlook for men with testicular tumours has improved beyond all belief. This can only be achieved, however, if patients with this unusual condition are treated in centres that specialize in it, and have gained skill and knowhow in managing each type of therapy.

MALE INFERTILITY

When couples seek advice because they have been unable to have a child, it is wise to begin by pointing out that in many instances something is wrong in both partners, and that at least half of the cases of infertility are caused by a disorder in the husband. It is to the urologist however that the man is usually referred.

General examination

Gross evidence of endocrine deficiency is usually obvious. When a young man comes up with normal physique and body hair, who shaves daily or grows a normal beard, there is no deficiency of testosterone and no point in giving him any.

Genetic disturbances may be more easy to miss, and the XXY *Klinefelter syndrome* may occur in an apparently normal, hairy, mesomorphic male, but his small testes and his positive buccal smear will give the diagnosis away. Cells in the buccal smear will show Barr's body—the pronounced knob of chromosome that indicates the additional X chromosome.

The examination of the testicles includes an estimation of their size and firmness. One must look carefully for previous evidence of *surgery* in the form of a scar in the groin from previous orchidopexy or hernia repair (at which the vas may have been damaged).

From time to time one will be unable to feel the *vas deferens* on either side, a condition that may go along with failure of development of the seminal vesicles, and a small semen volume. This physical examination will not be able to detect certain other congenital errors of development, equally important, such as failure of union of the vas with the epididymis, or a gap in the middle of the epididymis (Fig. 23.19).

Semen analysis

Semen for analysis should be produced by masturbation into a sterile plastic container, which has been previously tested to make sure that it does not inhibit sperm motility. The semen should be kept at about 20°C, not in the refrigerator, and not in the trousers pocket at body temperature.

Normal semen clots within a few minutes of ejaculation and then liquifies after another 20 minutes or so. It is examined after it has liquified.

Its *volume* is estimated in a calibrated cylinder. It varies from 1 to 8 ml. The greater part of the semen volume is contributed by the seminal vesicles, and when they are inflamed, absent, or diseased, one has a semen of very low volume. The absence of seminal vesicular function can be checked by measuring the fructose concentration in the semen.

Sperm density—a measurement is made of the numbers of sperm per ml using a haemocytometer and saline as one would for making a white blood count. The median figure of about 50×10^6 spermatozoa/ml must always be considered the peak of a very wide range: successful parents have been recorded with sperm densities less than 1×10^6.

The *motility* of the sperm is probably very important in predicting its value for the purpose of fertilizing an ovum: but this is also the quality of the semen that is the most difficult to measure with accuracy and with repeatable results. If sperm samples have been allowed to warm up to body temperature for more than one hour, or if they have been inadvertently placed in the refrigerator, one may obtain a grossly misleading motility score.

When sperms are present in low numbers, with a poor motility, one often finds that many of them, when stained and examined carefully, look quite

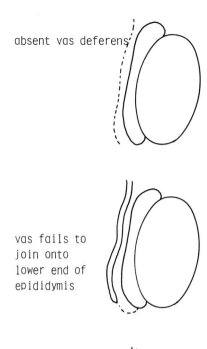

absent vas deferens

vas fails to join onto lower end of epididymis

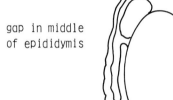

gap in middle of epididymis

Fig. 23.19. There are many different types of failure of development of the vas and epididymis: absence of the vas, failure of its uion with the epididymis, and a hiatus in the body of the epididymis are some of the more common varieties.

abnormal, with swollen heads or multiple tails. These evaluations of sperm *morphology* are notoriously subjective, and in any event one expects some 20–30% of sperms in the specimen from a fertile male to show these abnormal features.

Management

As a result of the semen analysis patients fall into three categories.

1. WITH NORMAL SPERM

In some of these men one can detect antibodies in the seminal plasma or the blood plasma that make the sperms stick together and prevent them swimming properly. There is some suggestion that the effect of these autoantibodies can be eliminated by steroids, or by injecting semen that has been washed and resuspended into the wife's cervix.

In most couples the next step is to examine the cervical mucus on the morning after coitus. One may find the sperms lying dead, lysed, or motionless in the cervical mucus. Much research is now being carried out in order to discover how to overcome this *cervical hostility*: at present there is no simple answer.

2. LOW SPERM DENSITY, MOTILITY AND/OR VOLUME—OLIGOZOOSPERMIA

At the time of revising this edition the author has sadly to record that earlier optimism in the possible benefits of various hormone and chemical treatments has been completely frustrated by the bleak results of controlled clinical studies. No single drug, hormone or other form of medication when tested by these strict methods has been shown to do any good at all for the man with infertility associated with a low sperm density. Steroids, testosterone, stilboestrol-rebound, chlomiphene, bromocryptine, arginine and innumerable other medications have all been given in the hope of doing good, and pregnancies are obtained every now and again which encourage the doctor and please the patient. Just as many pregnancies are obtained however by those given the dummy treatment.

One must include in this general condemnation the contemporary enthusiasm for *varicocelectomy*. Innumerable claims are made for the benefit of dividing the spermatic veins in men with varicocele. It is genuinely and widely believed to improve the semen density and motiblity, and even alter the sperm morphology from a 'stress effect' towards something that is more 'normal'. Alas few controls have even been used—and when they have, the results have been without any statistical significance at all.

3. NO SPERMS AT ALL

There are two possible causes: (a) the factory is no good; or (b) the delivery system is blocked.

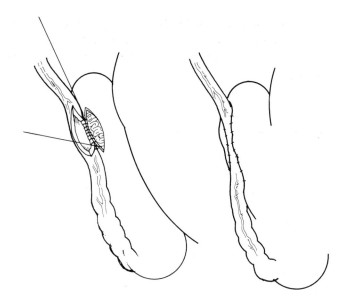

Fig. 23.20 Epididymovasostomy.

(a) may be determined by obtaining a tiny piece of the testis by *biopsy*, but this, albeit trivial operation, can for all practical purposes, be avoided when the plasma levels of follicle stimulating hormone and or luteinizing hormone (FSH and LH) are elevated. When the testicular germinal epithelium is hopelessly damaged, then these pituitary hormones are secreted in excess. If there is azoospermia and the FSH and LH levels are normal, one must consider the second possibility. To discover a blockage it may be necessary to explore the testicle. A testicular biopsy is usually performed before this, to double check that, despite normal FSH and LH levels, there really is spermatogenesis going on inside the testis.

At operation one may find sperms queuing up in the upper end of the epididymis (and this can easily be confirmed by aspirating some of them and examining the fluid on a microscope slide). It may be possible to see with the naked eye that there is a gap in the epididymis, or a gap between epididymis and vas. Or by injecting contrast towards the urethra up the vas, one may demonstrate a block in the groin or in the region of the ejaculatory ducts.

When the block can be overcome by anastomosing the side of the vas to the sperm-congested epididymis (*epididymovasostomy*) (Fig. 23.20) one may get a good result. Not at first—the sperms that appear in the ejaculate may be immotile and scanty for many months—but they may gain in numbers and motility and the occasional fortunate patient is able to sire a child. It must be admitted however that the results are as unpredictable as they are, in general, disappointing.

Testicular biopsy (Fig. 23.21)

Inside each tubule one finds Sertoli cells and germinal cells. The germinal cells

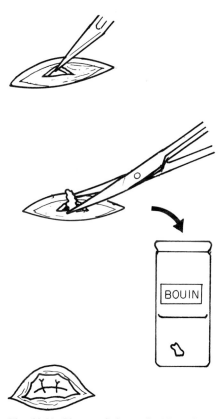

Fig. 23.21. Biopsy of the testis. Note that Bouin's fixative is used, not formalin.

are supposed to divide into more germinal cells and spermatocytes, the spermatocytes into spermatids and eventually to form mature sperms. This process does not go on uniformly throughout the testicle, but waves of spermatogenesis seem to pass up and down the tubules, so that one may, in a biopsy, catch one tubule that is nearly full of mature spermatids, another that is full of less mature spermatocytes and so on. Johnsen assigns an arbitrary number 1–10 to these phases of spermatogenesis, so that, for example, number 2 contains no spermatogenic cells, and number 7 will show many spermatids but no mature sperms. By counting all the tubules in the biopsy and getting an average of the score one has a more useful idea of the overall way the tubules are performing. Thus in a normal fertile male one expects to see more than 60% of the tubules in step 10 (mean score 9). In Klinefelter's syndrome (where there are hardly any germinal cells) the 'Johnsen mean score' will be as low as 1.2.

Such scoring requires however careful fixation of the testicular tissue or it cannot be done. For this purpose Bouin's fixative must be used—never ordinary formalin.

What to tell the patient

It always saves trouble if you can tell the patient the truth, but in the field of infertility, you should be exceedingly cautious before you proclaim that a given man is infertile. Never make this diagnosis only on the basis of a few semen analyses that purport to show 'oligozoospermia'—for there is a very considerable rise and fall in the sperm output in normal testes, and your sample may not be a representative one.

At the same time, give the couple the facts when you think you know that their chances are very poor, so that they can consider alternatives such as adoption or artificial insemination with donor semen. Temper the wind to the shorn lamb, dilute your frankness with gentleness and sympathy, and whenever you can, offer hope.

VASECTOMY FOR MALE STERILIZATION

Counselling

It is important that both husband and wife understand perfectly clearly that vasectomy may be irreversible, that there is a small chance of spontaneous recanalization (albeit a very small one) and that as in any other operation, there is a slight risk of postoperative complications which include haematoma and local wound infection. It is also most important that they fully understand that after vasectomy living sperms remain in the storage systems downstream of the testicle, i.e. in the ampulla of the vas and the seminal vesicle, and that until all these sperms have been cleared away, the patient is still capable of fathering a child.

Vasectomy should not affect a man's desire or his capability of making love, but occasionally men are seen who claim that their libido has vanished after the operation. This is certainly psychosexual, and if possible the counselling doctor should try to detect an unstable personality before agreeing to advise vasectomy. In the same way it is important to try to detect the man who is being bullied into the operation by a domineering wife, or the couple who are hoping that the operation will restore libido once it has been lost.

Physical examination of the patient asking for a vasectomy should note whether or not he has had previous hernia surgery which may have left the scrotum full of adhesions and make operation under local anaesthetic difficult to do.

Anaesthesia

Most vasectomies are performed under local anaesthetic, but where the surgeon anticipates difficulty from old adhesions, or where the patient is very anxious, a general anaesthetic is safer and easier.

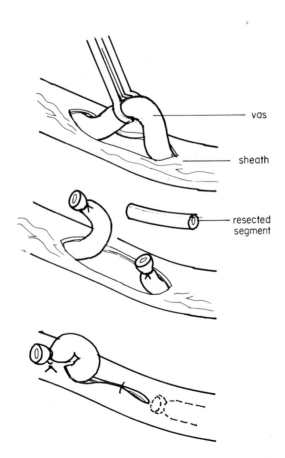

Fig. 23.22. One technique for vasectomy.

The operation

Most surgeons incise the sheath that encloses the vas, lift out the vas deferens, remove 1 cm of the tube, ligate each end with fine silk or catgut, and turn one end back on itself in the hope that this will frustrate the natural tendency of the tube to join itself together (Fig. 23.22).

There are many variations on this theme. Diathermy is sometimes used to seal off the cut ends of the vas.

Before the little incision or incisions in the scrotum are closed, great care is taken to make sure that all small bleeding vessels, (usually tiny veins) are controlled by ligature or diathermy. Even with this meticulous precaution, and despite great experience, haematomas still form. It is a sensible precaution to make a note in the operation sheet that exact haemostasis was secured.

Follow up

Because of the risk of reactionary haemorrhage many surgeons advise their vasectomy patients to rest quietly for 15 minutes or so (to give time for any local vasospasm to wear off) and then examine the scrotum for signs of haematoma before allowing them to go home. For the same reason, to prevent haematoma a scrotal support is worn which gives a little local pressure.

Complications

Haematoma is the most common and most frequently the cause of pain and litigation. If a large swelling develops then it should be probably be evacuated, for if allowed to remain, there is a significant risk of infection.

Infection occurs at the skin incision, and has recently been shown to occur only when there are organisms in the patient's own semen. It is treated on the usual lines.

Pain is common: it seems to occur in the epididymis and proximal end of the vas. It may well be the result of extravasation of sperms into the epididymal tubules or the soft tissues of the cord. Sometimes a distinct swelling can be felt at the site of ligature of the vas which on section will show *granuloma*. It occurs probably because the acid-fast material in the head of the sperm is very similar to the envelope of the *Mycobacterium tuberculosis* and gives rise to similar giant cell foreign body reactions. Occasionally this pain is very severe, but it is usually short lived.

MAKING SURE THE SPERMS HAVE DISAPPEARED FROM THE EJACULATE

In most men all the sperms have disappeared by about six weeks or after 10–20 ejaculations, but there remain a small number who still produce a tiny number of, usually, immotile sperms. Nobody knows for certain whether these are capable or not of fathering children. One can stain them with vital stains which will indicate that they are dead, not still alive. If large numbers of motile sperms are still present after 6–8 weeks, it means that either the vasectomy was incomplete (i.e. some structure other than the vas was divided) or there was a double vas on one side and only one channel was divided.

In a small number of well documented cases living sperms have reappeared in the vas many months after they had all disappeared. It is not possible to say for certain what this chance of *spontaneous recanalization* is in numerical terms—the information is wanting. My own estimate is that it occurs in less than 1% of patients. Nevertheless it is important that the hazard is understood by husband and wife, for if an unexpected pregnancy occurs, recriminiation and litigation may occur.

REJOINING THE VAS

From time to time a husband is separated, or a family tragically destroyed in some accident. The patient may remarry and want another family. The vasa may be found, freshened and joined together. About 80% can be reunited so that sperms reappear in the ejaculate, and about 50% of these men will father children again. Nevertheless the risk of failure is so great that no man ought to undergo vasectomy unless he and his wife are fully decided that they do not want any more children.

FURTHER READING

Allen T.D. (1976) Disorders of sexual differentiation. *Urology*, **7**, suppl. 1.

Barnes M.N. *et al.* (1973) One thousand vasectomies. *British Medical Journal*, **4**, 216.

Babaian R.J. & Johnson D.E. (1980) Management of Stages I and II nonseminomatous germ cell tumors of the testis. *Cancer*, **45**, 1775.

Blandy J.P. (1977) Testicular tumours. In Selwyn Taylor (ed.), *Recent Advances in Surgery 9*, Ch. 11, p. 244. Churchill-Livingstone, London.

Caldwell W.L., Kademian M.T., Frias Z. & Davis T.E. (1980) The management of testicular seminomas 1979. *Cancer* **45**, suppl. 1768.

Fonkalsrud E.W. & Mengel W. (eds) (1981) *The Undescended Testis*. Yearbook Medical Publishers Inc., Chicago, London.

Javadpour N. (1980) The role of biologic tumor markers in testicular cancer. *Cancer*, **45**, suppl. 1775.

Mostofi F.K. (1980) Pathology of germ cell tumors of testis: a progress report. *Cancer*, **45**, 1735.

Pugh R.C.B. (ed.) (1976) *Pathology of the Testis*. Blackwell Scientific Publications, Oxford.

Scorer C.G. & Farrington G.H. (1979) Congenital anomalies of the testes. In J.H. Harrison *et al.* (eds), *Campbell's Urology*, Vol. 2, 4th edn, p. 1549. W.B. Saunders Co., Philadelphia.

Setchell B.P. (1978) *The Mammalian Testis*. Paul Elek, London.

Stage K.H., Schoenvogel R. & Lewis S. (1981) Testicular scanning: clinical experience with 72 patients. *Journal of Urology*, **125**, 334.

Yeates W.K. (1976) Male infertility and vasectomy. In J.P. Blandy (ed.), *Urology*, pp. 1243 and 1271. Blackwell Scientific Publications, Oxford.

Chapter 24
Guide to the Management of Common Urological Problems

HAEMATURIA

History

When taking the history take note of the patient's occupation (remembering occupations that have a high risk of bladder cancer), whether there has been trauma, where in the stream the bleeding has occurred—if the patient notices, for example, that the blood only comes at the end of urination this usually means it originates in the bladder neck or urethra. Has the patient other evidence of inflammation in the bladder such as chills or a fever? Has he or she had a recent sore throat to raise the suspicion of nephritis?

Signs

Is the patient generally unwell? Fever, hypertension, oedema? Can you detect any enlargement of the kidney suggesting a tumour there, or a cyst perhaps? Can you detect an enlargement of the bladder, that would suggest outflow obstruction. Is there anything to suggest metastases in the pelvis?

Investigations

If there is an excess of protein, and especially if you see casts, then you should be thinking of a glomerulonephritis. Microscopy will confirm the stix test for haemoglobin in the urine (see page 11). The centrifuged fixed urine should be specially stained for malignant cells using the Papanicolaou technique. If your patient comes from Africa or the West Indies you might ask for a mid-day specimen to be examined for Schistosoma ova. Check for sickle cell disease.

EXCRETION UROGRAM

All your patients will need a IVU. If there is a space-occupying lesion in a kidney, this will require ultrasound examination. If it is trans-sonic, then it will need to be aspirated, to show that its fluid is free from malignant cells and that its wall is smooth when the fluid is partly replaced with contrast medium. If it contains echoes in the ultrasound examination, then it must be regarded as malignant until proved otherwise. Often there is no need to subject the patient to any more investigations, and you will go ahead with removal of the kidney. But if there is doubt, the diagnosis may be confirmed by a renal angiogram. Tumour circulation will show that the lump is malignant, and if necessary, the opportunity can be taken to inject gelfoam or chopped muscle into the renal artery to block it off and make subsequent surgical removal more easy (see page 118).

The IVU may not show a space-occupying lesion, but some other possible source of bleeding such as a calculus, an undrained pocket of stagnant urine (e.g. in a hydronephrosis or caliceal cyst) or filling defects in the renal pelvis, the ureter, or the shadow of the bladder.

In all these circumstances, as well as in the patient without any abnormality being found in the IVU, *cystoscopy* will be performed to rule out the presence of a tumour in the bladder. If a filling defect or abnormality in the ureter or kidney needs to be made more clear, then the opportunity is taken to pass a bulb-ended ureteric catheter into the ureter, to obtain a *ureterogram*.

Cystoscopy may show a bladder tumour or tumours and if so, a biopsy must be taken and a careful examination made to see how deeply the tumour has penetrated into the muscle of the wall of the bladder. According to the results of these findings, subsequent treatment will be planned (see page 188).

'Essential haematuria'

Finally there remain the very small number of real problem patients who have gone right through this entire investigation without any abnormality having been brought to light. They have no stone, infection or tumour. And yet they continue to show haematuria.

It is usual to follow up these patients with serial examinations of the urine, and occasional repeated urograms, to make sure that no neoplasm has been missed. In some of these patients one can discover some other significant abnormality—sickling, analgesic abuse, or perhaps recurrent, radiolucent, uric acid stones. Usually one finds nothing.

RETENTION OF URINE

Acute retention

1. WITHOUT WARNING

This may happen to any patient in hospital after almost any surgical operation, but especially one that confines him to bed and prevents him from passing urine standing up. In such patients a catheter is passed, the urine emptied out, and one expects the patient to resume a normal habit of micturition thereafter.

2. AFTER A CRESCENDO OF SYMPTOMS OF PROSTATISM

This is the usual story, and if an elderly patient develops retention of urine apparently 'out of the blue' you should always suspect that he does in fact have a previous story of prostatic outflow obstruction. In such a patient who is in agony and arrives in hospital frightened, confused and unprepared, the writer recommends the following plan. Have the patient given a large dose of a suitable pain-relieving drug e.g. 15–20 mgm of morphine, or 100 mgm pethidine. While this is having its effect, arrange for him to be given a comfortably warm bath (helped and supervised of course). Many a frightened patient will be able to void under these circumstances and the urgency is taken out of the clinical matter. During the 20 minutes that this is going to take, you go and have a cup of tea, having requested that the things you are likely to need for catheterization should be got ready for you. When you return you will, (a) find that your patient has passed water in the bath and is comfortable, and so you have nothing more to do; or (b) he has not, but is sitting tucked up and ready in bed for you to pass a catheter, the edge having been taken off his pain by the morphine.

Following the rules (see page 315) pass a small, soft, self-retaining catheter (e.g. 12–14 Ch) and leave it in the bladder connected with a sterile tube to a sterile plastic reservoir.

Having then completed your examination, and having ordered the appropriate investigations, arrange for your patient to have a transurethral resection by a specialist urologist on his next operating list. (Warn the patient that there is a 5% chance he may need an open procedure).

Chronic retention

In these patients the really important matter is the general assessment and investigation of the whole patient. He is not in pain, and a careful evaluation of his state of dehydration, his anaemia, and his cardiovascular status, takes precedence over the drainage of urine from his bladder. Indeed, in patients who are not uraemic or who do not have very distended bladders, there is no need to pass a catheter at all.

If your patient is uraemic and dehydrated, then pass the catheter using the precautions observed before (see page 315), making sure that you use only a narrow soft catheter and that strict aseptic precautions are taken at each step. Then turn your attention to his fluid balance. You may well agree that an enormously distended bladder should be allowed to decompress slowly, but you may find yourself confronted with a patient with a huge diuresis, with which his thirst mechanism cannot keep up. He may need large volumes of saline intravenously if he cannot drink them. His cardiovascular condition will need careful review, or else you run the risk of putting him over the edge into heart failure. As you rehydrate both his extracellular space and the circulating volume, you may disclose a more serious anaemia than your admission haemoglobin estimation gave you reason to suspect, and your patient may need blood transfusion before being ready for any kind of operation.

The elevated urea and creatinine should come slowly and steadily down as you rehydrate him, and his diuresis gets rid of his nitrogenous waste. An excretion urogram is interesting, but not really necessary, and, as in the patient with the acute retention, should not postpone the transurethral resection which should be carried out as soon as the patient's urea and creatinine have reached a level below which they will not fall. At this level you may find that he continues to run a very large diuresis and does not retain sodium—marks of irreversible loss of renal tubular function.

In this brief account the writer has assumed that the cause of the chronic retention is outflow obstruction from a prostate or a urethral stricture. When the time comes to examine him carefully it may be obvious that he has some neuropathy. In such a case urodynamic studies (see page 200) will be done before any type of surgical attack on the bladder outflow.

URETERIC COLIC

History

The patient gives a history of a sudden onset of severe pain, coming on in waves, waxing and waning. In its intensity he may be nauseated or vomit. The pain is difficult to localize, but as he writhes about, trying to seek relief, he indicates the loin and passes his hand towards the inguinal region or testicle. If he has previously passed a stone he is in no doubt at all that he is passing another one, and you do well to accept his expert testimony.

But, beware the drug addict who has been taught how to simulate ureteric colic. Beware the Munchausen, with belly criss-crossed with scars. And beware moreover, of other conditions which give rise to very similar pain, and sometimes deceive even the most experienced surgeons. Colicky pain sometimes ushers in the beginning of acute appendicitis: it certainly accompanies small bowel obstruction and torsion of the ovary, or rupture of an ectopic pregnancy may give rise to very similar symptoms.

Investigations

In cases of doubt you must confirm the diagnosis. A plain radiograph may not show a stone, or it may show so many misleading phleboliths that you are confused. Give the patient an adequate dose of contrast medium intravenously and have a 20 minute full length radiograph taken. (The radiographer will be upset because the tremendous amount of gas in the belly will spoil the picture and she has been taught to put off the IVU in such 'unprepared' patients.) If there is a stone you will see something odd in the side on which there is pain: there will be no excretion, a delayed nephrogram or even an appearance as if the kidney had ruptured, with contrast escaping into the fascia around the kidney (see page 161). If the ureter and renal shadow look completely normal, then the diagnosis is other than ureteric stone.

Unfortunately the drug addict and the Munchausen quickly learn to say that they are allergic to the IVU contrast medium. An isotope renogram—if you can get one done as an emergency—will show you if there is hold-up in the flow of urine on the affected side.

A very useful diagnostic investigation is to test for the presence of *red cells* in the urine. When a patient is actually passing a stone then red cells are almost invariably present. If your patient has a lot of pain and no red cells, then reconsider your diagnosis.

Management

Having made the diagnosis of ureteric colic the first job is to *relieve the pain*. Give your patient a good large dose of morphine or pethidine. Disregard the theoretical notion that morphine will make the smooth muscle of the ureter go into spasm: it does nothing of the sort. Nor does pethidine relax it. What the patient needs is relief of agonizing pain. Do not tease him with tiny doses of hyoscine or propantheline. They have no effect on the human ureter.

Do not oblige the patient to drink a lot of water. The stone will go down the ureter with or without a diuresis, and the diuresis will only increase the amount of urine that is extravasated around the kidney upstream of the obstructing stone.

The stone must be removed if the column of urine upstream of the stone is *infected*, and there is a risk of bacteraemia—though even here there is room for a measure of common sense. Many patients passing a tiny innocent stone have a little pyrexia and do not need to have it removed.

The stone must be removed if it is *too large* to go down the ureter, but otherwise it needs to be taken out only if it has made it perfectly clear that it cannot be passed naturally: i.e. there is increasing distension of the ureter and pelvis upstream of the stone, or it has been stuck in the same place for several weeks, giving rise to one attack after another of colic.

Finally, there is one very good reason for getting the stone out—*anuria*. Fortunately this is rare: but when it happens you should move fast. If the patient is too ill, for one reason or another to remove the stone when there is only one kidney and no urine is coming down, then one should consider perhaps the wisdom of a 'medical nephrostomy' (see page 19). This is much safer than a difficult ureterolithotomy and may buy you valuable time, during which you can correct other more serious disorders.

URINARY TRACT INFECTION

History

In a woman trace the history back to childhood if you do not want to miss the common reflux uropathy that presents in later life with scarred kidneys and recurrent infection. Enquire about bubble baths, the relationship of the attacks to coitus or the menses. Ask whether the patient has had a hysterectomy— which so often ushers in urinary tract troubles.

Examination

A physical examination usually shows nothing. Hypertension should be noted. The urine must be cultured, but remember that about half of the patients with real urinary infection will have urine that seems to be sterile on ordinary culture.

Investigations

If a patient has had a long story of recurrent infections and if there has been haematuria, an excretion urogram is always needed. This may show a stone in which the organisms are hiding from antibiotics and continuing to breed, a pool of stagnant urine in a caliceal or vesical diverticulum, a hydronephrosis, or a large residual urine. It may show the filling defect of a bladder cancer.

If your patient has had *haematuria*, then he or she must be cystoscoped. If not, then there is often not much point in doing the examination, except that it will confirm the diagnosis, show you follicular cystitis, and exclude rare causes of recurrent infection such as a vesicocolic fistula. It is certainly not needed in the straightforward patient who suffers from recurrent urinary infection.

If there is *sterile pyuria*, then matters are quite different. One must exclude cancer and tuberculosis. The former needs careful cystoscopy, supplemented, especially in middle-aged men, with biopsies from all four quadrants of the bladder to rule out carcinoma *in situ* (see page 194). The latter needs at least three early morning urine samples to be examined for acid-fast bacilli by the Ziehl–Neelsen stain, and cultured for *Mycobacterium tuberculosis* on a Loewenstein–Jensen slope (see page 88).

When an organism, such as *Escherichia coli* is found, and no underlying abnormality to keep it going has been discovered, then a five to seven day course of the appropriate antimicrobial is given. This is supplemented by advice about drinking a large volume of fluid and emptying the bladder frequently (see page 175).

In women past the menopause, atrophic changes in the vagina and lower urethra may give rise to local irritative symptoms that mimic bacterial infection. They may improve with local oestrogen creams, and rarely need oral oestrogen administration—best administered in consultation with a gynaecologist.

INCONTINENCE OF URINE

History

The patient's history will often establish the pattern of incontinence which may be intermittent or continuous. If intermittent it may be *urge incontinence*, whereby the patient has sudden severe urge to void, and if he or she cannot reach a toilet, they expel the contents of the bladder. It may be *overflow incontinence*, where there is a distended overfull bladder that dribbles a little urine when the patient laughs, exerts himself, or coughs. Or there may be *stress incontinence*, where a little urine similarly escapes, from an undistended bladder, under any conditions that increase the intra-abdominal pressure.

Any form of incontinence will be made worse if the lining of the bladder is rendered more irritable by infection, and so a history of urinary infection is exceedingly relevant.

Physical examination

A general physical examination will note other overt evidence of neurological disease such as multiple sclerosis, old spina bifida, etc. One will be aware of the possibility of neuropathy e.g. in diabetes. The local examination is directed: (a) to the possibility of chronic retention and a distended floppy bladder; and (b) to mechanical disorder at the neck of the bladder accompanying a herniation of the bladder base, so often seen in vaginal wall prolapse in parous women. Finally the possibility of a *urinary fistula* will be always borne in mind (see page 307).

Investigations

At this stage the diagnosis may be obvious. But usually it needs to be confirmed by further investigations. *Urography* will determine the state of the kidneys and ureters and will reveal the tell-tale evidence of duplex system leading to incontinence from an ectopic ureteric orifice, the grossly distended bladder of chronic outflow obstruction that so often leads to overflow dribbling, or the typical fir-tree bladder of gross neurological disease.

Urodynamic investigations (see page 200) are then usually carried out. They may show a hyper-irritable detrusor reflex, signifying either too much afferent stimulation, or an oversensitive reflex arc (see page 209). They may show an inert floppy detrusor. They may show that there is too low an outflow resistance in the region of the neck of the bladder. Pressure profile measurements may show that the internal, the external or both sphincters are too slack. Cystography may show exactly which sphincters are not operating, or, in the case of vaginal vault prolapse, how far they are being displaced when the patient strains or coughs. As a result of these investigations the cause of the incontinence can usually be established. According to what has been found, the treatment will vary.

Treatment of incontinence

When there is a mechanical cause for incontinence, e.g. displacement of the bladder neck and trigone in pelvic floor herniation then a repair operation will usually cure the patient. In the first instance a vaginal approach by a gynaecologist will give the simplest and least uncomfortable operation for the patient. If this has failed, then a Marshall–Marchetti–Krantz suspension, or a version of Millin's sling operation may be used (see page 214). The results are likely to be less good when the detrusor is very unstable, and one advantage of having discovered this by pre-operative cystometrography is that the patient can be warned, and will not be too disappointed with an imperfect result.

If one discovers a hyperactive detrusor reflex, and can get rid of its cause (e.g. severe cystitis) then the result is good. In most instances (in practice) the cause is incurable or unknown. One may try to pacify the jumpy detrusor with anticholinergic drugs (see page 215) and since they are to a slight extent sensitive to beta-adrenergic fibres, one may add a beta-blocker. Good results have been claimed from the operation of transection of the bladder: others distend it with a view to making it less irritable. The results are variable.

If the external sphincter has been destroyed in a surgical operation on the prostate, the patient must have recourse to a Cunningham clip or one of the prostheses such as those of Kaufman, Rosen, or Scott (see page 212) or manage with a urinal. *Incontinence appliances* for men are of two types: in the usual one,

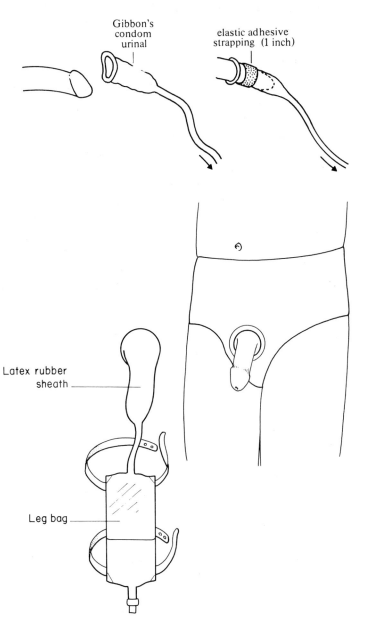

Fig. 24.1. The application of a urinal to the penis.

Fig. 24.2. Pubic pressure urinal.

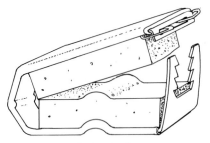

Fig. 23.3. Cunningham's clip.

a soft condom is stuck onto the penis (Fig. 24.1) and attached to a reservoir; in the other, a longer, looser condom is kept pressed up against the pubis with a pair of elastic pants (Fig. 24.2). None of them are entirely satisfactory. A Cunningham clip (Fig. 24.3) may be used to keep in the urine so long as there is no peripheral loss of sensation, and the patient is sufficiently alert and nimble-fingered to manage not to keep the clip on too long or too tightly.

If the bladder leaks only when it is overfull, whatever the cause, but especially where there is a neuropathy that has led to paralysis of the detrusor, then the patient may be kept dry and comfortable if he or she passes a catheter at regular intervals. *Intermittent 'clean' catheterization* is safe, provided it is done by the patient, whose own skin organisms are unlikely to cause inflammation if they colonize the patient's own bladder. Intelligent and cooperative patients can so keep themselves clean, comfortable and dry year after year.

An *indwelling catheter* is also useful. It is much frowned upon, because it inevitably becomes infected and becomes blocked from time to time, leading to back-pressure and urinary infection. But it is a wonderfully useful device. One should use as narrow a catheter as possible, and the silicone rubber ones have a very large internal diameter compared to the outside width. Catheters need to be changed regularly, before they get blocked. It may help to prevent blockage if the patient tries to keep her urine acid, e.g. with vitamin C and mandelamine, and it certainly helps to keep the urine dilute with a high fluid throughput.

Inevitably situations arise when the patient cannot, for one good reason or another, catheterize herself, when an indwelling catheter cannot be tolerated, or urine still escapes around it, or where in spite of incontinence, there is still sufficient back-pressure inside a neuropathic bladder to obstruct the ureters and threaten the kidneys. Then one must consider *urinary diversion*.

The method most commonly recommended today is the *ileal conduit*. The ureters are joined to an isolated segment of ileum (Fig. 24.4) which is led

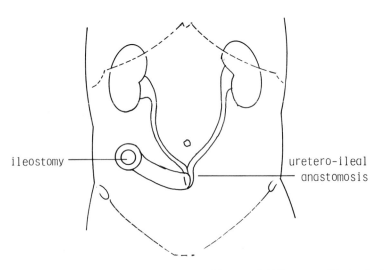

ileostomy

uretero-ileal anastomosis

Fig. 24.4. Ileal conduit. An adhesive bag is stuck over the stoma.

Chapter 24/*Common Urological Problems*

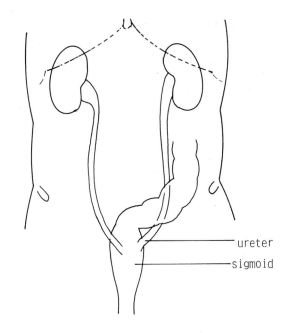

Fig. 24.5. Uretrosigmoidostomy.

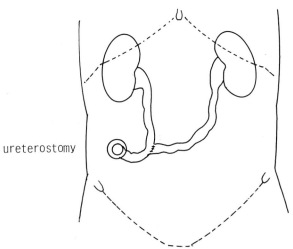

Fig. 24.6. Ureterostomy–en-Y.

through the skin of the abdominal wall where the urine can be collected in an adhesive appliance ('urostomy'). The alternatives include joining the ureters onto the sigmoid colon (ureterosigmoidostomy) (Fig. 24.5) or bringing the ureters onto the skin either through two separate openings, or through one opening, having anastomosed them together (ureterostomy-en-Y) (Fig. 24.6).

URINARY FISTULA

A fistula is an abnormal communication between one viscus and another, or to the exterior. In the urinary tract, fistulae may be *congenital* or acquired. Congenital ones include the patent urachus (see page 170) and the ectopic ureter that opens downstream of the sphincters and keeps the patient constantly wet day and night (see page 150). A number of very rare congenital fistulae are seen that join the urethra with the anal canal.

Acquired fistulae are common. Certain surgical principles have been known for many generations that keep fistulae patent:

1 *Obstruction downstream of the fistula.* If obstruction in the urinary tract (e.g. uncorrected outflow obstruction for a suprapubic fistula) remains, then pressure continues to be high inside the urinary tract and urine will continue to leak out.

2 *Epithelialization of the fistulous track.* When the track which is normally lined with granulation tissue, acquires a complete lining of skin or urothelium, then it may remain open, until the new lining is removed.

3 *Cancer* growing along the fistula may keep it open and prevent it from healing.

4 *Foreign bodies, and* this includes *calculi,* may be the cause of persistence of a fistula. This occurs in patients whose wounds have been sewn up with non-absorbable material such as silk or nylon close to where the urinary tract has been opened.

Bearing in mind these principles, certain of the more important types of fistulae need to be mentioned, with a brief outline of the way they are managed and investigated.

Often the cause of the fistula is obvious, e.g. there is a stone, or uncorrected obstruction to the urinary tract leading to build up of pressure in the system upstream of the problem. When the cause is not obvious contrast medium is injected into the visible opening of the fistula, to outline the track—a *sinogram* or *fistulogram.*

Vesicointestinal fistulae

The common one is a hole between the sigmoid colon and the bladder. It is caused by an abscess outside the colon caused by diverticular disease, or by breaking down of carcinoma of the colon. The abscess or the carcinoma erodes into the bladder. Faeces spill into the bladder, giving rise to severe and repeated attacks of acute bacterial cystitis (Fig. 24.7). Characteristically vegetable and other fibres from the diet may be found in the urinary deposit, which grows a wide range of intestinal organisms. Gas may be passed from the colon into the bladder and escape, like soda water, in the urine—a symptom called *pneumaturia,* about which patients are often so reticent that you must ask the question directly.

The differential diagnosis between carcinoma and diverticular disease is made by barium enema and colonoscopy and biopsy. The lining of the hole which can be easily seen in the bladder is usually made of oedematous, transitional epithelium and even when the cause is malignant, one cannot obtain confirmation of this by biopsy from the bladder.

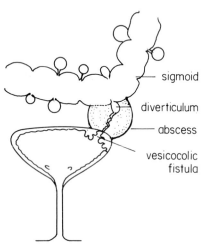

Fig. 24.7. Vesicocolic fistulae form when an abscess occurs in relation to a carcinoma or a patch of diverticular disease of the sigmoid colon.

sigmoid

diverticulum

abscess

vesicocolic fistula

Chapter 24/*Common Urological Problems*

The treatment is in the hands of the colorectal surgeon who will usually (nowadays) be able to perform a single stage resection of the diverticular disease or the cancer. If the pelvis is full of inflammatory adhesions, a three-stage operation is carried out: first the faeces are diverted from the bladder through a transverse colostomy, next the resection is performed, finally the colostomy is closed.

Similar, though much less common, vesicointestinal fistulae are caused by Crohn's disease or appendicitis.

Vaginal urinary fistulae

1. URETEROVAGINAL FISTULAE (Fig. 24.8)

If one or other ureter is damaged during hysterectomy, by being cut, crushed, or accidentally caught up in a ligature, urine will escape through the vault of the vagina. Often the urine does not appear for four to five days. The first step is to confirm the diagnosis by sending the fluid emerging from the vagina to the laboratory for urea estimation. If urine, the urea content will be higher than the plasma urea. Next, the exact site of the injury is confirmed by means of a cystoscopy and bulb ureterogram (see page 20). Finally the ureter is explored, freed, and reimplanted into the bladder using a Boari flap (see page 343).

2. VESICO-VAGINAL FISTULA

There are two types. The most common one in the West follows accidental injury or devascularization of the back of the bladder during a difficult hysterectomy. Urine escapes from the vagina and on cystoscopy a hole can be seen, usually 3–4 cms proximal to the interureteric bar (Fig. 24.9). If the hole is small, it may be closed by a vaginal operation, but if large, or if a previous vaginal operation has been tried unsuccessfully, the bladder is opened down the midline, the hole dissected cleanly, the vaginal vault closed, sealed with a plug made of greater omentum, and the bladder then closed (Fig. 24.10).

The more common form of vesico-vaginal fistula is seen in primitive communities where antenatal care is lacking and women are allowed to develop obstructed labour. Eventually—if they survive—it is found that a large ischaemic defect has formed where the baby's head had pressed for so long against the symphysis (Fig. 24.11). This usually involves much of the back of the bladder, often the lower ends of the ureters, and sometimes the external sphincter as well (Fig. 24.12). It may be possible to close this hole vaginally, especially by making use of a pedicled graft of the gracilis muscle, but in some cases the bladder is still incontinent thanks to damage to the external sphincter, and a diversion may be needed. A rather similar kind of ischaemic fistula is sometimes seen after very extensive radiotherapy to cancer of the uterus.

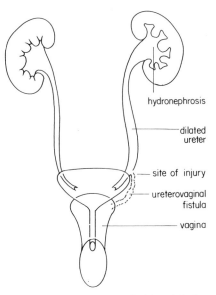

Fig. 24.8. When the ureter is injured during hysterectomy, a fistula forms between the ureter and the vaginal vault. On the injured side there is usually dilatation of the upper tract.

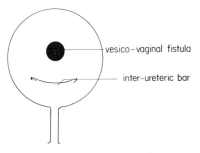

Fig. 24.9. Small vesico-vaginal fistula as seen on cystoscopy.

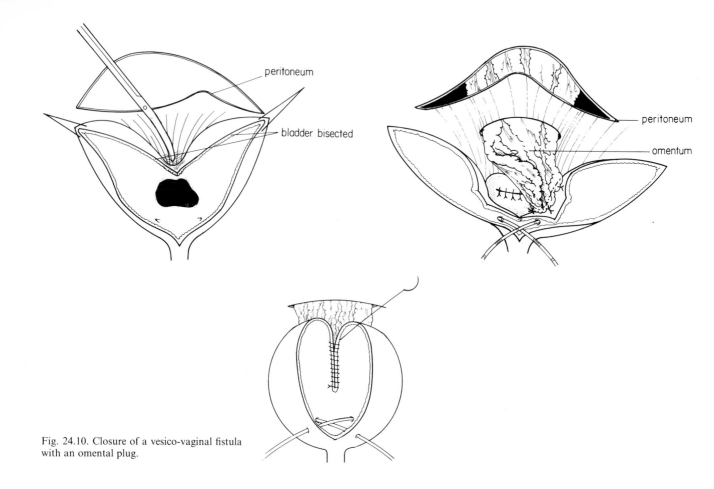

peritoneum

bladder bisected

peritoneum

omentum

Fig. 24.10. Closure of a vesico-vaginal fistula with an omental plug.

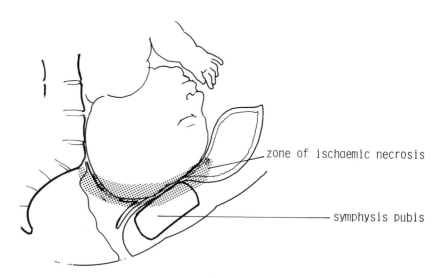

zone of ischaemic necrosis

symphysis pubis

Fig. 24.11. Mechanisms of the formation of a large vesico-vaginal fistula: prolonged pressure leads to ischaemic necrosis of the bladder, urethra and cervix which slough away.

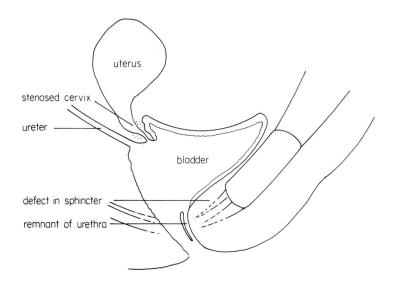

Fig. 24.12. Post-partum vesico-vaginal fistula. There is a kind of cloaca into which enter the ureters, the scarred cervix, and the back of the bladder and trigone. The sphincter may be completely destroyed.

Prostatorectal fistula

Fortunately this is very rare in Britain, perhaps because very few total prostatectomies are performed for cancer. When it happens faeces leak from the rectum into the prostatic urethra. The patient is troubled by severe ascending urinary infection as well as by the presence of urine in the rectum which often gives rise to incontinence. A small number of these are reported after open prostatic surgery where a carcinoma of the prostate has been found unexpectedly: it is very rare indeed after transurethral resection. When detected, a few

Fig. 24.13. Parks's operation for urethrorectal fistula.

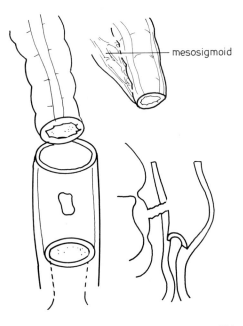
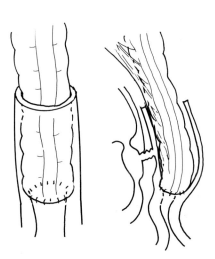

mesosigmoid

patients will heal up if a catheter is left in the bladder, but in most instances infection proceeds unchecked and calls for treatment. It is necessary to divert the faecal stream through a *colostomy* and then perform an operation to close the hole between the prostatic cavity and the rectum. Several operations have been devised for this. The most effective is that of Parks, who removes a sleeve of mucosa from the rectosigmoid down to the white line, and through the raw rectum he brings down the sigmoid, so that the hole is plugged by the full thickness of sigmoid (Fig. 24.13). Continence, determined by proprioception, is unimpaired since the appropriate end organs lie in the undamaged outer wall of the rectum.

**Chapter 25
Some of the
Common
Operations of
Urological
Surgery**

It is futile for the medical student to spend too much time on the details of surgical operations. Yet, like any craft, it can be fascinating, and it will not be long before he is a house-surgeon, and will be expected to prepare the patient for an operation and look after him afterwards. It is impossible, of course, to give a full account of all the procedures in the modern urological catalogue, but perhaps the following brief account will make it more interesting to follow your patient from the ward to the theatre, and explain why things are done the way they are.

UROLOGICAL ARMAMENTARIUM

Diathermy

The urologist cannot manage without a whole range of very special gadgets. Of these the most important is the *diathermy*. Since this uses a considerable amount of energy, it is a dangerous weapon and if disasters are to be avoided, one must at least know some of its underlying principles.

You will remember how Volta's first electric cell, when connected to a frog's leg to complete the circuit, made the leg twitch. When Galvani piled one Voltaic cell upon another, the leg twitched more violently, once when the current was applied, another when it was turned off. When Faraday devised the dynamo, giving alternating current, the frog's leg twitched twice for each revolution ('faradism') until the series of twitches merged into one sustained contraction.

However, if the rate of alternation of the current increased still further (and by using thermionic valves current frequencies in excess of 10 000 cycles/second could be used), a critical point was passed beyond which muscles would no longer twitch and nerves no longer be stimulated. A large current could now be passed through the body without causing pain or movement of muscles. This passage of electric current through the resistance of the body caused heat. If one terminal was very large, the heat produced under the contact would be negligible, but if the other were made small, as in the point of the diathermy electrode in common use, there would be very considerable heat indeed. At first the tissues would be poached, turning white like a boiled egg, later they would go brown and black, like a fried one, and finally they would (in air) catch fire. The combined effect of the distortion of blood vessels from coagulation and of clotting of the boiled blood inside them gave useful *haemostasis*.

If the current were increased still further an *arc* was struck, which disrupted the tissues as cleanly as if they were cut with a knife. This used more current, and very high frequences were needed. The availability of valve diathermy machines introduced a means of cutting and coagulating tissues under water, which meant that bladder tumours and prostatic adenomas could be removed transurethrally without the necessity for any incision in the skin.

However, this needed large currents. If by mischance (Fig. 25.1), the patient were to be connected to earth through a second small point of contact, the skin

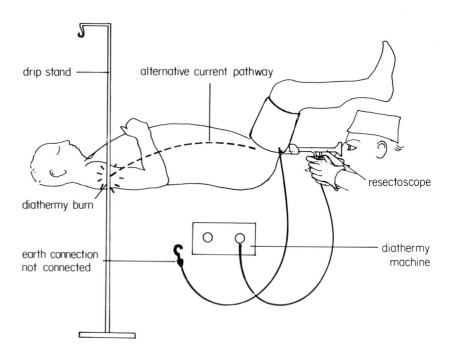

drip stand

alternative current pathway

resectoscope

diathermy burn

earth connection
not connected

diathermy
machine

Fig. 25.1. Diathermy burn caused by accidental 'earthing' of the patient through a small-area metal contact, when the proper earth has not been joined on.

making this contact would become hot, just like it did under the diathermy needle or the resectoscope loop. Hence the risk of diathermy burns. With modern diathermy machines a number of built-in safety measures ensure that the instrument will not work unless the earth plate is fixed to the patient, but it is still necessary that everyone concerned with the patient's welfare in the operating theatre (and that is why the people are all there) should feel personally responsible for ensuring that no unwanted contact with metal can possibly give him a burn.

Catheters and sounds

Essentially a catheter is a hollow pipe for letting urine out. It must be made of non-irritating material. Hence red rubber is not used, because it contains several irritating antioxidants. Pure latex rubber is used, or PVC or silicone rubber, of which the latter is the least irritating.

To keep a catheter inside the bladder a balloon is attached which can be inflated through a small side channel. However, this takes up some of the room inside the catheter (Fig. 25.2). On many occasions, it is useful to be able to keep the bladder continually washed out, and an additional third channel is added, which takes up even more room.

If a catheter fits exactly inside the urethra, then there is no room for the mucus secreted by its paraurethral glands to escape. The mucus can accumulate, may become infected, and cause a paraurethral abscess of which the end

Chapter 25/*Urological Surgery*

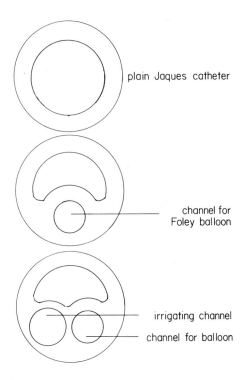

plain Jaques catheter

channel for
Foley balloon

irrigating channel

channel for balloon

Fig. 25.2. When any additional channel is added to a plain Jaques catheter, a good deal of its lumen is taken up.

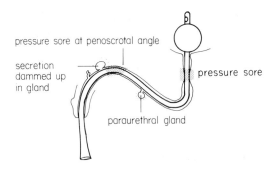

pressure sore at penoscrotal angle

secretion
dammed up
in gland

pressure sore

paraurethral gland

Fig. 25.3. Dangers of a snugly-fitting catheter: it gives rise to pressure sores inside the urethra; or it blocks off the openings of the para-urethral glands, inviting infection and abscess formation. Always use the smallest catheter that will do the job.

result may be a stricture (Fig. 25.3). Hence whenever possible the smallest catheter that will do the work is needed.

CATHETERIZATION

To get the catheter into the patient the urethra must be lubricated. This is done by filling the urethra with lubricating gel, and to help prevent carrying organisms from the open end of the urethra into the bladder, one usually employs gel containing 0.25% chlorhexidine antiseptic.

The urethra is very sensitive, and to make catheterization less unpleasant, the gel is medicated with 1% lignocaine. To get the mucosa numb will take

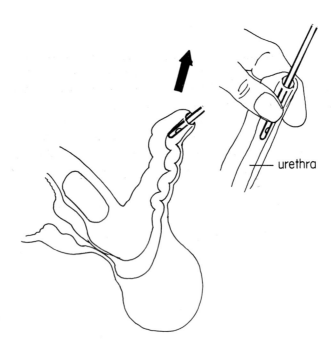

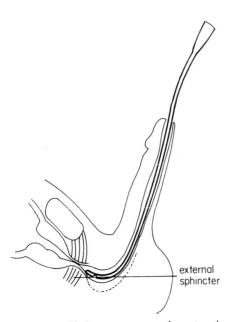

Fig. 25.4. Straighten out the urethra to straighten out its kinks.

Fig. 25.5. If the mucosa over the external sphincter is not well-anaesthetized, it may go into spasm. Never force the catheter past the unrelaxed sphincter.

about four minutes, so one must never be in a hurry between introducing the gel and passing the catheter.

In a *female*, the urethra is relatively short and straight, and so long as the catheter is soft, narrow and perfectly sterile, it may be passed straight into the lubricated anaesthetized urethra.

The urethra of a *male* is longer, and at rest, folded like an empty sock. To make it straight the penis must be gently pulled up (Fig. 25.4). The catheter is advanced, with aseptic precautions, so that the catheter never touches the patient's skin or that of the surgeon's hands, until its tip reaches the external sphincter. Here the patient experiences a twinge of discomfort unless the local anaesthetic has been left in the urethra for sufficient time (Fig. 25.5). If well anaesthetized, the catheter slips easily past the sphincter and on into the prostatic urethra. The tip of the catheter being soft and pliable, it readily adapts itself to the curve of the prostatic urethra, slips over the middle lobe if this is enlarged, and enters the bladder (Fig. 25.6).

Catheters come in many shapes and sizes. Many of the special curves given to catheters were devised on the supposition that force was needed to get the catheter into the bladder, and so the catheters were made somewhat stiff, and given an elbow bend (coudé) or double bend (bicoudé) to help negotiate the curve of the prostatic urethra. Neither bend is really necessary, unless it is required to lift the tip of the catheter up and over a ridge at the bladder neck, or out of a false passage. The lining of the urethra is very thin, very easily torn, and the first and last rule in passing a catheter is *never use any force at all*.

316

In the past urethral dilating instruments and catheters were assigned arbitrary sizes, according to how many different ones there were in a set. With the introduction of the metric system after the French Revolution, logic entered even into urology, and Charrière, a notable instrument-maker of Paris, calibrated his bougies and catheters according to their circumference in millimetres. This became the international system, Charrière, or French (Ch or F). Good old Charrière deserves to be remembered, particularly since there is an alternative French system, that of Béniqué (Bé) applicable to smaller catheters such as those used in the ureter.

The ordinary male adult urethra is about 26 Ch in its most narrow part (just inside the external meatus), but needless to say, men and their urethrae come in different sizes. For safety, in using a catheter merely to drain away the urine, nothing larger than 12 Ch or 14 Ch is needed, and gives plenty of room for mucus to escape alongside the catheter.

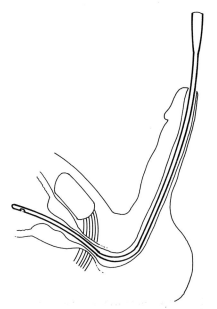

Fig. 25.6. Once past the external sphincter the catheter will find its way into the bladder so long as it is flexible and well-lubricated.

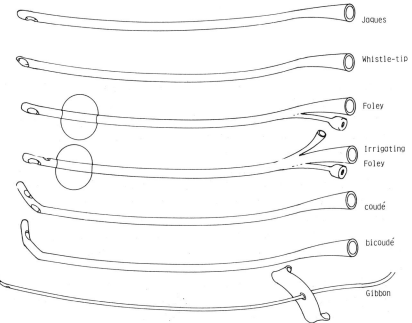
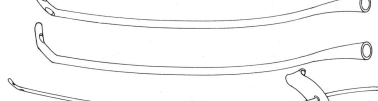

Jaques

Whistle-tip

Foley

Irrigating Foley

coudé

bicoudé

Gibbon

Fig. 25.7. Different types of urethral catheter.

Cystoscopes and endoscopic instruments

Modern cystoscopes utilize a remarkable invention of Professor Hopkins (of Reading University) which employs glass rods with air instead of glass lenses. These rods can be held and ground with the precision of a modern microscope. Blooming of the lenses prevents scattering of light and false reflections. To complement the wide field of view and the extreme optical resolution offered by modern cystoscopes, Hopkins added a fibre-light system which permitted a very intense light source to be housed outside the patient. Today one can get

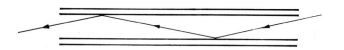

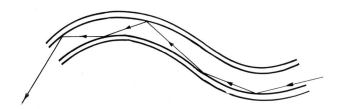

Fig. 25.8. Flexible fibre-lighting. Each thin glass fibre is coated with glass of different refractive index, ensuring total internal reflexion. Very powerful light sources can thus be sited at a distance from the patient.

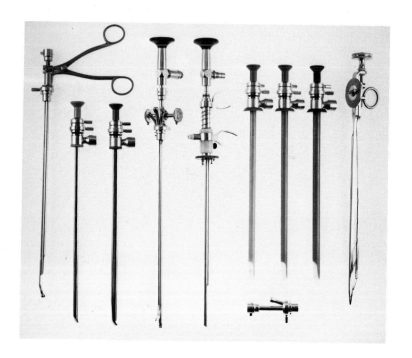

Fig. 25.9. Cystoscopic armamentarium.

enough light in and out of the cystoscope to make colour television or ciné film records (Fig. 25.8).

According to the design of the lens at the inner end of the telescope, one may look straight ahead or sideways, and so examine every millimetre of the inside of the bladder and urethra.

Not only can one examine it, one can take a biopsy from any part of it with special forceps, catheterize the ureteric orifices, coagulate small tumours, and remove large ones with a resectoscope loop armed with a cutting and coagulating diathermy current (Fig. 25.9). Thanks to these instruments, all

Chapter 25/*Urological Surgery*

adaptations of the cystoscope are manufactured to slip down the 24 Ch sized urethra and there is hardly a pathological condition in the urethra or bladder that cannot be treated endoscopically, and so there is, by the same token, almost no indication to open the bladder in modern urology.

CYSTOSCOPY

Indications

These are innumerable, but chiefly for *haematuria*. This being so, it is nearly always going to be necessary to do something as well as look inside the bladder: hence in recent years the 'routine cystoscopy' has been replaced by the 'cystourethroscopy and biopsy'. For the same reason cystoscopy under local anaesthetic has been more and more replaced by examination under anaesthesia, with the exception of patients having their bladders checked annually for recurrence of urothelial tumours, and some women with haematuria that will (almost) certainly prove to be of no consequence.

Preparation
If the urine is infected, a single dose of bactericidal antibiotic of the appropriate type is administered about one hour before the endoscopy.

Position on the table
Cystoscopic tables are available giving the patient the ideal position (Fig. 25.10) with the thighs flexed to about 45° and the legs horizontal. The right position for

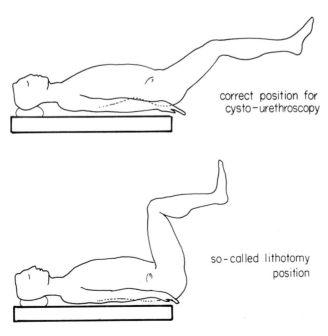

correct position for cysto-urethroscopy

so-called lithotomy position

Fig. 25.10. Cystoscopy position.

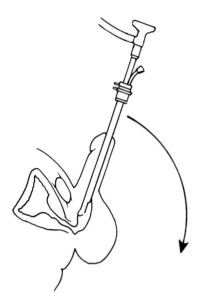

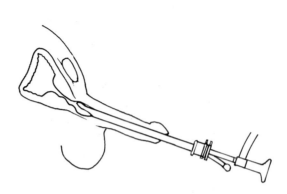

Fig. 25.11. Urethroscopy.

cystoscopy is quite different to the position for operations on the anus or the vagina ('lithotomy').

Urethroscopy

Today the urethra is always examined with a 0° or direct-viewing telescope (Fig. 25.11) *en route* to the bladder. This allows one to check the paraurethral duct openings, the presence of strictures, the state of the external sphincter and that of the prostatic urethra (in the male). The 0° telescope is then exchanged for one with a nearly right-angle view (usually its median ray is set at 70°).

Cystoscopy (Fig. 25.12)

By allowing the sterile water to flow in and out of the bladder, and by moving the telescope in and out, and rotating it through 360° all parts of the bladder are

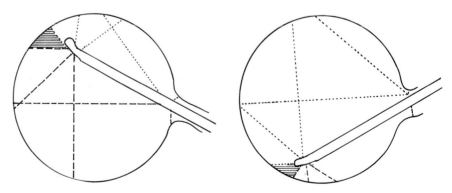

Fig. 25.12. Cystoscopy.

Chapter 25/*Urological Surgery*

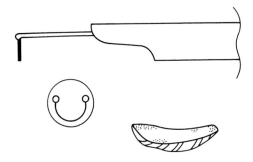

Fig. 25.13. Resectoscope.

carefully examined, and no part is invisible. If a biopsy is needed, cup forceps are inserted down the cystoscope. If the ureter has to be catheterized, or if a ureterogram is needed, a 'catheterizing slide' is used which is provided with a moveable lever (named after its French inventor, the Parisian surgeon Albarran). This makes it very easy to wriggle the catheter into the ureteric orifice. You can tell how far the catheter has gone by the rings that are marked every centimetre on its shaft. Most kidneys are about 25–30 cm up from the ureteric orifice. After biopsy, very small tumours may be coagulated with a flexible electrode introduced along the catheterizing slide. But more frequently nowadays the cystoscope is removed and replaced with the 'resectoscope' (Fig. 25.13).

The *resectoscope* allows the surgeon to move a tungsten loop to and fro. With a current of clear water, the view is kept crystal clear even when cutting tissue causes some bleeding. Using the resectoscope long half-cylinders of tissue are cut from the bladder tumour or the prostate. Small blood vessels are coagulated with the loop, but very large ones may need a bigger 'roly-ball' electrode.

If stones are present inside the bladder they can be crushed and the fragments irrigated away. Small stones can be dealt with using a visual lithotrite that allows the surgeon to see what he is doing, but larger stones need the stronger, old-fashioned, 'blind' *lithotrite*.

DILATATION OF A STRICTURE

Indications

For the patient whose stricture is well controlled, and who only needs to come to the clinic once or twice a year, the regular and gentle passage of a bougie offers an ideal method of treatment. Most new strictures will be examined by urethroscopy and probably treated in the first instance by optical urethrotomy.

1 *Bouginage*

No special premedication or precaution is needed unless the patient has found

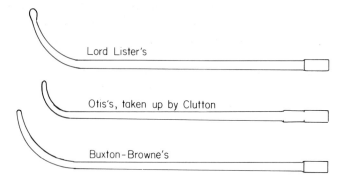

Fig. 25.14. Different curves of steel bougies or sounds: the Otis–Clutton curve is the type most generally useful.

that each instrumentation is followed by chills and fever, in which case an antibiotic is taken one hour before the instrumentation is due to be done, and continued for two to three days afterwards.

Local anaesthetic is instilled using a sterile nozzle, 1% lignocaine in 0.25% chlorhexidine gel. A penile clamp is applied for four minutes to allow the local to ooze the whole way along the urethra and have time to numb its lining.

Having carefully studied the previous notes of the patient, a straight (for the anterior urethra) or curved (for other parts) bougie is chosen of the size first used on the last occasion (Fig. 25.14). It is allowed to fall into the urethra by its own weight. There is never any need to push. If the instrument meets with resistance, it is very gently guided this way and that until its tip finds the opening of the urethral stricture.

Exceptionally, one is unable to find the hole in the stricture by blindly feeling with a steel bougie. A *filiform bougie* is chosen, its tip given a dog-leg, and then passed very gently down the urethra until the stricture is met (Fig.

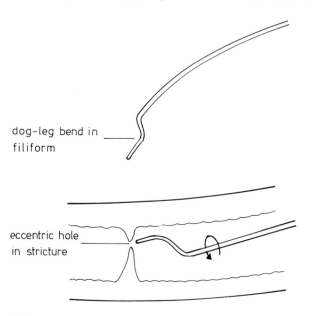

Fig. 25.15. Use of the filiform bougie.

Chapter 25/*Urological Surgery*

25.15). The filiform is then rotated so that the tip on its dog-leg moves around until it fetches up in the hole in the face of the stricture. *Followers* of flexible PVC are screwed into the female end of the filiform and the stricture gradually stretched.

Whether using flexible followers or rigid steel bougies, there must never be any force. It is futile to stretch a stricture roughly, or make the lining of the urethra bleed: this only invites extravasation through the lacerated mucosa and this will make the subsequent scarring worse.

2 *Optical urethrotomy*

Using a specially modified cystoscope armed with a sharp blade (Fig. 25.16), the stricture is divided from within under direct vision. After the urethra has been slit, a catheter is left indwelling. Nobody knows how long one needs to leave the catheter *in situ*. It seems as if four days is as good as four weeks. Some urologists claim that instilling steroid cream into the urethra may prevent the return of strictures. This has never been tested against adequate controls.

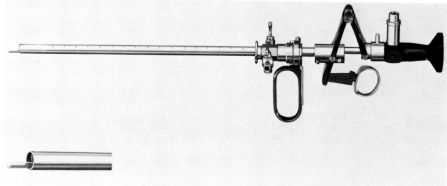

Fig. 25.16. Storz–Sachse optical urethrotome.

OPERATIONS ON THE KIDNEY

Nephrectomy

1. FOR REMOVAL OF A SMALL DESTROYED KIDNEY

Many of these kidneys are infected, and it is wise to avoid the hazard of bacteraemia with a suitable pre-operative dose of antimicrobial. Always check the side that is to be removed. Make sure that this is understood by yourself, the surgeon and the patient, and mark the correct side with an indelible cross on the skin.

Two units of blood should be cross matched.

Profound general anaesthesia will be needed, and because of the risk of

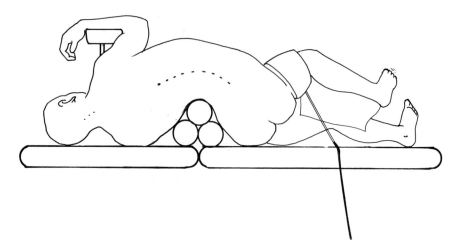

Fig. 25.17. Nephrectomy position.

inadvertently opening the pleura, the anaesthetist will need to pass an endotracheal tube.

The patient is placed in the full lateral position (Fig. 25.17) with the table broken or an inflatable cushion under the patient. Extreme arching of the back may compress the vena cava, and so when the patient is in the final position, the blood pressure must be checked.

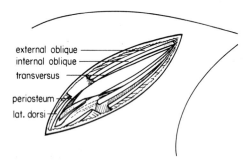

external oblique
internal oblique
transversus
periosteum
lat. dorsi

Fig. 25.18. 12th rib-tip incision.

The incision is carried from the tip of the 12th rib forwards, severing the latissimus dorsi, external and internal obliques and splitting the transversus muscle in the line of its fibres (Fig. 25.18). The fascia of Gerota around the kidney is incised and the fatty packing of Zuckerkandl dissected off the kidney, to which it is often very adherent when there has been much previous infection. Careful dissection of the renal hilum enables a ligature to be passed around the renal artery and renal vein separately. Each of these large vessels is ligated twice. Catgut is used where there is infection, otherwise non-absorbable ligature material may be used. The ureter is ligated with catgut (Fig. 25.19).

In a straightforward easy nephrectomy no drain is needed. The wound is closed either in layers or in a single layer.

Postoperatively one nearly always gets considerable pain, and unless this is relieved the patient has difficulty in coughing and ridding the basal segments of

Chapter 25/*Urological Surgery*

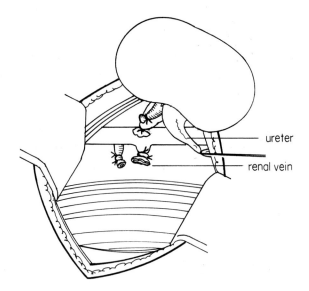

ureter

renal vein

Fig. 25.19. Nephrectomy for a small kidney.

his or her lungs of accumulated sputum. Postoperative atelectasis is common and infection often needs physiotherapy and antibiotics.

Complications to watch for

Haemorrhage into the wound usually occurs from muscle vessels pricked during closure of the wound. It is seldom severe. Fortunately haemorrhage from a slipped ligature on the renal pedicle, much dreaded in a former era, is of extreme rarity today. Since many nephrectomies are performed for kidneys that have been damaged by infection, wound infection is common.

Late sequelae

Nephrectomy incisions, however made, are notoriously painful. Often, and especially when there has been a difficult dissection to get the kidney out, the subcostal nerves of the 11th and 12th thoracic segment are stretched or bruised and there is weakness of part of the abdominal wall on that side: it usually recovers, but there may be a permanent bulge. If the tip of the rib has had to be removed there may be a discrete herniation there.

2. NEPHRECTOMY FOR CANCER OF THE KIDNEY

More blood is necessary in these cases and 4 units should be cross matched. If the renal artery has been embolized before operation the patient will already require considerable pain medication.

The patient is supine on the table. A long transverse or paramedian incision is made, entering the peritoneum. The colon is mobilised medially to expose the hilum of the kidney (Fig. 25.20).

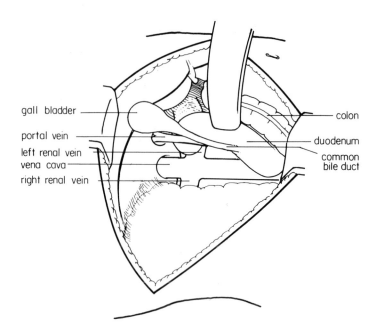

gall bladder

portal vein

left renal vein

vena cava

right renal vein

colon

duodenum

common bile duct

Fig. 25.20. Transabdominal nephrectomy.

On the right side the renal vein is short, and the right renal artery is approached by retracting the vein, until a ligature has been placed on the renal artery to cut the blood off from going into the kidney (Fig. 25.21). This manoeuvre is somewhat easier on the left side. Only when the renal artery has been safely obstructed by a ligature is the renal vein divided. If one can feel tumour inside the renal vein, the vena cava is taped above and below the entry

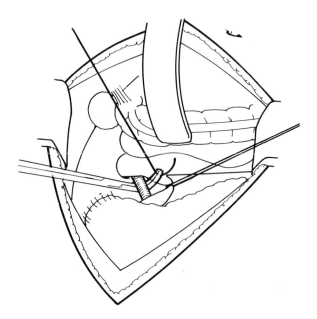

Fig. 25.21. Ligature of the right renal artery.

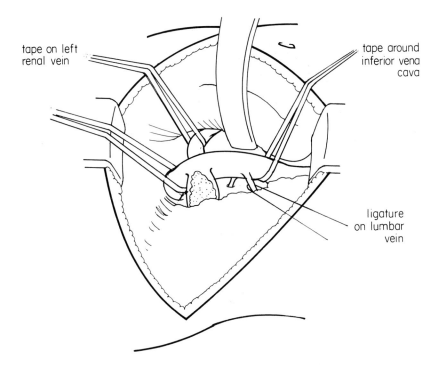

tape on left
renal vein

tape around
inferior vena
cava

ligature
on lumbar
vein

Fig. 25.22. Removing a malignant thrombus
from the vena cava.

of the renal vein, so that any tumour inside the lumen of the cava can be removed (Fig. 25.22). The cava is closed with a vascular suture.

Once the renal artery or arteries have been divided, the tissues lateral to the aorta (on the left) or the cava (on the right) are dissected *en bloc* down as far as the common iliac vessels, and laterally in the plane outside Gerota's fascia. The dissection is taken up to the liver and includes the adrenal gland.

After securing haemostasis the wound may be drained if there is any ooze. The bowel is carefully replaced, and the wound closed with the usual precautions against dehiscence.

Complications to watch for

As with any major abdominal operation, one expects a few days of ileus during which the patient is fed intravenously and his stomach is kept empty by nasogastric aspiration. If a difficult dissection has been necessary under the diaphragm then one must anticipate difficulty in coughing and breathing so that adequate pain relief may be supplemented by physiotherapy and antibiotics according to the sputum flora.

These are usually big tumours and they have a prodigious blood supply, so that it is easy to underestimate the amount of blood that has been lost at the time of operation. Careful estimations of the postoperative haematocrit should be made, and blood given as necessary.

Stone in the kidney

A. EASY STONE IN THE RENAL PELVIS (PYELOLITHOTOMY)

Any stone that is obviously too big to go down the renal pelvis ought to be removed. Precautions to cover the patient against bacteraemia if the urine is known to be infected, and 2 units of blood cross-matched precede the operation. The patient is in the nephrectomy position, the back arched on a break in the table or an inflatable cushion.

The kidney is approached through the 12th rib-tip incision without resecting any part of the rib. The abdominal muscles are incised in the line of the rib avoiding the subcostal bundles of the 11th and 12th ribs. Care is taken to avoid opening the pleura or the peritoneum (if possible).

When the kidney is relatively normal and the stone easily felt, minimal dissection is necessary. After feeling the stone on the posterior aspect of the kidney, two stay sutures are placed in the renal pelvis which is opened, the stone removed, and after closing the pelvis the wound closed with drainage (Fig. 25.23).

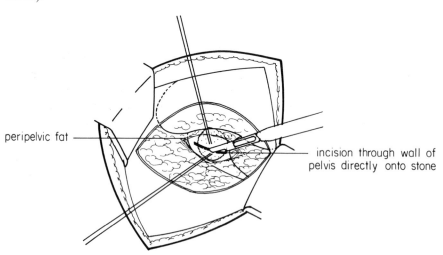

peripelvic fat

incision through wall of
pelvis directly onto stone

Fig. 25.23. Pyelolithotomy.

The difficulty arises if the stone is small and difficult to find, or the kidney very stuck with many and very vascular adhesions. In such a case a longer incision is needed, which usually passes through the bed of the 12th rib (12th rib-bed incision) without however needing to resect any bone (Fig. 25.24).

The kidney is fully dissected out from its stiff covering of adherent Zuckerkandl's fat. If the stone can still not be felt, an X-ray may be taken at this stage. Otherwise one proceeds as for a staghorn calculus, by entering Gil-Vernet's blood plane in the renal sinus (see below).

B. DIFFICULT AND STAGHORN STONES IN THE KIDNEY

The approach to the difficult kidney stone must be far more cautious. First, the

Chapter 25/*Urological Surgery*

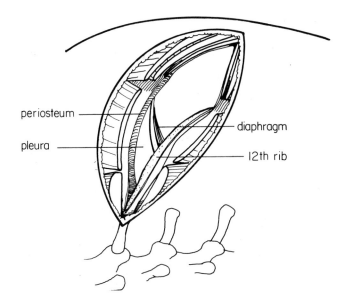

periosteum

pleura

diaphragm

12th rib

Fig. 25.24. 12th rib-bed incision.

incision must be a long one, for the most important aid to safety is adequate exposure. The incision is carried along the 12th rib. Its periosteum is stripped off the superior border, opened, and the incision carried forward between the 11th and 12th neurovascular bundles cutting through the muscles of the abdominal wall. The kidney is then dissected out completely. When particularly stuck, the peritoneum is opened as a safety measure so that the colon and/or duodenum can be seen and avoided. The renal artery is dissected and taped.

By following up the bloodless plane between the muscle of the ureter and its adventitia, the scissors lead up into Gil-Vernet's space, lying between the renal pelvis and parenchyma (Fig. 25.25). This is enlarged until the necks of the

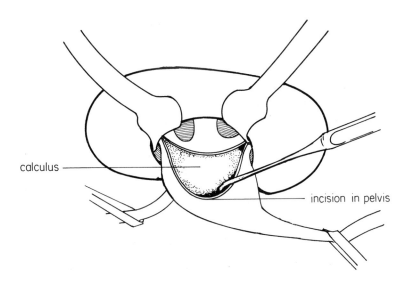

calculus

incision in pelvis

Fig. 25.25. Gil-Vernet's bloodless plane in the renal sinus.

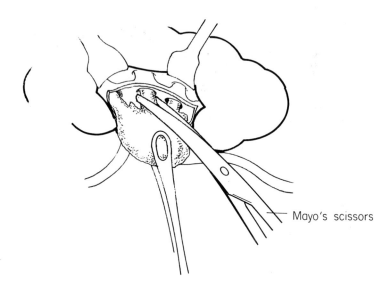

Mayo's scissors

Fig. 25.26. Breaking off the 'mushroom' extensions of a staghorn stone.

calices can be seen. The major part of the body of the stone is then removed, if necessary, breaking off the necks of its extensions going out into the calices (Fig. 25.26).

When large mushroon-shaped extensions of stone are left out in the calices, they are approached through radially placed incisions that avoid the renal arteries (Fig. 25.27). (One may mark out the position of the renal arteries with the Doppler probe at the time of operation if necessary, and cut between the marks.)

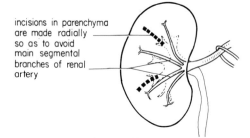

incisions in parenchyma are made radially so as to avoid main segmental branches of renal artery

Fig. 25.27. Radial incisions in the renal parenchyma avoid the segmental arteries of the kidney.

If the parenchyma is very thin over these peripheral mushrooms, insignificant loops of blood occurs. If the parenchyma is very thick and vascular, then the renal artery is occluded with a DeBakey clamp, the kidney is cooled, and the parenchyma incised in a bloodless field. Before closing the parenchyma any vessel that has been cut across is carefully closed by suture-ligature.

To cool the kidney one may use a pair of sterile coils through which coolant is circulated at 4°C, or immerse the kidney in sterile ice slush, or irrigate it with sterile saline or water at 4°C. Reducing the temperature of the kidney to this level affords 60–90 minutes of safe operating time—more than enough to get the stone out and X-ray the kidney to make sure it is all clear (Fig. 25.28).

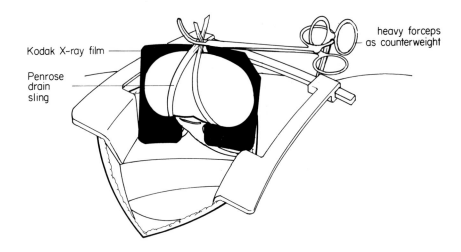

Kodak X-ray film

Penrose
drain
sling

heavy forceps
as counterweight

Fig. 25.28. Taking an X-ray of the kidney *in situ*.

Such a kidney operation is always likely to leak urine and the wound must be drained. If there is any doubt about the renal function on the other side, a nephrostomy tube is put into the kidney as a safety measure.

Complications to watch for

The main hazards are those of ileus and chest infection. Secondary haemorrhage is rare, but may occur if nephrotomies have been made through very thick kidney tissue. Wound infection from inoculation of the raw surfaces of the wound by *Proteus* or *E. coli* in the kidney and the stone is very common.

If the renal function on the other side is precarious, the handling of the kidney, especially if one has had to occlude the renal artery, may bring about temporary renal failure, so that in such a patient the operation should not be undertaken unless one can be sure of being able to take care of a period of renal failure afterwards with dialysis and other appropriate measures.

Pyeloplasty

Most examples of hydronephrosis are caused by narrowing at the pelviureteric junction of unknown aetiology. Before embarking on the pyeloplasty it is often wise to make sure that the rest of the ureter is normal by means of a ureterogram (see page 20).

In slim people and children, the pyeloplasty is most easily done through an anterior horizontal incision which can be made relatively inconspicuous by siting it in a skin crease. In muscular young males however this gives a very poor exposure and a 12th rib approach is better.

After dissecting out the kidney from Zuckerkandl's fat, the anatomy is displayed. One may find the lower pole artery and vein crossing very near, and seeming to pinch the pelviureteric junction, hence the origin of the notion that

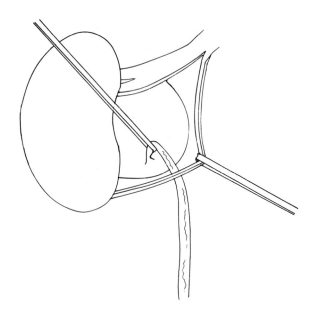

Fig. 25.29. Anatomy of the pelviureteric junction when dissected during the operation for hydronephrosis.

the 'aberrant artery' caused the trouble. A little dissection will usually show that the vessels are lying a long way off the narrow bit in the ureter (Fig. 25.29).

A flap is formed from the redundant renal pelvis, in such a way that it hangs down without any tension, and can be inserted into the slit up the ureter, to permanently enlarge the pelviureteric junction (Fig. 25.30).

How this flap is formed leads to endless discussion among urologists, and

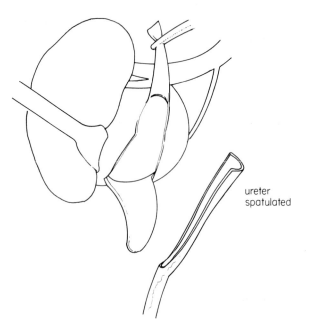

ureter
spatulated

Fig. 25.30. In pyeloplasty a V-shaped gusset of pelvis is let into the narrow part of the ureter.

Chapter 25/*Urological Surgery*

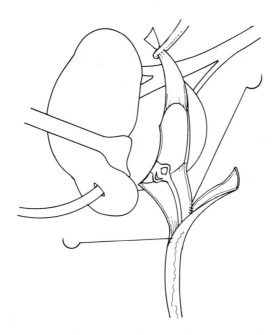

Fig. 25.31. Use of a splinting Cummings tube in pyeloplasty.

several names are given to the variations on what is all essentially the same theme. In Britain the operation is usually named after Anderson and Hynes: but if the ureter is not cut right off, then the procedure is named after the late Dr Ormond Culp. In practice one looks at the anatomy and does what is obviously needed.

The anastomosis between the flap of pelvis and the ureter must be sewn with catgut. If non-absorbable sutures are used, they will give rise to stones. The anastomosis is usually protected with a nephrostomy tube, and a splint to keep it straight while it is healing (Fig. 25.31).

The wound is closed with drainage.

COMPLICATIONS TO WATCH OUT FOR

Most pyeloplasties go smoothly, but if there is much extravasation of urine one may get prolonged ileus and even a collection of undrained urine (urinoma) that may have to be left out through a separate incision after a week or so. Wound infection may occur especially if the urine inside the hydronephrosis was infected.

LATE FOLLOW UP

A pyelogram is always taken at three months after the operation and the patient is followed for five to ten years to make sure that the other side does not develop a similar pelviuretic junction obstruction. Hypertension has been recorded as a late sequel to hyronephrosis and this is monitored at each out-patient visit. Stones sometimes form, perhaps on the catgut of the sutures.

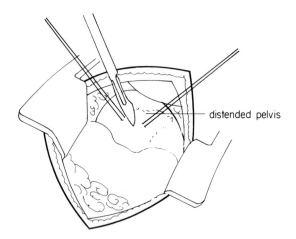

distended pelvis

Fig. 25.32. Nephrostomy.

Fig. 25.33. Nephrostomy tube in position.

Nephrostomy

Fortunately nowadays the 'medical nephrostomy' (see page 19) has made it only very seldom necessary to perform an open nephrostomy, for it can be a very difficult and quite dangerous operation under the circumstances when it is required.

One cannot enumerate the indications for nephrostomy, they are all unusual, and comprise the sorts of occasion when one anticipates recovery of ureteric continuity, but the patient is too ill to undergo the definitive operation. Nephrostomy is seldom, if ever, justified as a permanent method of diversion, for changing the nephrostomy tube is always unpleasant, the tube often becomes caked with calculus, and the intubated kidney is invariably infected.

The patient is in the full lateral position. Approaching the kidney through a 12th rib-tip incision, without resecting any rib, the peritoneum is dissected off the front of the distended kidney (Fig. 25.32). As soon as one is sure that the renal pelvis is reached, it is opened between stay sutures, and an angled forceps

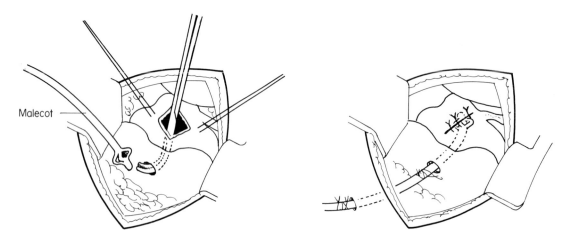

Malecot

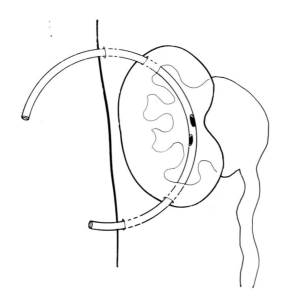

Fig. 25.34. Tresidder's ring nephrostomy.

or malleable probe passed retrograde-fashion through the parenchyma from pelvis outwards. To this probe is attached the tip of a suitable catheter, which is then brought so that its tip lies inside the kidney (Fig. 25.33).

Most surgeons use a soft Malecot catheter for nephrostomy, but if it is anticipated that the tube may have to remain in position for any length of time, and so might have to be changed when it becomes clogged up with stone, then Tresidder's ring nephrostomy method is used (Fig. 25.34). This allows the tube to be changed by attaching the new tube to the old one.

Renal transplantation

The donor kidney having been obtained, it will be (as a rule) lying in a polystyrene container surrounded by ice, and kept sterile by being wrapped in

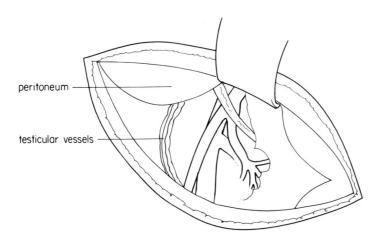

peritoneum

testicular vessels

Fig. 25.35. Preparation of the iliac fossa for a renal transplant.

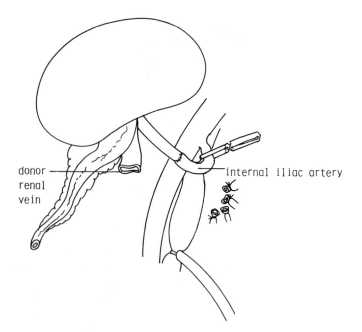

Fig. 25.36. Renal transplantation: the donor renal artery is anastomosed here to the internal iliac artery after ligating its distal branches.

two sterile nylon bags. If the donor kidney is coming from a living donor, it will have been flushed through with Collins solution, and will be ready in an ice cold bowl of sterile saline.

An oblique incision is made in the loin, extraperitoneally, to expose the external iliac artery and vein, which are cleaned and dissected back to the bifurcation of the common iliac artery (Fig. 25.35).

If the donor artery is a single one, and if the recipient has not got gross atheroma in the internal iliac artery, the latter is divided, irrigated with heparinized saline, and anastomosed to the donor artery (Fig. 25.36). If there

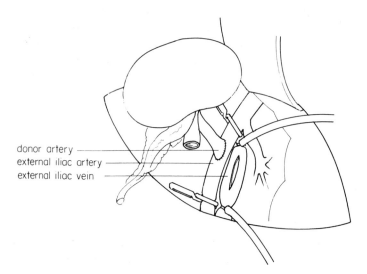

Fig. 25.37. The donor renal artery/arteries may be placed end-side onto the external iliac artery.

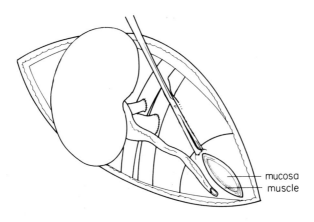

Fig. 25.38. The ureter is anastomosed to the bladder in an anti-reflux tunnel.

are several donor arteries on a Carrel patch of donor aorta, this is attached to a slit in the side of the external iliac artery (Fig. 25.37). The donor renal vein is anastomosed to the side of the external iliac vein. When the clamps are taken off, care is taken to make sure that the kidney is well perfused, and that the arterial and venous anastomoses are unobstructed and unkinked. Then the donor ureter is led through an anti-reflux tunnel made in the detrusor muscle (Fig. 25.38) and anastomosed over a splint (some surgeons dispense with any splint) to the mucosa of the bladder. The bladder is drained with a catheter and the wound is closed with suitable extraperitoneal drainage.

Postoperative complications after transplant operations would require a book to themselves. There are many things that can go wrong. If there is no urine coming from the kidney, one has to decide whether this is because the donor kidney has undergone renal failure (e.g. from inadequate cooling or late removal from the cadaver); or there is obstruction at the vascular anastomosis; or acute rejection. If the patient develops fever, one has to discover whether this is caused by infection (which is apt to occur because the patient's immune defences have been suppressed) or by rejection. If cadaver kidneys are used, they seldom function perfectly from the beginning, and are often more or less damaged by tubular damage. In living donor transplantation this hazard is minimized and one expects the kidney to pour out urine from the first moments in its new site.

OPERATIONS ON THE URETER

Stone in the ureter

STONE IN THE UPPER THIRD OF THE URETER

Here the main problem is that the stone may slip back into the kidney. A radiograph is taken between the patient leaving the ward and arriving in the

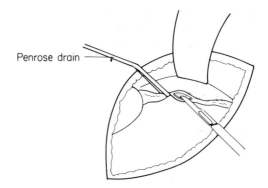

Penrose drain

Fig. 25.39. Removal of a calculus from the upper third of the ureter.

operating theatre. If the stone has slipped back, it may be more prudent to put off the operation.

With the patient in the lateral kidney position a small 12th rib-tip approach is used. Very gently feeling along the back of the peritoneum, as soon as Gerota's fascia has been opened, the finger touches the stone. A Deaver's retractor is gently slid along the back of the finger, and the peritoneum lifted up and away (Fig. 25.39). The ureter can now be seen. Without dislodging the stone, with a right-angled forceps a silastic sling is passed round the ureter upsteam of the stone, to stop it from slipping upwards. An incision is made down onto the stone, which is separated from the jelly-like nest of ureteric oedema which clings to it (Fig. 25.40). A ureteric catheter is slid up to the kidney and down to the bladder to make sure there are no more stones in the ureter and the wound is closed with a tube drain down to the incision in the ureter. Some surgeons close the ureter with a 5-0 catgut suture. Others leave it open. The writer closes a ureter that seems to gape but not otherwise.

Draining the ureterotomy

The drain is left in position for four days, then it is shortened for half its length

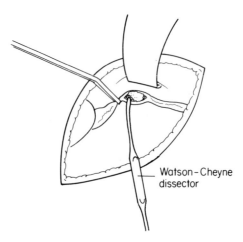

Watson-Cheyne dissector

Fig. 25.40. The stone is often stuck by oedema to the wall of the ureter.

Chapter 25/*Urological Surgery*

and removed on the sixth day. If the drain is left, as is customary with surgical drains, 'until it has stopped draining', you will wait for ever. The drain need only be left in just long enough for a firm tube of granulation tissue to form along its track to prevent extravasation and urinoma formation.

Postoperative complications

Persistent leakage of urine from the drainage hole sometimes occurs, and may mean that there is an uncorrected obstruction downstream such as a missed stone. If this can be excluded, one can usually guarantee that the fistula will close, but after three weeks this process may be judiciously speeded up by retrograde passage of a catheter, which can be left in for the two or three days needed to ensure closure of the fistula.

STONE IN THE MIDDLE THIRD OF THE URETER

This is the ideal position in which to remove a stone from the ureter, but just because it is easy, should not tempt one to remove a stone that will almost certainly pass on its own, given a little more time.

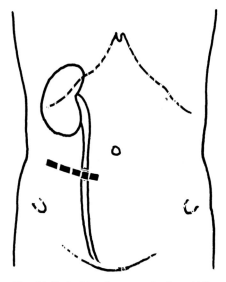

Fig. 25.41. Incision for stone in the middle third of the ureter.

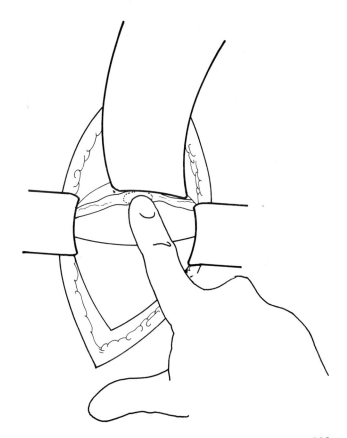

Fig. 25.42. Removal of stone from the middle third of the ureter.

The patient lies supine, with a soft support under the buttock on the side where the stone is. A crease incision is made just over where the X-rays (taken *en route* to the theatre) confirm that the stone is lying (Fig. 25.41). Entering the extraperitoneal fat well in the lateral aspect of the wound, a finger once more gently feels along the back of the peritoneum (where the ureter is always caught up) until the stone is felt (Fig. 25.42). Thence forward the operation is as described above.

STONE IN THE LOWER THIRD OF THE URETER

In contrast to the stone in the middle third, the removal of a stone in the lower third of the ureter can be a very miserable operation indeed, unless the surgeon knows the secret. The secret is to start by dividing the *superior vesical pedicle* between ligatures before tackling the ureter (Fig. 25.43).

A Pfannenstiel incision is the easiest to use. After sweeping the peritoneum upwards and the bladder medially, the finger follows the unmistakable cord of the 'obliterated' umbilical artery down towards the side wall of the pelvis. This

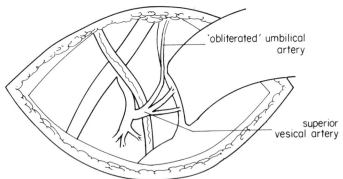

Fig. 25.43. The key to the approach to a stone in the lower third of the ureter is division of the superior vesical vessels.

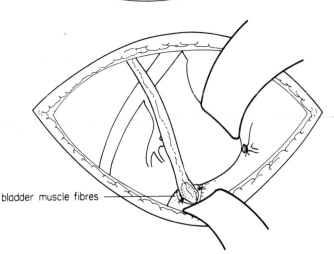

Fig. 25.44. Removing the stone at the lower end of the ureter.

Chapter 25/*Urological Surgery*

cord will lead him to the internal iliac artery and its sturdy leash of vessels that form the superior vesicle pedicle.

Once this pedicle has been divided, the ureter is traced from where it crosses in front of the division of the common iliac artery down towards the bladder. Several other tiny vessels often cross it and need to be divided, but once the main superior pedicle is divided, the ureter is released and this dissection is easy. Soon one comes across the stone, incises upon it, releases it, and the operation is over (Fig. 25.44).

It is never necessary to open the bladder for a stone in the lower end of the ureter unless there are impenetrable adhesions in the perivesical space.

USE OF THE STONE-DISLODGING BASKET

Baskets are available of various shapes and kinds. The writer prefers Pfister's modified Dormia instrument. It is only for stones that are less than 5 mm in diameter and less than 5 cm from the ureteric orifice. It should never be used just because the patient is in a hurry, when it is obvious that with a little more time the stone will pass.

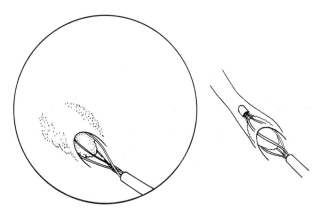

Fig. 25.45. Using the Pfister or Dormia stone-basket to retrieve a stone in the lower 5 cm of the ureter.

The basket is used like a ureteric catheter. It is slid up the ureter past the expected site of the stone. The fibres are then opened by manipulating the handle, and the basket is then slowly and gently withdrawn (Fig. 25.45). If luck is on the side of the surgeon, the stone will be trapped in the basket and drawn out through the ureteric orifice. If it is stuck at the opening because of a tight fibrous ring there, the ureteric orifice is incised with a fine diathermy electrode taking care not to touch the wire with the arc, or it will be severed (Fig. 25.46). A catheter may be left in for 24 hours, but is usually unnecessary.

Reimplantation of the ureter

1. FOR VESICOURETERIC REFLUX

In children with severe reflux and persistent infection, the ureter may be

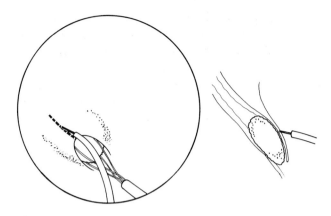

Fig. 25.46. If the stone in the basket is jammed in the ureteric orifice it may be incised with a diathermy knife.

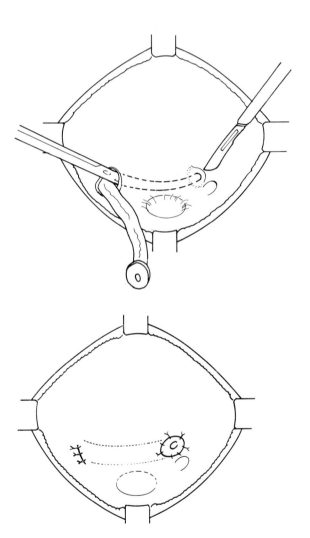

Fig. 25.47. Reimplanatation of the ureter for reflux using Cohen's method.

reimplanted with Cohen's technique as follows (Fig. 25.47). Through the open bladder, the ureteric orifice on the affected side is circumcised with a fine knife, and then drawn down into the bladder. Fine adhesions between the ureter and the detrusor have to be divided. When about 6 cm of ureter have thus been drawn into the bladder, a new tunnel is made for the ureter across the trigone, the ureter is drawn through this tunnel, and its orifice sewn into the new position. Now, when the pressure is raised with micturition, there is a long valve to prevent reflux. It is possible to perform this operation on both ureters at the same time, crossing them over.

2 FOR AN INJURED URETER—THE BOARI FLAP (Fig. 25.48)

After dissecting the ureter free from its surroundings, the distance between the free, opened-out ureter and the bladder is measured. The bladder is filled with saline, and a flap carefully marked out on its surface with stay sutures that will more than bridge the gap. It is given a wide base to provide a good blood supply.

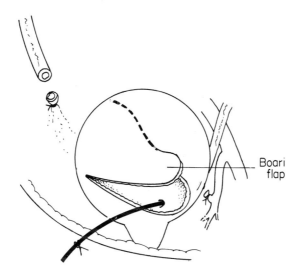

Fig. 25.48. Reimplantation of the ureter with a Boari flap: first step, making the flap of the detrusor muscle.

The ureter is then led through a short, submucosal tunnel in the Boari flap, and splinted. The flap is then sewn into the form of a tube, tethered to the tendon of Psoas minor (if there is any tendency for it not to lie straight) and the wound is closed with drainage (Fig. 25.49).

Nephroureterectomy

This is now almost restricted to cases with urothelial carcinoma of the kidney and ureter. Some surgeons prefer to place the patient in the full lateral position, others (the writer included) in the supine position. The kidney is approached

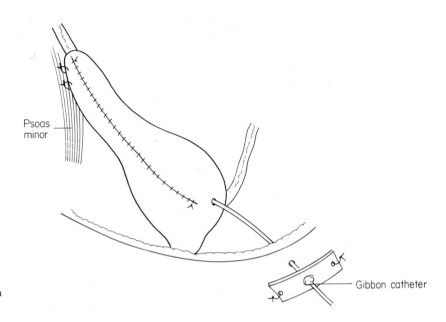

Fig. 25.49. Anastomosis of the ureter to a Boari tube over a suitable splint.

Psoas minor

Gibbon catheter

through a transverse extraperitoneal incision, its pedicle divided, and its surrounding fat removed *en bloc* together with the ureter (Fig. 25.50).

Through a second Pfannenstiel incision the bladder is exposed and opened, and an ellipse of full-thickness bladder wall incised around the ureteric orifice, drawing the ureter into the bladder until (as in the reimplant operation) the ureter is freed. Then the ellipse of bladder on the ureter is withdrawn along with

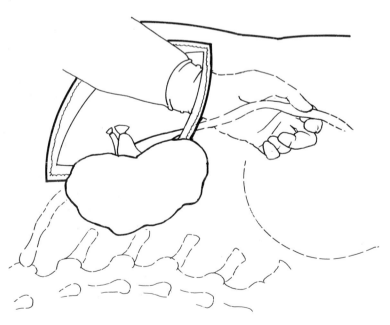

Fig. 25.50. Incisions for nephroureterectomy.

Chapter 25/*Urological Surgery*

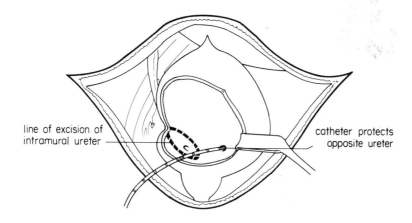

line of excision of intramural ureter

catheter protects opposite ureter

Fig. 25.51. Removal of an ellipse of the bladder around the ureteric orifice.

the kidney through the uppermost incision (Fig. 25.51). Both incisions are closed with drainage to the lower one.

If the cuff of bladder is not taken around the ureteric orifice there is a tendency to leave some of the intramural ureter behind from which new tumours may arise.

Urinary diversion

A. ILEAL CONDUIT

There are many indications for making an ileal conduit (see page 306), of which the most common and most important is the need to divert the urinary stream after total cystectomy for cancer.

Mechanical preparation of the bowel prevents some postoperative distension. The writer prefers antibiotics in most of his patients because their urine is nearly always infected.

The terminal ileum is examined, and viewed through transmitted light so that the vessels of the mesentery can be clearly seen. One tries to make sure that there are at least two large branches of the ileocolic artery supplying the chosen loop of ileum. An isolated loop of ileum is prepared, and the gap in the mesentery closed after anastomosing the ends of the ileum together end to end in the usual two layers (Fig. 25.52).

The contents of the ileal loop are washed out, and 1% neomycin used to irrigate it clean. The ureters are brought together so that their ends lie side by side (Fig. 25.53). This will mean that the left ureter must be brought behind the mesosigmoid to reach the right side easily. The distal ends of each ureter are slit up for 2 cm and their adjacent edges sewn together with catgut. These flat conjoined ends of the ureters are then sewn to one end of the ileum over two suitably sized nasogastric tubes to serve as splints. The other end of the ileum is brought through the abdominal wall and everted on itself and sewn to the skin like any other bowel stoma (Fig. 25.54).

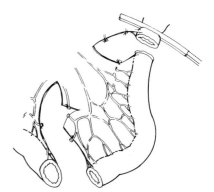

Fig. 25.52. Preparation of an isolated ileal loop. The small bowel continuity is restored by end-to-end anastomosis.

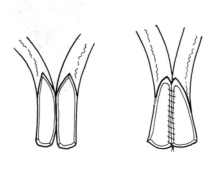

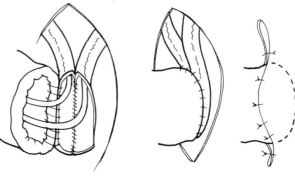

Fig. 25.53. The ureters are spatulated, sewn side to side, and both joined on to the open end of the ileal loop by Wallace's method over suitable splints.

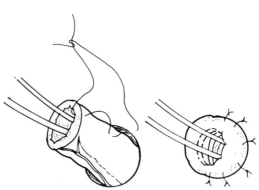

Fig. 25.54. Formation of the urinary ileal stoma. This may be flush, or everted.

There are many complications after making an ileal loop, particularly when it is done after total cystectomy. Prolonged ileus is the chief worry, but leakage of urine from the anastomosis may require reoperation. Intestinal obstruction, wound infection and wound dehiscence all occur in the elderly and irradiated patient, but in the young person, when an ileal diversion is done for incontinence, these complications are very uncommon.

B. URETEROURETEROSTOMY-EN-Y

When the ureters are very dilated one may make one of them into a useful and

Chapter 25/*Urological Surgery*

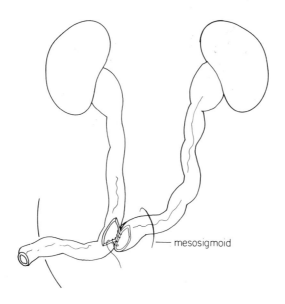

Fig. 25.55. Ureterostomy-en-Y. One ureter is joined end-to-side to the other, over suitable splints. Here the left ureter is led behind the mesosigmoid to be joined to the right. The right is led through the skin.

effective stoma, and join the other to its side in the pelvis (Fig. 25.55). Both ureters are temporarily splinted. The wider one is led out onto the skin and sewn to a Z incision in the skin to help prevent subsequent stenosis (Fig. 25.56). It is a most useful procedure after cystectomy, when feasible, and avoids the complications that occur when an ileal loop and a bowel anastomosis are added to those that complicate cystectomy anyway.

The chief complication is stenosis of the ureterostomy stoma and one must be prepared, if necessary, to convert the ureteric stoma to an ileal loop.

C. URETEROSIGMOIDOSTOMY

There is still a useful operation, though its drawbacks always need to be considered. Urine is absorbed after a ureterosigmoidostomy from the large expanse of colonic mucosa offered to urine, and if urine is absorbed in large amounts, this will lead to acidosis and renal failure. Typically the patient has low potassium, high chloride and acidosis. They complain of weakness, nausea and vomiting. In addition to the metabolic hyperchloraemic acidosis, reflux of faeces occurs from the colon to the kidneys and results in interstitial nephritis and renal scarring, adding to the problems already caused by the absorption of urine. Its main advantage is that the patient need not wear a bag on an external abdominal stoma. The chief drawback in elderly people is incontinence from urine in the rectum which they find as difficult to control as they do when afflicted with diarrhoea.

After mechanical cleansing of the intestine, the mobilized ureters are led through the mesocolon and brought out near the wall of the bowel, which is then incised down to the submucosa, so that the ureter lies in a comfortable

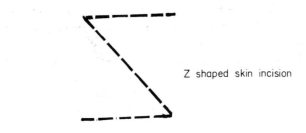

Z shaped skin incision

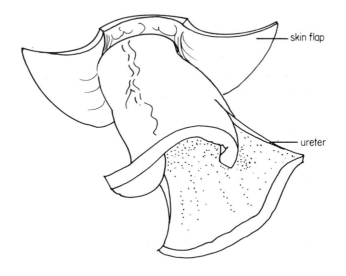

skin flap

ureter

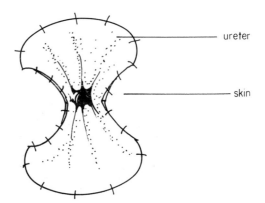

ureter

skin

Fig. 25.56. Eckstein's method of ureterostomy: a Z shaped incision in the skin forms two V shaped skin flaps that are inserted into incisions in the ureter to prevent stenosis at the suture-line.

Chapter 25/*Urological Surgery*

loose tunnel (Fig. 25.57). There the spatulated ureter is anastomosed to an elliptical hole in the colonic mucosa. The ureter is then covered with a tunnel formed by a series of sutures in the wall of the colon, placed over a thin rubber tube so as not to squeeze the ureter too tightly.

Early postoperative complications include leakage of urine from the wound, wound infection, and urinary infection. In times past when this operation was done more often, there were many leaks at the site of anastomosis, probably because pre-operative irradiation had impaired the blood supply to the wall of the ureter.

OPERATIONS ON THE BLADDER

Cystostomy or cystotomy

To open the bladder merely to deal with something wrong inside it is today very rarely necessary, since most bladder conditions can be dealt with endoscopically. Very large calculi may require an open operation, and so may the removal of some foreign bodies. It should be avoided when there is cancer in the bladder in view of the real (if rare) chance of implanting tumour in the wound. If one must open the bladder for cancer, then some pre-operative irradiation must be given to the wound to minimize the risk of implantation.

To make it easier, the bladder should be catheterized and filled with saline or water.

One may make a Pfannenstiel or vertical incision. The peritoneal reflexion must be carefully swept up from the dome of the bladder. The bladder is opened between pairs of stay-sutures (Fig. 25.58). The stone is lifted out (if that is why

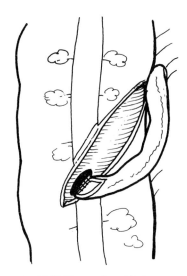

Fig. 25.57. Ureterosigmoidostomy.

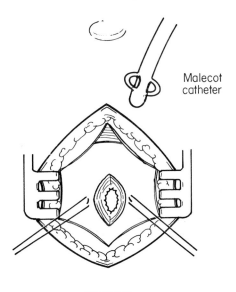

Fig. 25.58. Suprapubic cystotomy. The bladder is incised between stay sutures.

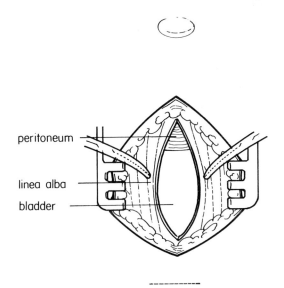

peritoneum

linea alba

bladder

Malecot catheter

the bladder is being opened) and if necessary a biopsy is taken from the place the stone has been rubbing to make sure there is no squamous metaplasia present. The bladder is closed in two layers and drained with the catheter.

Total cystectomy

Although the place of total cystectomy in the management of bladder cancer is still controversial, we are obliged to perform this operation from time to time. At the time of writing the policy in our department is to attempt to cure the bladder cancer with radical radiotherapy, and to reserve cystectomy for those patients in whom the cancer fails to disappear, who develop intractable symptoms afterwards, or who develop complications as a result of irradiation, such as haemorrhage or a contracted bladder. Widely used is an alternative approach, namely to offer patients a combination of 2000 or 4000 rads radiotherapy followed by cystectomy. Which of these two policies will give the better results is simply not known today. There is however a very significant difference in the operative difficulty of cystectomy: after radical radiotherapy the operation is very much more hazardous. Planes of cleavage are lost, fibrosis is more dense, and landmarks are confused. After 2000 rads tissues are oedematous and dissection rendered, if anything, more easy.

PRECAUTIONS BEFORE OPERATION

This is such a dangerous and difficult operation that every possible precaution must be taken to bring the patient to the table in the best possible condition. Anaemia must be fully corrected: infection must be controlled: the bowel must be prepared both mechanically and with antibiotics.

POSITION ON THE TABLE

In most instances today one will be removing the urethra along with the bladder and prostate since recurrence in the urethra occurs rather frequently in long term survivors. If the operation is being done only for palliation (e.g. because of severe symptoms) there is no point in removing the urethra.

If setting out to perform urethrectomy the patient is placed as for cystoscopy with the legs slightly flexed and held in Lloyd-Davies supports.

A catheter is passed connected to closed drainage and left in the bladder.

INCISION

A long paramedian or midline incision is made. Having ensured that there are no distant metastases to make the operation unworthwhile, the peritoneum is incised and the sigmoid and ascending colon mobilized to give access to the bifurcation of the aorta and the iliac vessels. The ureters are divided at a convenient distance, well clear of the tumour. There are three main groups of

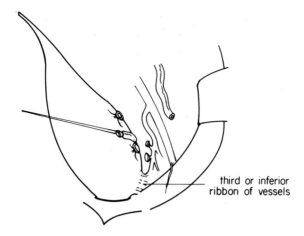

third or inferior
ribbon of vessels

Fig. 25.59. Total cystectomy: three main vascular pedicles must be divided in order to liberate the bladder.

blood vessels that supply the bladder, all entering it from laterally on the wall of the pelvis (Fig. 25.59). Each is ligated and divided in turn. As each pedicle is divided, the bladder is rendered progressively more mobile. Once the most inferior leash of vessels has been cut and secured, the urethra is dissected out through a second perineal incision, which is carried upwards through the gap between the corpora cavernosa, securing the arteries to the bulb and the main dorsal veins of the penis. The urethra is removed through a short incision because it can be evaginated from the penis (Fig. 25.60).

Once the bladder is removed great care is taken to ensure haemostasis. Bleeding tends to persist from vessels in the tissues on either side of the rectum

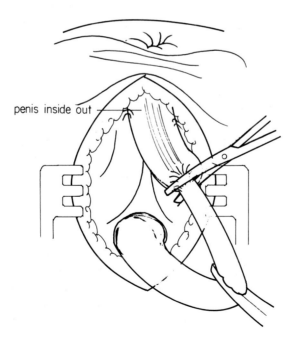

penis inside out

Fig. 25.60. Urethrectomy in continuity with the bladder through a midline incision in the perineum.

and from behind the symphysis. Metal clips are of great help in securing these vessels.

The ureters are then brought to the surface in a ureterostomy-en-Y or anastomosed to an isolated loop of ileum.

COMPLICATIONS TO WATCH FOR

Blood loss that is uncorrected on the table must be replaced as soon as possible, and one must measure the haematocrit carefully during the first 24 hours postoperatively. Ileus is prolonged and severe, and the patient is much better if his calorie intake is kept up with parenteral hyperalimentation using a high calorie fat compound. Wound infection and wound dehiscence are regretably common complications against which more than usual care is taken in closing the incision. Prolonged drainage of lymph from the inferior perineal incision is often thought at first to be drainage of urine. If in doubt, the urea content can be measured to settle the question.

Intestinal obstruction from kinks and adhesions in the pelvis may prolong the paralytic ileus and give great confusion in the postoperative management. Whenever possible they should be treated conservatively—in which parenteral hyperalimentation has proved to be a great help.

OPERATIONS ON THE PROSTATE

Transurethral resection for benign enlargement of the prostate

The precautions needed before TUR include all those proper to any other major operation. In particular, blood must be available: blood loss is proportionate to the amount of prostatic tissue resected and may be sudden and severe, just when least expected. Two units of blood should be available for every TUR. Antibiotic cover is given only when the urine is known to be infected.

After preliminary cystourethroscopy during which the urethra is carefully examined for stricture, the prostate for its size, and the bladder to exclude stones, the cystoscope is changed for the resectoscope to peer inside diverticula, and to exclude cancer.

There are many different details of transurethral resection of a benign gland (Fig. 25.61), but every surgeon who performs this operation aims to remove all the adenoma and leave the capsule intact. He has the great advantage over anybody doing the operation by one of the open techniques in that he can see the verumontanum and external sphincter and can make sure he avoids injury to them.

After removing all the chips of ademona, care is taken to stop the bleeding from all the arteries. Small veins can be controlled with traction on a catheter with a balloon. A narrow (say 22 Ch), three-way irrigating catheter is left in the

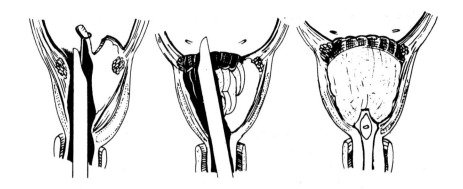

Fig. 25.61. Transurethral resection of the prostate gland. With a series of slices of the resectoscope loop, the adenoma is taken out leaving the 'capsule' intact.

bladder. This is irrigated slowly and continuously with sterile physiological saline for 24 hours or until the bleeding has stopped.

The catheter is removed as a rule after 48 hours—sometimes a little longer if the resection has been difficult or the bleeding is a little slow to stop.

Patients are allowed home about the fourth or fifth postoperative day, but must take care to avoid straining which might dislodge the clots that seal the openings of the prostatic vessels, and start bleeding. Secondary haemorrhage around the 12th postoperative day often causes a little bloodstaining of the urine, and in about 1% of patients, is enough to require clot evacuation.

COMPLICATIONS TO WATCH OUT FOR

If the catheter is blocked in the immediate postoperative period the cause may be a small fragment of prostate caught in the eye of the catheter, or a small blood clot. One must try to dislodge it with a bladder syringe, but if this does not succeed, the catheter must be changed.

Pyrexia may occur out of the blue, and signify bacteraemia. It may happen to the patient with sterile urine who has therefore not been given antibiotics, probably from organisms arising in the prostate itself. It needs intensive treatment along the usual lines adopted for bacteraemia (see page 83).

Haemorrhage occurs on the table or within the first 20 minutes afterwards, and if it is severe, the patient should be brought back to the operating theatre. It rarely occurs later on. If in doubt, and if the bleeding is severe, it is far safer to have the patient anaesthetized and to look inside the bladder to stop any bleeding vessel than to go on wasting time washing out clots and hoping that something magical will happen to cause the bleeding to stop.

Retropubic prostatectomy

If the surgical team are not experienced in transurethral work, or if the prostate is so big that TUR is not feasible or safe, the adenoma is removed by Millin's retropubic technique. After preliminary cystoscopy at which the bladder is emptied, the patient is opened through a Pfannenstiel incision, the rectus sheath

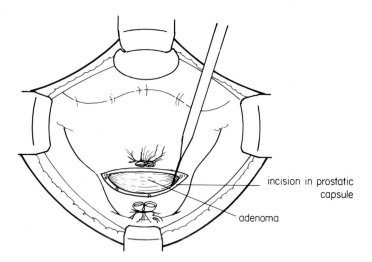

Fig. 25.62. Retropubic prostatectomy.

is parted, and the peritoneum swept upwards to expose the front of the bladder. Fat in front of the prostate is carefully dissected away to expose the large veins lying there, which are divided between two stout sutures (Fig. 25.62). An incision is made with a diathermy needle directed downwards towards the anus, just about where the prostate adenoma can be felt to merge with the detrusor of the bladder. The incision is made slowly and as many bleeding vessels are sealed with the diathermy as possible.

This incision exposes the glistening white outer surface of the adenoma. A plane of cleavage is developed with the curved scissors between the adenoma and the capsule first over one lateral lobe and then the other, until each lateral lobe is almost freed (Fig. 25.63). Then the lateral lobes are parted from each other, by breaking through the anterior commissure with the finger, which enters the cleft of the prostatic urethra, and immediately searches for the

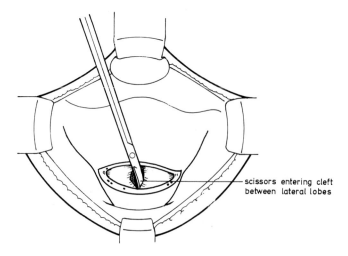

Fig. 25.63. The plane of the cleavage between the adenoma and capsule is developed, sparing the verumontanum and a strip of mucosa along the back of the prostatic urethra.

Chapter 25/*Urological Surgery*

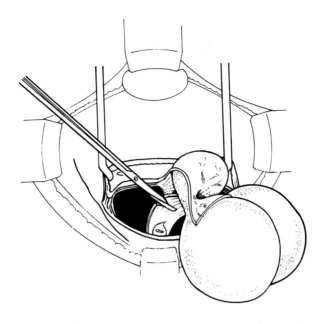

Fig. 25.64. Lateral and middle lobes are removed in one lump by dividing their remaining attachment to the prostatic urethra, preserving the verumontanum.

shallow pimple of the verumontanum. Recognizing the verumontanum, a cleft is made to one side of it, again entering the plane between adenoma and capsule, to join the original plane over the lateral lobe. The same is done on the other side. And so both lateral lobes are freed entirely, and can be lifted out into the wound (Fig. 25.64). The middle lobe has only to be dissected from the trigone with the diathermy needle and the removal of the adenoma is complete. Most of the haemorrhage is now seen to issue from the prostatic arteries at the corners of the incision in the capsule. These are secured with stout sutures. When haemostasis has been secured (and a few other small vessels may need to be underrun) a catheter is placed in the bladder. A three-day foley is now usual, but some surgeons prefer a plain catheter and leave in a suprapubic one through which, if necessary, irrigation can be carried out.

The catheters are usually removed on or about the fourth day, and the patient can usually go home about the eighth or ninth day if all is well.

COMPLICATIONS TO WATCH OUT FOR

Obstruction of the catheter by clot is the most tiresome problem after this, and any form of prostatectomy. But with all open operations on the prostate, there are additional hazards from pulmonary embolism and chest infections.

Wound infection is unfortunately rather common in patients who arrive with infected urine and an indwelling catheter. Epididymitis is now rare, but when it occurs, requires intensive and prompt antibiotic treatment. Secondary haemorrhage, stricture and incontinence are also seen, though only in a small percentage of cases.

Chapter 25/*Urological Surgery*   355

Transsvesical prostatectomy

This is the oldest of all forms of prostatectomy. It is still in use, though seldom indicated. Through an opening in the bladder the mucosa around the bulging lobes of the prostate is incised with scissors or diathermy, and the plane of cleavage between adenoma and capsule that was formed in the Millin operation, formed here but more blindly, and usually with the finger-tip. Eventually the lateral lobes are 'enucleated' (Fig. 25.65).

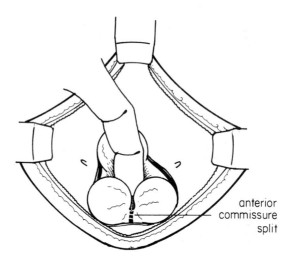

anterior
commissure
split

Fig. 25.65. Transvesical prostatectomy.

The difficulty here is that the crucial part of the operation, the preservation of the sphincter apparatus adjacent to and just downstream of the verumontanum, has to be done completely by feel. Worse, haemostasis is difficult because the access to the vessels is so indirect across the open bladder. Because of this, various big haemostatic sutures are used in the corners of the hole left by the prostate, or as a purse-string around the catheter to serve as a tamponade. It has all the disadvantages of any open procedure but is fortunately extremely easy and quick.

The one advantage of the transvesical operation is that it can be combined with other procedures that call for an opening into the bladder, such as the (rare) open removal of a huge calculus or the excision of a vesical diverticulum.

Urethral operations

Dilatation and internal urethrotomy have been described above (see page 256). They remain the mainstay of urethral surgery, but have in recent years been supplemented by a number of open plastic operations—urethroplasty. There are several different versions. The following are those in use in the writer's practice.

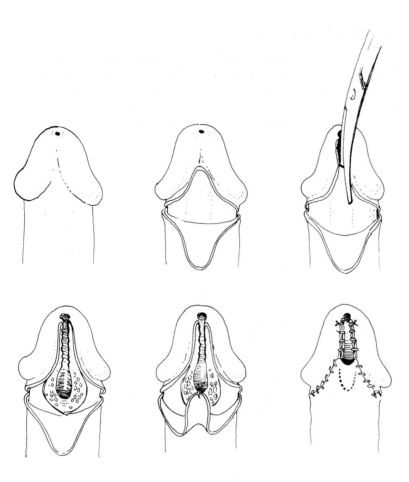

Fig. 25.66. Meatoplasty.

MEATOPLASTY (Fig. 25.66)

Through a short, U-shaped flap, the tight distal meatal stricture is slit open until one comes into normal urethra. The flap is then let into the urethral incision as a gusset to keep it permanently widened. The end result is an oval meatus a little further back from the tip of the penis than the normal one, but it does not undergo stenosis. Unfortunately patients find that the stream sprays a bit afterwards and they must relearn how to control it.

ANTERIOR URETHRAL STRICTURES

These are now all dealt with by the island patch urethroplasty (Fig. 25.67). The patch of skin is marked out on a bougie to ensure that it is neither too big nor too small. It is provided with a pedicle of dartos to maintain viability. A splinting narrow silicone catheter is left in position for 14 days.

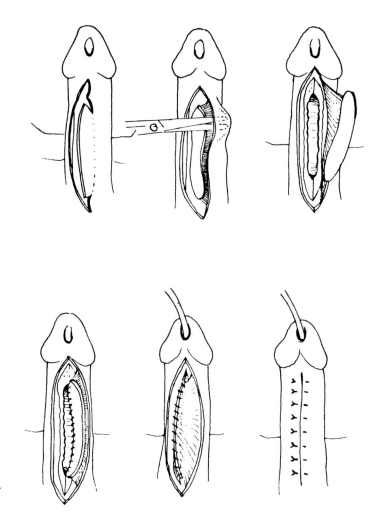

Fig. 25.67. One-stage, island-patch urethroplasty.

POSTERIOR URETHRAL STRICTURES

If uncomplicated by fistulae and infection, these are all dealt with by a modification of the island patch, in which the patch of skin is taken from the tip of a scrotal U shaped flap (Fig. 25.68).

After dividing the stricture right through the patch of skin on its little 'mesentery' of dartos, it is sewn into the defect with 3-0 chromic catgut, and a silicone catheter is left in position for 14 days.

When the strictures are complicated by sinuses and infection, one cannot rely on this one-stage operation, and it is still occasionally necessary to perform the urethroplasty in two stages. At the first (Fig. 25.69) the stricture is laid open and as many of the sinuses and fistulae and abscesses laid open too, while the defect is bridged with a generous U-shaped flap of scrotal skin. This is left in

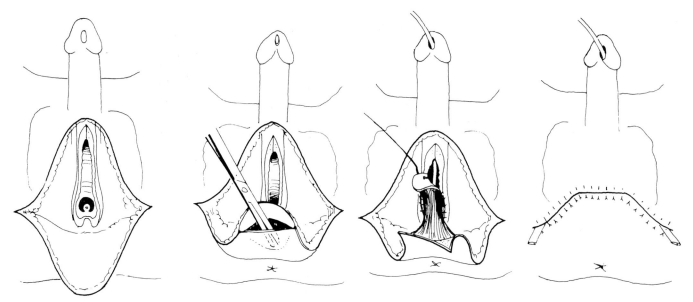

Fig. 25.68. One-stage, island-patch urethroplasty for posterior strictures, based on the tip
of a scrotal flap.

Fig. 25.69. Method of dealing with posterior
strictures—two-stage, scrotal flap urethroplasty for stricture of the posterior urethra.

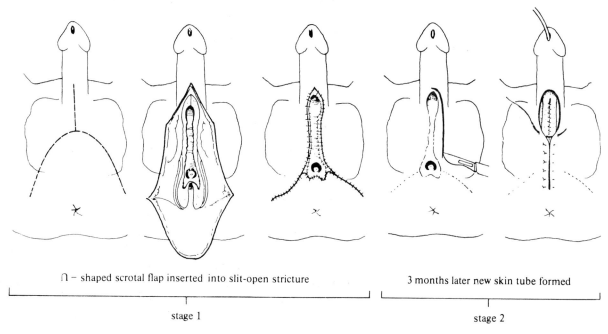

∩ – shaped scrotal flap inserted into slit-open stricture

3 months later new skin tube formed

stage 1

stage 2

position as a kind of perineal urethrostomy for several months until all the scrotal and perineal induration have resolved. When the skin is all supple and healthy, the urethral tube is reconstituted at a second stage.

Operations on the testicle

ORCHIDOPEXY (Fig. 25.70)

Through an incision in the skin crease sited over the internal inguinal ring

Fig. 25.70. Orchidopexy.

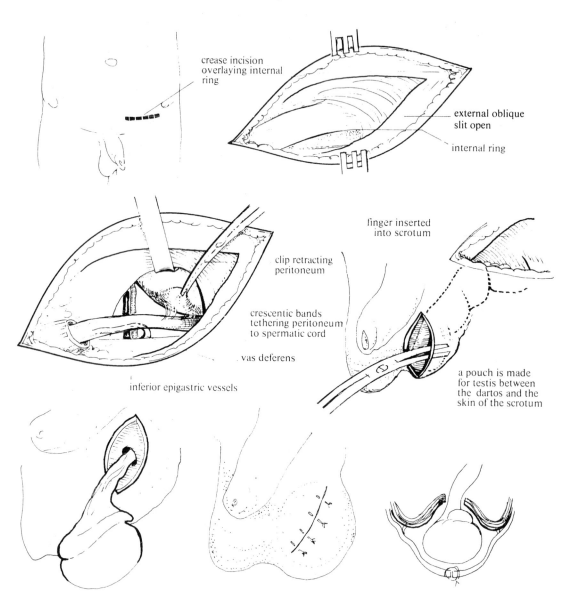

Chapter 25/*Urological Surgery*

(where the major part of the dissection is to be carried out) the external oblique is slit along its fibres to reveal the spermatic cord. On the anterior aspect of the cord is found the processus vaginalis of the peritoneum, and the hernial sac if one is present. The processus is dissected off the cord, and the plane between them continued right up behind the main abdominal peritoneum, carefully dividing the crescentic bands of 'adhesions' that stick the spermatic vessels firmly to the peritoneum. When these are all liberated, one usually has plenty of length in the spermatic cord to allow the testicle to be placed in the scrotum. To

Fig. 25.71. Orchidectomy.

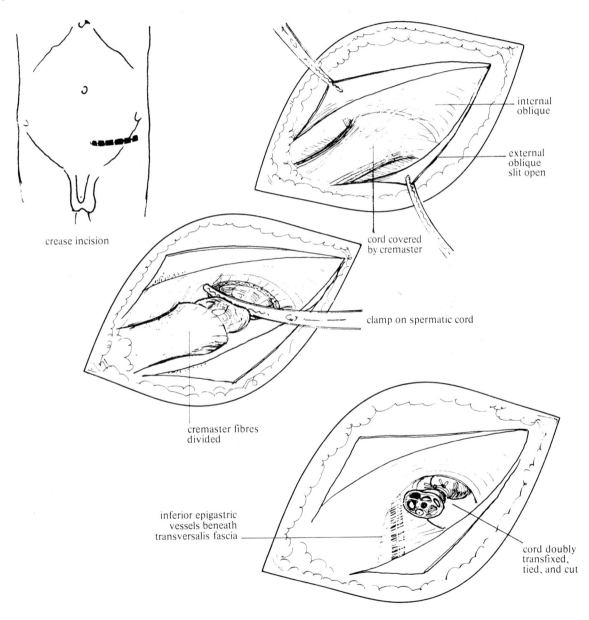

crease incision

internal oblique

external oblique slit open

cord covered by cremaster

clamp on spermatic cord

cremaster fibres divided

inferior epigastric vessels beneath transversalis fascia

cord doubly transfixed, tied, and cut

keep it there a little pouch is formed in the plane between the skin and the dartos at the bottom of the scrotal sac. Rubber bands and traction are not necessary if the preliminary liberation of the spermatic vessels has been complete.

ORCHIDECTOMY FOR TESTICULAR TUMOUR (Fig. 25.71)

The scrotal skin must not be incised for fear of allowing testicular tumour to get into the lymphatic catchment system of the scrotum and hence into the inguinal nodes. Instead, a transverse incision is made in the skin crease over the internal inguinal ring, the external oblique is opened, and a clamp placed on the spermatic cord to occlude all its vessels before any manipulation of the testicle begins. Then the testicle is delivered up from the scrotum, with the help of a little counterpressure over the scrotum. Usually the diagnosis is all too obvious and one proceeds at once to transfix and ligate the spermatic cord upsteam of the clamp before cutting it across. If there is doubt about the diagnosis the wound area may be towelled off and the testicle incised, and a frozen section obtained to confirm what is usually all too tragically evident.

SUBCAPSULAR ORCHIDECTOMY FOR PROSTATIC CANCER (Fig. 25.72)

Through a small incision in the scrotum, first one testis and then the other is squeezed into the wound, the tunica vaginalis is incised, the soft testicular tubules wiped away with gauze, and with a running 3-0 catgut suture the testicular vessels and then the tunica vaginalis are oversewn to stop bleeding and to close the tunica. A haematoma forms inside the tunica which, for a time, resembles the testis, but gradually shrinks away.

In certain cases a plastic prosthesis may be inserted inside the tunica before closing it.

TESTICULAR BIOPSY (Fig. 25.73)

Through a small scrotal incision, the tunica vaginalis is punctured with a sharp

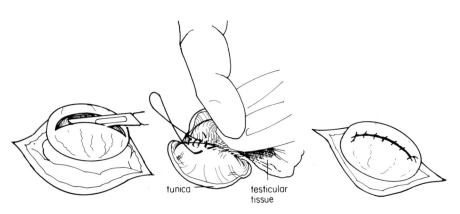

tunica   testicular
tissue

Fig. 25.72. Subcapsular orchidectomy for cancer of the prostate.

Chapter 25/*Urological Surgery*

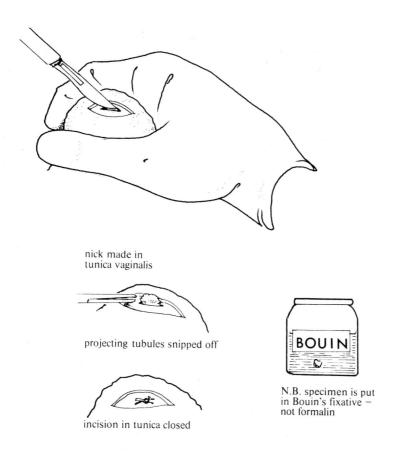

nick made in
tunica vaginalis

projecting tubules snipped off

incision in tunica closed

BOUIN

N.B. specimen is put
in Bouin's fixative –
not formalin

Fig. 25.73. Biopsy of the testis.

knife. Tubules well out of the incision are snipped off with very sharp fine-pointed scissors, and are plunged at once into a pot of Bouin's fixative. The biopsy must not be prodded or pinched with forceps or the tubules will be distorted and formalin must never be used as a fixative.

The tiny hole is closed with a 4-0 chromic catgut suture.

Operations for Hydrocele

TAPPING A HYDROCELE

This is still a useful manoeuvre that can be repeated when the hydrocele fills up again and is much less dangerous to a sick and elderly patient than a curative operation (Fig. 25.74).

It is essential to provide yourself with a sharp trochar and cannula, and since these are so hard to come by today, a disposable 'intracath' as used for intravenous injections, is next best. Shine a bright light through the scrotum to check that the site you select for insertion of the needle is well away from the testis and any large subcutaneous veins. Inject a drop or two of 1% lignocaine into the skin after cleansing it with povidone-iodine. Nick the skin with a

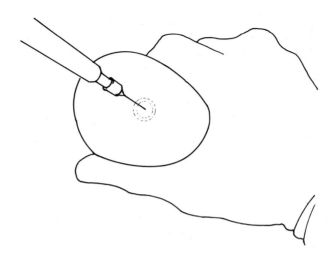

Fig. 25.74. Tapping a hydrocele.

sharp-pointed knife, and then plunge the intracath into the lumen of the hydrocele, aiming it away from the testis. Withdraw the trochar and allow the fluid to escape from the hydrocele into a sterile receiver. When the hydrocele is all emptied out, compress the lips of the little puncture firmly for one minute and apply a drop of collodion or spray dressing.

Complications to watch out for include haemorrhage into the hydrocele (haematocele) if you have inadvertently opened a vein, infection, and laceration of the testicle (which will give pain).

RADICAL CURE OF A HYDROCELE

Many elderly men are content with occasionally having their hydroceles tapped, and this is safe and sensible surgical practice. But in young men where the fluid soon fills up the sac, or in anyone who finds the procedure irksome or

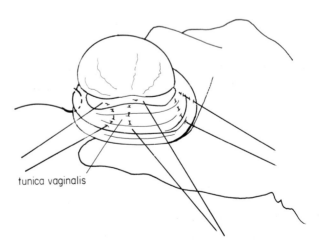

tunica vaginalis

Fig. 25.75. Lord's operation for hydrocele.

Chapter 25/*Urological Surgery*

painful, a radical cure can be offered. If the hydrocele wall is thin, Lord's operation is quick and reliable. Through a very short scrotal incision the wall of the hydrocele is seized, opened, its fluid expelled, and then with a series of rucking-up, catgut sutures, the surplus hydrocele wall is bunched into a frill, all around the testicle (Fig. 25.75). The testicle is then firmly replaced and the skin closed. If the hydrocele is thick and of long-standing it is not possible to bunch it up in this way and the sac is removed, care being taken to oversew the thick wall of the sac all the way round to stop haemorrage (Fig. 25.76).

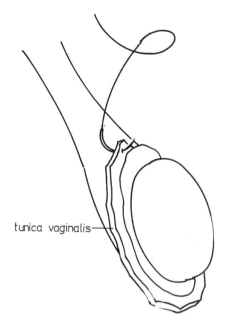

tunica vaginalis

Fig. 25.76. Radical cure for a hydrocele.

COMPLICATIONS TO WATCH OUT FOR

All operations on the scrotum are likely to be followed by haematoma, for its veins are so thin and the tissues so slack there is nothing to prevent blood oozing from veins however slightly they may have been breached. Hence the most obsessional care must be taken to prevent haemorrhage on the table, to stop it when it occurs, and to keep the scrotum firmly supported afterwards. The usual method is to strap the scrotum tightly onto the groin with adhesive plaster or tape for the first 12 postoperative hours.

Vasectomy

Vasectomy for sterilization is becoming a common procedure, but its complications are becoming increasingly the subject of bitter and expensive litigation. It is most important that great care is taken to select only those patients who are stable and mature (see page 294) and who understand fully the implications—the risk of haematoma, the chance of late recanalization, the occasional postoperative sepsis and pain, and the need to use other methods of contraception until no more live sperms can be found in the ejaculate.

A general anaesthetic should be used where the patient is apprehensive, or has had previous surgical procedures done in the groin such as orchidopexy or hernia repair.

In other cases one may use a local anaesthetic. Through a midline incision, or two small ones at the neck of the scrotum on each side, the vas is seized in specially curved forceps (Fig. 25.77), infiltrated with anaesthetic, slit along its sheath, and then drawn out, doubly clamped, cut, and one end turned back on itself. It is usual to send a small portion of vas for histological confirmation that it was the vas deferens that was in fact removed. Meticulous haemostasis must be used throughout (see page 296).

REJOINING VASA AFTER VASECTOMY

This is a much more difficult operation and needs a general anaesthetic. A larger exposure is necessary in order to dissect out the healthy vas on either side of the previous vasectomy. A firm lump usually marks the site of one or both cut ends. This is traced up to the healthy vas, and on the testicular end, to a dilated lumen

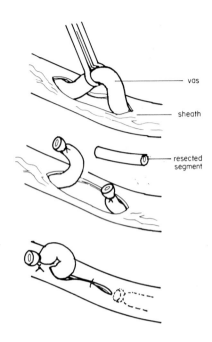

Fig. 25.77. Vasectomy.

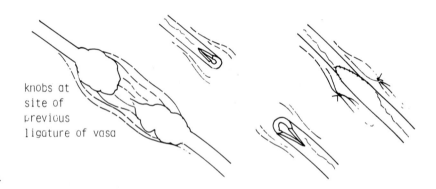

knobs at
site of
previous
ligature of vasa

Fig. 25.78. Reanastomosis of the vas deferens.

out of which turbid sperm-rich fluid can be seen to ooze. Using the help of a magnifying loupe or dissecting microscope the ends are sutured together using 8-0 prolene or similar, very fine, suture material. The tension is taken off the anastomosis by bringing together the fibrous sheath of the vas with heavier suture material (Fig. 25.78).

EPIDIDYMOVASOSTOMY (Fig. 25.79)

Through a scrotal incision the vas and epididymis are displayed, and the part of

Chapter 25/*Urological Surgery*

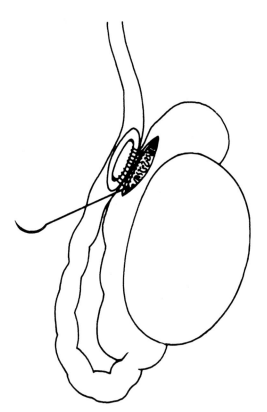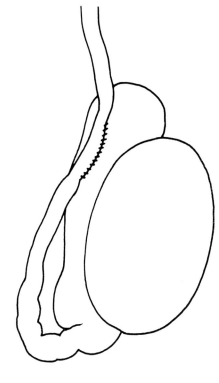

the epididymis which is obviously seen to be stuffed with sperm-filled tubules is selected. The selection is confirmed by aspirating sperms from this area with a fine syringe and checking them under a microscope in the operating theatre. Using loupe or operating microscope a longitudinal incision is made in the vas deferens, until the lumen is opened for about 4 mm. The patency of the urethral end of the vas may be confirmed by injecting methylene blue, and showing that it issues from a urethral catheter or by filling the vas with contrast and obtaining a vasogram radiograph. The slit in the vas is then anastomosed to the selected site in the epididymis using 8-0 fine suture material of stainless steel nylon or polypropylene. Some surgeons like to leave a splint in position: the writer prefers not to.

Fig. 25.79. Epididymovasostomy.

FURTHER READING

Blandy J.P. (1978) *Operative Urology*. Blackwell Scientific Publications, Oxford.
Blandy J.P. (1978) *Transurethral Resection*, 2nd edn. Pitman Medical, Tunbridge Wells.
Marston A., Chamberlain G.V.P. & Blandy J.P. (eds) (1979) *Contemporary Operative Surgery*. Northwood Books, London.
Mitchell J.P. (1981) *Endoscopic Operative Urology*. Wright, Bristol.

Albarran, Joaquin (1860–1912). Cuban urologist working in Paris. Described pedunculated 'middle lobe' of prostrate and invented the Albarran lever on the catheterizing cystoscope.

ampulla. Latin, a flask.

Anderson–Hynes. Method of pyeloplasty devised by James Christie Anderson, urologist, Royal Hospital, Sheffield and Wilfred Hynes, plastic surgeon, United Sheffield Hospitals. (See Anderson (1963). *Hydronephrosis*. William Heinemann Medical Books, London.)

Avicenna (1037). Abu Ali Hussein Ibn Sina. Iranian physician. Used soft catheters of leather, and of silver. (See Hanafy M.H. *et al.* (1976) *Urology*, **8**, 63.)

balanitis. Greek, βάλανος, the glans penis, xerotica obliterans (Greek, dry; Latin, obliterating).

Behçet, Hulúsi (1889–1948). Turkish dermatologist. Described a syndrome including ulceration of mouth, genitalia, uveitis, iridocyclitis.

Belfield, W.T. American urologist who probably did the first open prostatectomy intentionally. (See Belfield W.T. (1887) *J. Am. med. Ass.*, **8**, 303.)

Bellini, Lorenzo (1643–1704). Anatomist of Pisa. Described, among many other things, the straight collecting tubules of the renal papilla.

Benedict, Stanley Rossiter (1884–1936). Biochemist of Cornell University, USA. Described test for sugar in the urine.

Bertin, Exupère Joseph (1712–81). Associate anatomist at the Academy of Sciences in Paris.

Bigelow, Henry Jacob (1818–90). Surgeon of Boston, USA. (See Bigelow H.J. (1879) Lithotrity by a single operation. *Boston Med. Surg. J.* (later *New Eng. J. Med.*), **98**, 259 and 291.)

Bilharz, Theodor Maximilian (1825–62). German physician working in Cairo who first described *Schistosoma haematobium*; hence Bilharziasis.

Boari, Achille (1894). Italian urologist who devised bladder flap procedure for bridging gap at lower end of ureter.

bougie. French, candle (wax 'bougies' were often used to dilate urethral strictures).

Bouin, Paul (1870). Histologist of Strasbourg. Described fixative for testicular biopsies containing picric acid, acetic acid and formalin.

Bowman, Sir William (1816–92). Ophthalmic surgeon of London. Described the capsule of the glomerulus and recognized that it was extruded from the end of the renal tubule.

Braasch, W.F. Urologist of the Mayo Clinic. Described many urological conditions and invented many instruments, of which the bulb-ended ureteric catheter is best known today.

Bricker, Eugene M. Professor of Surgery, Washington University School of Medicine, St. Louis. Described ileal conduit. (See Bricker E.M. (1950) Bladder substitution after pelvic evisceration. *Surg. Clin. N. Am.*, **30**, 1511.)

Bright, Richard (1789–1859). Guy's Hospital Physician.

Browne, Sir Denis (1892–1967). Paediatric surgeon at Great Ormond Street Hospital for Children. Invented operation for hypospadias. (See *Postgrad. med. J.* (1949), **25**, 367.)

Brown–Buerger. One of the best cystoscopes was devised by Tilden Brown and Leo Buerger. (See A new combination observation catheterizing and operating cystoscope. *N.Y. Med. J.*, Aug. 25, 1917.)

von Brunn, A. (1841–1895). Professor of Anatomy, Göttingen. Described cell nests in chronic cystitis. (See *Arch. Mikr. Anat.* (1893) **41**, 294.)

Buck, Gordon (1807–77). New York surgeon who described the deep fascia of the corpora cavernosa of the penis.

Calix. Greek κύλιξ, cup; 'confused by modern scientific writers with Graeco-Latin *calyx* and written calyx' (OED).

calyx. Greek κάλυξ, from root καλύπτειν. Often confused with calix. The whorl of leaves forming the outer covering of the flower while in the bud.

Carr, R.J. Contemporary radiologist, Bradford. Described his tiny concretions and worked with Henry Hamilton Stewart in studying the 'stone nest theory' of calculus formation.

Charrière, Joseph (1803–76). Instrument maker of Paris. Made instruments for Civiale (1792–1867) and many other celebrated French surgeons. Made the first effective lithotrite. Devised the French (logical) metric system of catheter sizes, the number signifying the circumference of the instrument in millimetres.

Chevassu, M. Urologist of Paris. Made many contributions including a useful bulb-ended catheter for the ureter. His thesis (Paris, 1906) first clearly distinguished between seminoma and teratoma and urged early and radical orchidectomy.

chordée. A painful downward concavity of the penis. Originally associated with inflammation of the corpora cavernosa from gonorrhoea (chaudepisse cordée) it is now used more often for the bend associated with hypospadias.

Clutton, Henry (1888). The curved steel bougies named after him were copied from those recommended by Otis (q.v.) and Clutton never pretended otherwise.

Glossary of Urological Eponyms and Jargon

Colles, Abraham (1773–1843). Professor of Surgery in Dublin. Described the tough layer of superficial fascia of the perineum. (See *A Treatise on Surgical Anatomy*, Edinburgh, 1811.)

Collings, C.W. Early exponent of TUR: knife named after him. (See *J. Urol.* (1926) **16**, 545.)

coudé. French, elbowed—a shape of catheter invented by Mercier of Paris.

Cowper, William (1666–1709). Anatomist and surgeon of London who described the glands sandwiched in the levator ani behind the bulbar urethra.

Culp, Ormond. Chief of Urology, Mayo Clinic.

Cushing, Harvey Williams (1869–1939). Surgeon of Boston, the father of modern neuro-surgery.

Denonvilliers, Charles Pierre (1808–72). Surgeon and anatomist of Paris. Remembered for the fascia formed by fusion of the layers of peritoneum between rectum and prostate. (See L'anatomie du Perinée. *Bull. Soc. Anat. Paris* (1836), **12**, 106.)

Dietl, Joseph (1804–78). Pathologist of Cracow. Described the episodes of pain of intermittent hydronephrosis—the so-called Dietl's crises.

dilate. Latin, dilatare, whence *dilatation*. The shorter 'dilation' is wrong.

Dormia, Enrico. Contemporary assistant Professor of Urology, Milan. Devised his basket for dislodging stones, and now celebrated for methods for dissolving calculi with continuous ureteric irrigation.

Ducrey, Augosto (1860–1940). Dermatologist of Rome. Described the *Haemophilus ducreyi* which causes soft chancre.

Duplay, Simon (1836–1921). Surgeon of Paris. Devised an operation for urethral stricture similar to that of Denis Browne. (See Injuries and disease of the urethra. *Int. Encycl. Surg.* (1886), **6**, 487.)

enuresis. Greek ἐνουρεῖν, incontinence of urine. Today generally applied to bed-wetting, which should strictly be called nocturnal enuresis.

epididymis. Greek, ἐπι upon, and δίδυμοι, twins (testes).

epispadias. Greek, ἐπι and σπάδον, a rent or tear.

Escherich, Theodor (1857–1911). Paediatrician of Munich who described *Bacillus coli*, now named *Escherichia coli* in his memory.

extrophy, Greek ἐξ and τροφή, nutrition.

Fallopius, Gabriel (1523–62). Polymath of Padua, favourite pupil of Vesalius.

Fenwick, Hurry (1856–1944). Surgeon at St Peter's and The London Hospital. Introduced the new-fangled electric cystoscope to England, founded the International Society of Urology and pioneered retrograde urography.

Foley, Frederic Eugene Basil (1891–1966). Urologist of Minneapolis–St. Paul. Devised self-retaining balloon catheter and a method of pyeloplasty.

fossa. Latin, ditch.

Fournier, Jean Alfred (1832–1914). Venereologist and dermatologist at Hôpital St. Louis, Paris. Described Fournier's gangrene.

fraenum, fraenulum. From Latin, fraenum, a bridle.

Freyer, Sir Peter J. (1851–1921). Surgeon at St. Peter's Hospital. Brilliant Irish surgeon. Won international fame by litholapaxy in children in India and later perfected the method of transvesical prostatectomy now named after him.

Fuller, Eugene (1858–1930). New York urologist. Made many contributions to urology including the transvesical operation. (See *J. cutan. genit. Dis.* (1895) **13**, 229.)

fundus. Latin, bottom. The bottom or the part furthest from the orifice.

Gerota, Dumitru (1867–1939). Anatomist of Budapest. Described the posterior fascia of the kidney. (See *Arch. Anat. Leipsig* (1895), 265.)

Gersuny, Robert (1844–1924). Surgeon of Vienna. Attempted to devise method of urinary bladder substitution using rectum for urine, and bringing faecal stream through anal sphincter (his case died).

Gibbon, Norman. Contemporary urological surgeon, Sefton Hospital, Liverpool. Devised narrow plastic catheter for use in paraplegics.

Gil-Vernet, J.M. Contemporary Spanish surgeon of Barcelona. Devised extended pyelolithotomy through renal sinus.

Giraldes, Joachim (1808–75). Professor of Surgery, Paris. (See *C.R. Soc. Biol. Paris* (1859), 123.)

Grawitz, Paul Albert (1850–1932). Pathologist of Greifswald. (See *Virchow's Archiv.* (1883), **93**, 39.)

gum elastic. Catheters formerly made of silk, woven and impregnated with gum. Invented by Bernard (a Parisian jeweller) in 1779.

Guthrie, Sir George James (1785–1856). Hero of Waterloo and Surgeon to the Westminster Hospital. Pioneer of TUR.

Harris, Samuel Henry (1880–1937). Urologist of Sydney, Australia, who published first safe and antiseptic transvesical, one-stage prostatectomy series. (See *Brit. J. Surg.* (1933), **21**, 434.)

Helmstein, Karl. Contemporary Swedish urologist, Stockholm.

Henle, Freidrich (1809–85). Anatomist of Berlin.

Henoch, E. (1820–1910). Paediatrician, Berlin.

Hopkins, Professor Harry. Contemporary Professor of Optics, University of Reading. Devised modern rod-lens system, and flexible fibre-optic cable used throughout modern urology.

Hunner, Guy Leroy (1868–1951). Gynaecologist at Johns Hopkins Hospital, Baltimore. Described interstitial cystitis. (See Hunner G.L. *Boston Med. Surg. J.* (1914), 660.)

hyaline. Greek ὕαλος, glass.

hydatid. Greek ὕδωρ, drop of water.

hydrocele. Greek κήλη, swelling, like κοίλακος, belly: often misspelt hydrocoele, from confusion with κοίλος, hollow, hence coelom: means watery swelling.

hypospadias. Greek ὑπο, below, σπάδον, a rent or tear.

Jaboulay Mathieu (1860–1913). Surgeon of Lyons.

Jacques, Frère Jacques de Beaulieu (1651–1714). Itinerant lithotomist through lateral approach. (See Barrett (1949) *Ann. Roy. Coll. Surg. Eng.*, **5**, 275.)

Jaques, James Archibald (1815–1878). Works manager, William Warne and Co. Ltd., Barking, Essex. Improved and patented soft rubber catheter.

Johanson, Bengt. Contemporary surgeon, Stockholm. Pioneer of urethroplasty.

Kidd, Frank, S. (1878–1934). London Hospital surgeon. Invented the 'big-ball' diathermy cystoscope.

Klinefelter, E.W. Contemporary radiologist, Massachusetts General Hospital.

Kolff, W.J. Contemporary nephrologist. Pioneer of first effective artificial kidney in Holland during Nazi occupation, 1944. Now at Cleveland.

Leadbetter, Wyland (1911–74). Distinguished urologist of Boston.

Leydig, Franz von (1821–1908). Anatomist and zoologist of Bonn.

litho. Greek λίθος, stone, *-tripsy*, Greek τρίβειν, wear away, τομή cut, λάπαξις, evacuation.

Littre, Alexis (1658–1726). Anatomist of Paris.

Loewenstein–Jensen. Culture medium for tuberculosis. Ernst Loewenstein (1878), pathologist of Vienna and Carl Oluf Jensen (1864–1934), pathologist of Copenhagen.

Lowsley, O.S. (1884–1955). New York urologist.

McCarthy, Joseph Francis (1874–1965). New York urologist. Inventor of the foroblique lens, and the 'panendoscope'.

malakoplakia. Greek μαλακός, soft and πλακεία, plaque.

Malécot, Achille Etienne (b. 1852). Described his winged self-retaining catheter in 1892. (See Outwin E.L. (1955), The development of the modern catheter. *J. Am. Surg. Tech.*, **1**, 8.)

Malpighi, Marcello (1628–94). Anatomist, physician, polymath of Rome and Bologna. Described just about everything.

Marchetti, A.A., see below.

Marshall, Victor F. Contemporary urologist at New York Memorial Hospital. (See Marshall V.F., Marchetti A.A. and Krantz K.E. (1949) The correction of stress incontinence by simple vesicourethral suspension. *Surg. Gynec. Obstet.*, **88**, 509.)

Marion, Georges (1869–1960). French urologist of Paris. Described many conditions, especially 'prostatisme sans prostate', i.e. bladder neck stenosis, which is sometimes called after him, though it was described by John Hunter, Morgagni, Valsalva and Ambroise Paré beforehand.

meatus (pl. meatus). Latin, a passage or channel.

micturition. From Latin, micturire, derived from mingere, to mix (originally meant the desire to make water, implying 'a morbid frequency in the making of urine: often erroneously the action of making water'. OED).

Millin, Terence. Contemporary urological surgeon. Described retropubic prostatectomy. (See Livingstone E. & S. (1947) *Retropubic Urinary Surgery*. Edinburgh.)

Morgagni, Giovanni Battista (1682–1771). Anatomist and pathologist of Padua.

Morris, Sir Henry (1844–1926). Surgeon trained at Guy's Hospital, London, worked at the Middlesex Hospital. Did the first deliberate removal of a calculus from the kidney. (See *Invest. Urol.* (1973), **11**, 170.)

Müller, Johannes (1801–58). Physiologist of Berlin. Described the paramesonephric ducts and the organs (Müllerian this and Müllerian that) which are derived from them.

navicularis. Latin, having the shape of a small boat.

Neisser, Albert Ludwig Siegmund (1855–1916). Dermatologist of Breslau. (See *Centr. med. Wiss.* (1879), **17**, 497.)

neph. νέφρος, Greek, kidney; -ectomy, -itis, -stomy, etc.

nexus. Latin, a tying together (like connected, knitted, etc.).

Nitze, Max. Professor of Urology in Berlin, invented the first incandescent lamp cystoscope in 1877.

nocturia. The discharge of an abnormally large quantity of urine at night.

Otis, Fessenden Nott (1825–1900). American urologist who devoted his life to the study of the urethra.

Paget, Sir James (1814–99). Surgeon, St. Bartholomew's Hospital, London. (See *St. Barts. Hosp. Rep.* (1874), **10, 87.**)

Papanicolaou, G.N. (1883–1962). Greek pathologist working in New York. (See Cytology of the urinary sediment in neoplasms of the urinary tract. *J. Urol.* (1947), **57, 375.**)

papilloma. Latin papilla, a nipple, and Greek -oma, tumour.

Politano. Victor. Contemporary urologist, Miami, Florida.

Peyronie, François de la (1678–1747). Surgeon of Paris.

Pfannenstiel, Hermann Johann (1862–1909). Gynaecologist of Breslau. Described the lower abdominal incision named after him.

polyuria. Greek poly, much, and uria. An increase in the amount of urine excreted, usually implies frequency.

Queyrat, L. Dermatologist of Paris. (See Queyrat, L. (1911) Erythroplasie du gland. *Bull. Soc. Franç. Derm. Syph.* **22, 378.**) Described carcinoma *in situ* of penis, already described by Paget (1874).

Randall, Alexander (1883–1951). Urologist of Philadelphia. Made many contributions including the description of the various lobes of the prostate and the 'bar at the neck of the bladder', as well as the Randall's plaques on the renal papillae.

Rehn, Ludwig (1849–1930). Surgeon of Frankfurt. Noticed workers in factory making fuchsin got bladder cancer.

Riches, Sir Eric. Contemporary Consulting Urologist, Middlesex Hospital.

Rovsing, N.T. (1862–1927). Professor of Surgery, Copenhagen.

Scarpa, Antonio (1747–1832). Professor of Anatomy at Pavia, Italy.

Sertoli, Enrico (1842–1910). Physiologist of Milan.

Stewart, Henry Hamilton (1904–70). Urologist of Bradford. One of the pioneers of punch resection in England; inventor of numerous, ingenious, plastic, urological procedures for urethral stricture, hydronephrosis, etc.

strangury. From Greek στράγξ, drop squeezed out, and οὖρον, urine. Slow and painful emission of urine.

teratoma. From Greek τέρας, monster.

testis. Latin, witness.

Thompson, Sir Henry (1820–1904). Great stone-crusher. (See *Invest. Urol.* (1973), **11, 263.**)

Tiemann, G., and Co. Instrument makers of New York.

trichomonas. θρίξ, a hair, μονος, unit (though it has three to five hairs!).

urethra. Greek, οὖρηθρα.

utriculus. Latin, small bag.

vas. A vessel, deferens, carrying.

verumontanum. Latin veru, a spit; montanus, mountainous.

vesicle. Latin, a little bladder.

vulva. Latin, a wrapper.

Wilms, Max (1867–1918). Surgeon of Heidelberg. Nephroblastoma was previously described by Rance (1814).

Wolff, Kaspar Friedrich (1733–94). German anatomist and embryologist, working in St. Petersburg.

xanthogranuloma. ξανθός, Greek, yellow.

Young, Hugh Hampton (1870–1945). Urologist of Baltimore. Inventor of the first cold punch, and a method of perineal prostatectomy.

Ziehl–Neelsen. Method of staining the tubercle bacillus, named after Franz Ziehl (1859–1926), physician of Lübeck, and Friedrick Karl Adolph Neelsen (1854–94), pathologist of Dresden.

Zuckerkandl, Emil (1849–1910). Anatomist of Vienna.

Index

Index